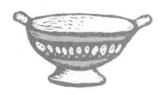

500 More
Low-Carb Recipes

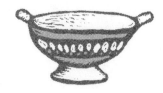

500 More
Low-Carb Recipes

500 All-New Recipes from Around the World

Dana Carpender

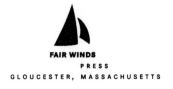

FAIR WINDS
PRESS
GLOUCESTER, MASSACHUSETTS

First published in the USA in 2004 by
Fair Winds Press
33 Commercial Street
Gloucester, MA 01930

08 07 06 05 04   2 3 4 5

ISBN 1-59233-089-4

Library of Congress Cataloging-in-Publication Data available

Cover design by Mary Ann Smith
Book design by Leslie Haimes

Printed and bound in Canada

*This book is dedicated to all of the people who contributed to it —
the folks who sent recipes, and the folks who diligently tested those recipes
and gave me vital feedback. As you page through this book, you'll see a
whole lot of names — this book is dedicated to every single one of them.
It is only through their hard work, creativity, and generosity that this work
was possible — and it is because of that same hard work, creativity, and
generosity that this book is far more interesting, diverse, and complex
than I ever could have made it myself. These folks are the heart and
soul of the growing low-carb community, and I'm proud and
grateful to be among them.*

*And, once again, to my husband Eric Schmitz, who worked fourteen-hour
days right alongside me, getting this book done on time. When I say I
couldn't have done it without him, it's just the simple truth.*

c o n t e n t s

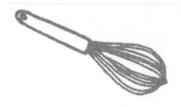

9		Introduction
19	Chapter 1	Ingredients You Need To Know About
41	Chapter 2	Snacks, Party Nibbles, and Other Incidental Food
77	Chapter 3	Eggs, Cheese, and the Like
105	Chapter 4	Breads, Muffins, Cereals, Crackers, and Other Grainy Things
135	Chapter 5	Hot Vegetables and Other Sides
185	Chapter 6	Side Salads and Dressings
217	Chapter 7	Chicken and Turkey
261	Chapter 8	Fish and Seafood
291	Chapter 9	Beef
343	Chapter 10	Pork and Lamb
379	Chapter 11	Main Dish Salads
403	Chapter 12:	Soups
439	Chapter 13:	Sauces, Seasonings, and Other Incidental Stuff
453	Chapter 14:	Cookies, Cakes, Pies, and Other Sweets
527	Chapter 15:	The BONUS CHAPTER!
541	Appendix A	A Refresher on Measurements
543	Appendix B	Where to Find a Few Less-Common Ingredients
545		Index

Introduction

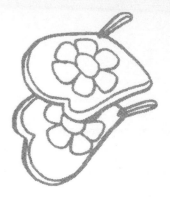

Some of this Introduction will seem familiar to those of you who have my previous cookbooks! However, you still might want to read it—I've updated quite a few things.

How Do I Get Into These Things?!

After putting together *500 Low-Carb Recipes* on a killer-tight schedule during the winter of 2001–2002, I swore I was never writing a book that big in that little time again.

Hah. Just try writing a best seller. Just try! Your readers and your publisher will never let you sleep again. I had no idea that *500 Low-Carb Recipes* would do as well as it did, but it turned out to be the most popular low-carb cookbook of 2003 (and thank you all very much!). Next thing I knew I was appearing on national talk shows (Hey! I met Wayne Brady!), taping for the Food Network, and finding the bookstore buyers, the readers, and my publisher all clamoring for a sequel as soon as possible!

I started in October of 2003—only to have my hard drive crash and eat all my work in mid-December ("Back up early and often" is the moral of that story.) So I started again, and had just over five months to come up with 500 recipes! YIKES!

All of which is by way of explaining why this book is even more of a collaborative effort than the first one: There was simply no way I was going to come up with enough recipes by my deadline without considerable help. So I put out the call to the readers of *Lowcarbezine!*, my Internet newsletter, telling them that I needed recipes, and plenty of them!

The response was overwhelming, as you will appreciate as you page through this book—fully half the recipes come from *Lowcarbezine!* readers. Bless them, one and all, for their generosity in sharing their best recipes with me, and through me, with the whole low-carb community.

Not only did my *Lowcarbezine!* readers send recipes, but they sent a lot of really great recipes. Indeed, as they flooded into my inbox, over and over, I had the thought, "Geez, how am I going to come up with anything better than these?" I'm humbled by the talent of my readership, some of whom could teach me a thing or two about cooking. If you find this book varied, interesting, useful, and fun, a great deal of the credit goes to the people whose names you will find all through this book. Thank them in your heart, they deserve it.

However . . .

My readers, for the most part, don't write cookbooks for a living. Often their recipes came in with wording such as "1 package frozen spinach" or "1 can green chilies" instead of exact measurements. We've generally gone with the most common-sized packaging, or what made instinctive sense to my cook's brain. And some recipes came with no quantities given—in these cases we relied heavily on our testers' feedback.

Ditto with the instructions; often they simply said "Cook"—without specifying skillet or saucepan, high heat or low. And more than half the recipes came in with no suggestion as to how many servings they made. Again, we went with testers' feedback, and my experience.

Some recipes came in with specific products recommended; whenever possible we went with a generic recommendation, but where a specific product seemed like it would really make a difference, we kept it. And there are certain ingredients we simply won't use around here, among them hydrogenated shortening and the very well known fake whipped topping that comes in a tub. We've substituted more wholesome ingredients in those cases.

Too, I reworded recipes for clarity wherever I felt it was needed, though I think you'll be able to hear a lot of my readers' voices coming through, as well.

For any errors made in this process, any recipes that have undergone a sea change, and anything that just seems to the original creator like it's just not the same recipe anymore, I take full responsibility, and apologize.

Why Is There Such a Wide Range of Carb Counts in the Recipes in This Book?

Just as with *500 Low-Carb Recipes*, not all of the recipes in this book are of the very-low-carb Atkins-induction variety. You'll find recipes with no carbs at all, and you'll find recipes with as much as 12 or 15 grams of usable carbohydrate per serving—and the whole range in between.

Let me say it loud and clear: I am a huge believer in low-carbohydrate eating. I am forever opposed, however, to NO-carbohydrate diets. Indeed, people who decide that, if low carb is good, no carb must be better, make me want to beat my head against a wall. When people do this, it's almost invariably because they figure if they eat this way, they'll lose their weight fast-fast-fast. Why do they want to lose their weight fast-fast-fast? Because they're looking forward to the day that they can *go off the diet*. I confidently predict that that day is the day they start to gain their weight back, along with their insulin-related health problems.

Please, get it through your head: *There is no finish line.* Whatever you do to lose weight is what you must continue to do for the rest of your life to keep it off. Whatever you do to improve your health you must continue to do forever if you want to keep your new found energy, reduced blood pressure, stable blood sugar, and improved cholesterol and triglyceride numbers.

So stop trying to lose weight at a ridiculous rate. (I've actually had people write to me about how discouraging it is that they're losing "only" two pounds per week. Heck, at that rate, you'd lose 104 pounds in a year! Two pounds a week is quick weight loss.) Instead, focus on making your low-carbohydrate lifestyle just as enjoyable as it can possibly be—which is darned enjoyable! Try new dishes; budget money for low-carb extravagances like expensive cheeses or macadamia nuts. Get comfortable here, because this is the rest of your life.

That being said, carb tolerance varies widely. Only you can know, through trial and error, how much carbohydrate you can eat in a day and still lose weight, and whether you also need to keep an eye on your calorie count. (By way of example, I need to eat no more than 50 grams per day of usable carb, and no more than 2,000 calories per day, or I start to gain. If I stay below 30 or 40 grams, and 1,800 calories, I lose slowly.) Further, you may have allergies, sensitivities, or religious dietary restrictions this book is not meant to deal with. It is up to you to pick and choose among the recipes in this book, with an eye to the carbohydrate counts provided, your own tastes, and any other limiting factors, and put together menus that will please your palate and your family, while staying within that critical carb level.

However, I do have this to say: Always, always, always the heart and soul of your low-carbohydrate diet should be meat, fish, poultry, and eggs; healthy fats; and low-carb vegetables. You will find a boggling array of ways to combine these things in this book—use them! Don't just find one or two recipes that you like and make them over and over. Try at least one new recipe every week, so that within a few months you'll have a whole new repertoire of familiar low-carb favorites!

You will find recipes in this book for what are best considered low-carb or reduced-carb treats. Do not take the presence of a recipe in this book to mean that it is something that you can eat every day, in unlimited quantity, and still lose weight. I can tell you from experience that even low-carb treats, if eaten frequently, will put weight on you. Recipes for breads, cookies, muffins, cakes, and the like are here to give you a satisfying, varied cuisine that you can live with for life—not to become the new staples of your diet. *Do not try to make your low-carbohydrate diet resemble your former standard American diet.* That's the diet that got you in trouble in the first place, remember?

One other thought: it is entirely possible to have a bad reaction to a food that has nothing to do with its carbohydrate count. Gluten, a protein from wheat that is essential for baking low-carb bread, causes bad reactions in a fair number of people. Soy products are problematic for many folks, as are nuts. Whey protein, used extensively in these recipes, contains lactose, which some people cannot tolerate. Surely you've heard of people who react badly to artificial sweeteners of one kind or another. And I've heard from diabetics who get bad blood-sugar spikes from eating even small quantities of onions or tomatoes.

Yet all of these foods are just fine for many, many low-carb dieters, and there is no way I can know which foods may cause a problem for which people. All I can tell you is to pay attention to your body! If you add a new food to your diet, and you gain weight (and you're pretty certain it's not tied to something else, like your menstrual cycle or a new medication), or find yourself unreasonably hungry, or tired, or whatever, despite having stayed within your body's carbohydrate tolerance, you may want to consider avoiding that food. One man's meat is another man's poison, and all that.

"Usable Carb Count"

You may or may not be aware of the concept of the usable carb count, sometimes called the effective carb count—some low-carb books utilize this principle, some do not. If you're not familiar with the concept, here it is in a nutshell:

Fiber is a carbohydrate, and is—at least in American nutritional breakdowns—included in the total carbohydrate count. However, fiber is a form of carbohydrate made of molecules so big that you can neither digest nor absorb them. Therefore, fiber, despite being a carbohydrate, will not push up your blood sugar, and it will not cause an insulin release. Even better, by slowing the absorption of the starches and sugars that occur with it, fiber actually lessens their bad influence—this is very likely the reason that high-fiber diets look so good when compared to "American normal."

For these reasons, many, if not most, low-carb dieters now subtract the grams of fiber in a food from the total grams of carbohydrate, to get the number of grams of carbohydrate that are actually a problem—"usable" carbs, or the "effective carb count." These nonfiber grams of carbohydrate are what we count, and limit. Not only does this approach allow us a much wider variety of foods, and especially lots more vegetables, but it also actually encourages us to add fiber to things like baked goods. I am very much a fan of this approach, and give the usable carbohydrate count for these recipes. However, you will also find the breakdown: total carb count and fiber count both.

As I explain later on in this introduction, the food processors have dramatically expanded the concept of the effective carb count, which they tend to call "net carbs" or "impact carbs." I am unconvinced that this is a good idea, as I'll explain.

What's a "Serving"?

I've gotten a couple of queries from folks who bought *500 Low-Carb Recipes*, wanting to know how big a serving size is, so I thought I'd better address the matter.

To be quite honest, folks, there's no great technical determination going on here. For the most part, a "serving" is based on what I think would make a reasonable portion, depending on the carbohydrate count, how rich the dish is, and, for main dishes, on the protein count. You just divide the dish up into however many portions the recipe says, and you can figure the carb counts on the recipes are accurate. In some cases I've given you a range—"3–4 servings" or whatever. In those cases, I've told you how many servings the carb counts are based on, and you can do a little quick mental estimating if, say, you're serving four people when I've given the count for three.

Of course, this "serving" thing is flukey. People are different sizes, with different appetites. For all I know you have three children under five, who might reasonably split one adult-sized portion. On the other hand, you might have one seventeen-year-old boy who's shot up from five foot five to six foot three in the past year, and what looks like four servings to me will be a quick snack for him. You'll just have to eyeball what fraction of the whole dish you're eating, and go from there.

I've had a few people tell me they'd rather have specific serving sizes—like "1 cup" or the like. I see a few problems with this. First of all, it sure won't work with things like steak or chops—I'd have to use weights instead, and then all my readers would have to run out and buy scales. Second, my recipes generally call for things like, "1 head cauliflower" or "2 stalks celery." These things vary in size a bit, and as a result, yield will fluctuate a bit, too. Also, if one of my recipes calls for "1 1/2 pounds boneless, skinless chicken breasts" and your package is labeled "1.65 pounds," I don't expect you to whack off that final 0.15 of a pound to get the portions exact.

In short, I hate to have to weigh and measure everything, and I'm betting that a majority of my readers feel the same way, even if some do not.

So I apologize to those who like exact measures, but this is how it's gonna be, for now, at any rate.

How Are the Carbohydrate Counts in These Recipes Calculated?

The carbohydrate counts have been calculated using MasterCook software, a very useful program that allows you to enter the ingredients of a recipe and the number of servings it makes, and then spits out the nutritional breakdown for each serving. MasterCook has wonderful flexibility, in that the program allows me to enter low-carb specialty ingredients like vanilla whey protein powder or Splenda into the database.

The carb counts for these recipes are as accurate as we can make them. However, they are not, and cannot be, 100 percent accurate. MasterCook gets its nutritional information from the USDA Nutrient Database, and my experience is that the USDA's figures for carbohydrate content tend to run a bit higher than the food count books. This means that the carbohydrate counts in this book are, if anything, a tad high—which beats being too low!

Furthermore, every stalk of celery, every onion, every head of broccoli is going to have a slightly different level of carbohydrate in it, because it grew in a specific patch of soil, in specific weather, with a particular kind of fertilizer. You may use a different brand of vanilla whey protein powder than I do. You may be a little more or a little less generous with how many bits of chopped green pepper you fit into a measuring cup.

Don't sweat it. These counts are, as the old joke goes, near enough for government work. You can count on them as a guide to the carbohydrate content in your diet. And do you really want to get obsessed with getting every $1/10$ of a gram written down?

In this spirit, you'll find that many of these recipes call for "1 large rib of celery," "half a green pepper," "a clove of garlic." This is how most of us cook, after all. These things do not come in standardized sizes; they're analyzed for the average. Don't sweat it! If you're really worried, use what seems to you a smallish stalk of celery, or green pepper, or clove of garlic, and you can count on your cumulative carb count being a hair lower than what is listed in the recipe.

Low-Carb Specialty Foods

As you are no doubt aware, in the past year or so, low carb has exploded onto the American scene. It is now estimated that over half of American women, and something like a third of men, are watching their carbs.

True to American tradition, business has hastened to exploit our new concern with a vast array of new "low carb" specialty products. I see this proliferation of low-carb specialty products as a double-edged sword. On the one hand, anything that helps carbohydrate-intolerant people remain happily on their diets is a good thing. On the other hand, most of these specialty products are highly processed foods and do not equal genuine foodstuffs in nutritional value. I fear that too many people are eating these things as staples of their diet, displacing the real foods that should be the bedrock of any healthy low-carb diet.

Worse, the food processors, in order to come up with the lowest possible "net carb" or "impact carb" number, have dramatically expanded the concept. Originally, the effective carb count was simply the total carb count minus the grams of fiber. Then the food merchants decided for us that we could completely discount polyol sweeteners (aka sugar alcohols—maltitol, lactitol, sorbitol, xylitol, isomalt, erythritol, etc.) because they are only partially and slowly absorbed. Now they've decided that any carbohydrate with a low glycemic index—that is, a low blood-sugar impact—doesn't "count."

I consider all of this to be *hopelessly* optimistic. There's no doubt that low glycemic index carbs are easier on your body than high glycemic index carbs are, but they're still carbs, and they're still absorbed. I know from experience that adding even quite low-impact carbs back to my diet in any frequent quantity—like, say, a slice or two per day of 100 percent whole-grain rye bread—will make me gain weight. If the same holds true for you, eating low-carb specialty stuff loaded with polyols, inulin, low glycemic cornstarch, and the like, with any frequency, may very well torpedo your diet. Worse, because the food processors so kindly subtract those carbs out for you, it may be difficult for you to keep track of how many grams of those "negligible" low-impact carbs you're getting.

But what concerns me most is that many of the low-carb specialty products on the market are highly processed foods, with lots of additives and objectionable ingredients. Entenmann's bakery has started putting out a line of "low carb" cookies, coffee cakes, and the like. Invariably, the predominant ingredient is polyol sweetener, and they contain both refined white flour and hydrogenated oils, worse than which it is difficult to get. These products may have a somewhat less disastrous effect on your body, but they are still a nutrition-free zone, and they are not, are not, are not good for you.

(I should mention here, however, that there are some low-carb products out there that really are minimally processed, with few or no additives. I buy a great granolalike product called Flax 'n' Nut Crunchies that pretty much consists of nuts and seeds, with a little Splenda and flavoring added. Good stuff, and it sure jazzes up a bowl of yogurt. If you find a product you like that's *not* full of refined and processed junk, enjoy.)

This proliferation of low-carb junk concerns me especially because it is unclear how much of the health benefits of a low-carbohydrate diet, historically speaking, have been due solely to reduced carbohydrate intake and insulin control—which are, no doubt, powerful factors—and how much has been due to the fact that, until recently, a low-carbohydrate diet forced you to eat real, unprocessed foods, with few additives, no hydrogenated oils, and with all the vitamins and minerals intact.

In other words, if we've decided we can eat all the low-impact carbs we want— a very iffy proposal right there—we should be eating them primarily as fruit and whole grains, not brownies, chips, and coffee cakes.

Low-carb specialty foods also tend to be very expensive. I'd hate for you to start basing your diet on specialty products, and then decide that a low-carb diet is too expensive and go back to eating junk. So use these products wisely—to add a little variety, as an occasional treat, and to fight off cravings, not as staples of your diet. But remember: forever and for always, the heart and soul of your low-carb diet should be meat, poultry, fish, eggs, cheese, and other minimally processed dairy products, vegetables, low-sugar fruits, nuts and seeds, and healthy, unprocessed fats. Low-carb junk is still junk, and a bag of low-carb chips and a low-carb brownie are never a substitute for a big salad and a steak or a piece of chicken. Neither, for that matter, is a protein bar. Eat real food, would you?

Where to Find Low-Carbohydrate Specialty Products

Availability of low-carbohydrate specialty products varies a very great deal. Health food stores are a good place to start looking, but while some will carry these products, others still are caught up in low-fat, whole-grain mania, and shun them. Some carry things like fiber crackers and protein powder but refuse to carry anything artificially sweetened, because they pride themselves on carrying only "natural" products. Still, you'll want a good health food store as a source of many ingredients in this book, especially those for low-carb baking, so you may as well go poke around any health food stores in your area and see what you can find.

Little specialty groceries often carry low-carbohydrate products as a way to attract new repeat business. In my town, Sahara Mart, a store that has long specialized in Middle Eastern foods, has become the best source for low-carb specialty products as well. Generally, if a store carries a broad line of products specifically for low-carb dieters, they'll advertise it with signs in the windows—keep your eyes open.

If you can't find a local source for such things as sugar-free chocolate, low-carb pasta, brownies, or whatever you want, your best bet is to go online. Hit your favorite search engine, and search under "low-carbohydrate products," "sugar-free candy," or whatever it is you're looking for. There are a whole lot of low-carb "e-tailers" out there; find the ones with the products and prices you want! If you don't care to use your credit card online, most of them have toll-free order numbers you can call; others have the ability to take checks online as well as credit cards. A few companies I've done business with happily are Carb Smart, Low Carb Grocery, and Synergy Diet, but there are tons of them out there. Go look!

On the Importance of Reading Labels

Do yourself a favor, and get in the habit of reading the label on every food product, and I do mean every food product, that has one. I have learned from long, hard, repetitive experience that food processors can, will, and do put sugar, corn syrup, corn starch, and other nutritionally empty, carb-y garbage into every conceivable food product. I have found sugar in everything from salsa to canned clams, for heaven's sake! (Who it was who thought that the clams needed sugaring, I'd love to know.) You will shave untold thousands of grams of carbohydrate off your intake in the course of the year by the simple expedient of looking for the product that has no added junk.

There are also a good many classes of food products out there to which sugar is virtually always added—the cured meats come to mind. There is almost always sugar in sausage, ham, bacon, hot dogs, liverwurst, and the like. You will look in vain for sugarless varieties of these products—one good reason why you should primarily eat fresh meats instead, by the way. However, you will find that there is quite a range of carb counts among cured meats, because some manufacturers add more sugar than others. I have seen ham that has 1 gram of carbohydrate per serving, and I have seen ham that has 6 grams of carbohydrate per serving—that's a 600 percent difference! Likewise, I've seen hot dogs that have a gram of carbohydrate apiece, and I've seen hot dogs that have 5 grams of carbohydrate apiece.

If you're in a position where you can't read the labels—for instance, at the deli counter at the grocery store—ask questions. The nice deli folks will be glad to read the labels on the ham and salami for you, and can tell you what goes into the various items they make themselves. You'll want to ask, too, at the meat counter, if you're buying something they've mixed up themselves—Italian sausage or marinated meats, or whatever. I have found that if I state simply that I have a medical condition that requires that I be very careful about my diet—and don't come at the busiest hour of the week!—folks are generally very nice about this sort of thing.

This advice to always read labels holds doubly true when you're buying products labeled "low carb." The amount of sheer junk flooding onto the market that says it has only, say, 2 net carbs, when it's really loaded with polyols, corn starch, inulin, and other carbohydrates, is alarming. And remember, reduced-carb refined, processed junk is still refined, processed junk.

In short, become a food sleuth. After all, you're paying your hard-earned money for this stuff, and it is quite literally going to become a part of you. Pay at least as much attention as you would if you were buying a car or a computer!

Using This Book

I can't really tell you how to plan your menus. I don't know if you live alone or have a family, if you have hours to cook or are pressed for time every evening, or what foods are your favorites. I can, however, give you a few suggestions.

- You'll find a lot of one-dish meals in this book—main dish salads, skillet suppers that include meat and vegetables both, hearty soups that are a full meal in a bowl. I include these because they're some of my favorite foods, and to my mind, about the simplest way to eat. I also think they lend a far greater variety to low-carb cuisine than is possible if you're trying to divide up your carbohydrate allowance for a given meal among three or four different dishes. If you have a carb-eating family, you can appease them by serving something on the side—whole-wheat pitas split in half and toasted with garlic butter, brown rice, a baked potato, or some noodles. (You can't imagine I'll recommend that you serve them something like canned biscuits, Tater Tots, or Minute Rice, can you?)

- However, when you're serving these one-dish meals, remember that most of your carbohydrate allowance for the meal is included in that main dish. Unless you can tolerate more carbohydrate than I can, you probably don't want to serve a dish with lots of vegetables in it with even more vegetables on the side. Remember, it's the total usable carb count you have to keep an eye on.

- Simple meat dishes—roasted chicken, broiled steak, pan-broiled chops and the like—are the dishes you'll want to complement with the more carbohydrate-rich vegetable side dishes.

- Break out of your old ways of looking at food! There's no law on the books insisting that you eat eggs only for breakfast, have tuna salad for lunch every day, and some sort of meat and two side dishes for dinner. Both time and money are short? Serve eggs for dinner a couple of nights a week—they're fast, cheap, and unbelievably nutritious. Having family video night or game night? Skip dinner and make two or three healthy snack foods to nibble on. Can't face another fried egg at breakfast? Throw a chop or a hamburger in the electric tabletop grill while you're in the shower, for a fast and easy breakfast. Sick of salads for lunch? Take a protein-rich dip in a snap-top container and some cut-up vegetables to work with you.

- Please note that we have provided metric conversions for all ingredients. Metric conversions appear inside parentheses; for example, "1 cup (130 g) chopped onion."

chapter one

Ingredients You
Need To Know About

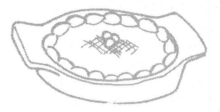

This is by no means an exhaustive rundown of every single ingredient used in this book, just the ones I thought you might have questions about. I've grouped them by use; within those groupings they're in alphabetical order.

Black Soy Beans

Most beans and other legumes are too high in carbohydrate for many low-carb dieters, but there is one exception: Black soy beans have a very low usable carb count, about 1 gram per serving, because most of the carb in them is fiber. Several recipes in this book call for Eden brand canned black soy beans. Many health food stores carry these; if yours doesn't, I'll bet they could special-order them for you. Health food stores tend to be wonderful about special orders.

If you can't find canned black soy beans, you may be able to find them dry and uncooked; if so, you'll have to soak them and then cook them for a looooong time until they soften—soy beans can be stubborn. I'd recommend using your slow cooker.

I would also recommend not eating soy bean recipes several times a week. I know that soy has a reputation for being the Wonder Health Food of All Existence, but there are reasons to be cautious. Soy has been known for decades now to be hard on the thyroid, and if you're trying to lose weight and improve your health, a slow thyroid is the last thing you need. More alarmingly, there was a study done in Hawaii in 2000 that showed a correlation between the amount of tofu subjects ate in middle age and their rate and severity of cognitive problems in old age. Since scientists suspect the problem lies with the soy estrogens that have been so highly touted, any unfermented soy product, including our canned soy beans, is suspect.

This doesn't mean we should completely shun soy beans and soy products, but it does mean we need to approach them with caution, and eat them in moderation. Since many low-carb specialty products are soy-heavy, you'll want to pay attention there, too.

Personally, I try to keep my soy consumption to 1 serving a week or less.

Eggs

There are a few recipes in this book that call for raw eggs, an ingredient that is currently frowned upon by officialdom because of the risk of salmonella. However, I have it on pretty good authority that only 1 out of every 16,000 uncracked, properly refrigerated eggs is actually contaminated. As one woman with degrees in public health and food science put it, "The risk is less than the risk of breaking your leg on any given trip down the stairs." So I use raw eggs now and again, and don't worry about it, and we've never had a problem around here.

However, this does not mean that there is no risk. You'll have to decide for yourself if this is a worry for you—among other things, I generally use very, very fresh eggs from local small farmers, which may well be safer than eggs that have gone longer distances, with more risk of cracking or of refrigeration problems.

One useful thing to know about eggs: While you'll want very fresh eggs for frying and poaching, eggs that are at least several days old are better for hard-boiling. They're less likely to stick to their shells in that maddening way we've all encountered. So if you like hard-boiled eggs—they're certainly one of the most convenient low-carb foods—buy a couple of extra cartons of eggs and let them sit in the refrigerator for at least three or four days before you hard-boil them.

Fats and Oils

Bland Oils

Sometimes you want a bland oil in a recipe—something that adds little or no flavor of its own. In this case, I recommend peanut oil, sunflower oil, or canola oil. These are the oils I would recommend when a recipe calls for simply "oil." Avoid highly polyunsaturated oils like safflower; they deteriorate quickly both from heat and from contact with oxygen, and have been associated with an increased risk of cancer.

Butter

When a recipe says butter, use butter, will you? Margarine is nasty, unhealthy stuff, full of hydrogenated oils, trans fats, and artificial everything. It's terrible for you. So use the real thing. If real butter strains your budget, watch for sales and stock up—butter freezes beautifully. Shop around, too—in my town, I've found stores that regularly sell butter for anywhere from $2.25 a pound to $4.59 a pound. Big difference, and worth going out of my way for.

Coconut Oil

Coconut oil makes an excellent substitute for hydrogenated vegetable shortening (Crisco and the like), which you should shun. You may find coconut oil at health food stores, in Asian markets, and in the international food aisle of many big grocery stores—my grocery store carries it in the "ethnic foods" section, with Indian foods. My health food store keeps coconut oil with the cosmetics—they're still convinced that saturated fats are terrible for you, so they don't put it with the foods, but some folks use it for making hair dressings and soaps. Coconut oil is solid at room temperature—except in the summer—but melts at body temperature. Be aware that for baking recipes, it is essential that your coconut oil be in its solid state—if it's melted when you add it to the recipe, the texture of your finished product will be way the heck off. Surprisingly, coconut oil has no coconut flavor or aroma; you can use it for sautéing or in baking without adding any "off" flavor to your recipes.

Olive Oil

It surely will come as no surprise to you that olive oil is a healthy fat, but you may not know that there are various kinds. Extra-virgin olive oil is the first pressing. It is deep green, with a full, fruity flavor, and makes all the difference in salad dressings. However, it is expensive, and also is too strongly flavored for some uses. I keep a bottle of extra-virgin olive oil on hand but use it exclusively for salads.

For sautéing and other general use, I use a grade of olive oil known as "pomace." Pomace is far cheaper than extra-virgin olive oil, and has a milder flavor. I buy pomace in gallon cans at the same Middle Eastern grocery store where I buy my low-carb specialty products. These gallon cans are worth looking for; it's the cheapest way to buy the stuff. If you can't find gallon cans of pomace, feel free to buy whatever cheaper, milder-flavored type of olive oil is available in your grocery.

Be aware that if you refrigerate olive oil it will become solid. No big deal; it will be fine once it warms up again. If you need it quickly, you can run the bottle under warm water or microwave it for a minute or so on low power, if the container has no metal and will fit in your microwave.

Flour Substitutes

As you are no doubt aware, flour is out, for the very most part, in low-carb cooking. Flour serves a few different purposes in cooking, from making up the bulk of most baked goods, to creating stretchiness in bread dough, to thickening sauces, to "binding" casseroles. In low-carb cooking we use different ingredients for these various purposes. Here's a rundown of flour substitutes you'll want to have on hand for low-carb cooking and baking.

Brans

Because fiber is a carbohydrate that we neither digest nor absorb, brans of one kind or another are very useful for bulking up (no pun intended!) low-carb baked goods. I use different kinds in different recipes. You'll want to have at least wheat bran and oat bran on hand; both of these are widely available.

Cake-Ability

Cake-ability is a product by Expert Foods designed to improve the baking qualities of ground nuts and other low-carb flour substitutes. It's made of soluble fiber, baking soda, and dried, powdered egg white, and I know of no substitute. Cake-ability is used in only one recipe in this book, so whether you need to seek it out will depend on whether you want to make that recipe, but if you do, you can obtain Cake-ability through many of the low-carb online merchants, or "e-tailers." I know that my friends at CarbSmart carry it.

Ground Almonds and Almond Meal

Finely ground almonds and almond meal are wonderful for replacing some or all of the flour in many recipes, especially cakes and cookies. Packaged almond meal is becoming easier to find; the widely distributed Bob's Red Mill brand makes one. It's convenient stuff, and you certainly may use it in any of the recipes that call for almond meal.

However, I have gone back to making my own almond meal by grinding shelled almonds in my food processor, using the S-blade. It takes only a minute or so to reduce them to the texture of corn meal, after which I store the meal in a tightly lidded container. Why do I bother?

Because the carb count is lower. How on earth can that be? Because I grind my almonds with the brown skins still on them, while commercial almond meal is made from almonds that are "blanched"—have the skins removed. Since the skins are practically pure fiber, the fiber count of my homemade almond meal is higher, and the usable carb count per cup is accordingly lower. The carb counts in this book reflect my homemade, high-fiber almond meal; if you use purchased almond meal you'll want to revise your estimated carb count a gram or two higher per serving.

It's good to know that almonds actually expand a little during grinding—something that surprised me; I thought they'd compress a bit. Figure that between $2/3$ and $3/4$ cup of whole almond kernels will become 1 cup of meal when ground.

Guar and Xanthan Gums

These sound just dreadful, don't they? But they're in lots of your favorite processed foods, so how bad can they be? What the heck are they? They're forms of water-soluble fiber, extracted and purified. Guar and xanthan are both flavorless white powders; their value to us is as low-carb thickeners. Technically speaking, these are carbs, but they're all fiber. Nothing but. So don't worry about it.

You'll find guar or xanthan used in a lot of these recipes. Don't overuse it to get a thicker product! Why? Because in large quantities they make things gummy; the texture is not terribly pleasant. But in these tiny quantities, they add oomph to sauces and soups without using flour.

Those of you who read *500 Low-Carb Recipes* know that I used to recommend putting your guar or xanthan through the blender with part or all of the liquid in the recipe, to avoid lumps. You may now happily forget that technique. Instead, acquire an extra salt shaker, fill it with guar or xanthan, and put it by the stove. When you want to thicken something, simply sprinkle a little of the thickener over the surface while stirring, preferably with a whisk. Stop when your sauce, soup, or gravy is a little less thick than you want it to be—it'll thicken a little more on standing.

Your health food store may well be able to order guar or xanthan for you—I slightly prefer xanthan, myself—if they don't have them on hand. You can also find suppliers online. Keep either one in a jar with a tight lid, and it will never go bad—I bought a pound of guar about fifteen years ago and it's still going strong!

Some of my readers' recipes call for a product called ThickenThin Not Starch, from Expert Foods. ThickenThin is a blend of various soluble fibers and can be used interchangeably with guar or xanthan. ThickenThin is also available through online low-carb stores.

Oat Flour

One or two recipes in this book call for oat flour. Because of its high fiber content, oat flour has a lower usable carb count than most other flours; even so, it must be used in very small quantities. Oat flour is available at health food stores. In a pinch, you can grind up oatmeal in your blender or food processor.

Pumpkin Seed Meal

A few recipes in this book call for pumpkin seed meal—I started experimenting with it after getting a fair amount of e-mail from folks who couldn't make my baked goods because of an allergy to nuts, and I've found it works quite well. (If you're allergic to nuts and want to make any of my recipes that call for almond meal, I'd try substituting pumpkin seed or sunflower seed meal.)

It's very easy to make pumpkin seed meal. Just buy raw shelled pumpkin seeds at your health food store (or, for that matter, at any market that caters to a Mexican-American population)—sometimes they'll be labeled "pepitas." Then put your pumpkin seeds in your food processor and grind them with the S-blade until they reach a cornmeal consistency. That's all.

(Do not try this with the salted pumpkin seeds in the shell that are sold as snacks! You'll get salty food with a texture like wood pulp.)

By the way, when I first published my recipe for Zucchini Bread, which calls for pumpkin seed meal, a few *Lowcarbezine!* readers wrote to tell me that their bread was tasty, but that it had come out green. I assume this is because of the green color of the seeds. I haven't had this problem, but it's harmless.

Rice Protein Powder

For use in savory recipes—entrees and such—you need protein powder that isn't sweet, and preferably one that has no flavor at all. There are a number of these on the market, and some are blander than others. I've tried several kinds, and I've found that rice protein powder is the one I like best. I buy Nutribiotic brand, which has 1 gram of carbohydrate per tablespoon, but any unflavored rice protein powder with a similar carb count should work fine. Your health food store should be able to order Nutribiotic Rice Protein for you. For that matter, I see no reason not to experiment with other unflavored protein powders, if you like.

Rolled Oats

Also known as old-fashioned oatmeal—you know, oat grains that have been squashed flat. Available in every grocery store in the Western Hemisphere. Do not substitute instant or quick-cooking oatmeal.

Soy Flour

In *500 Low-Carb Recipes* there were some recipes that called for soy powder—not soy flour, soy powder. Barely a day has gone by since that I haven't gotten an e-mail from someone asking plaintively where they can find the stuff, what brand I use, and if what they bought was the right thing. Accordingly, there is not a single recipe in this book calling for soy powder.

Moreover, none of my recipes call for soy flour; I prefer not to use a lot of soy (see the "Black Soy Beans" section earlier for an explanation of why). But some of the contributed recipes do call for soy flour, which is made from whole raw soy beans, ground fine. You should be able to find soy flour at any health food store. It is not the same thing as soy protein powder or soy protein isolate.

Wheat Gluten

Gluten is a grain protein; it is the gluten in flour that makes bread dough stretchy so that it will trap the gas released by the yeast, letting your bread rise. We are not, of course, going to use regular, all-purpose flour, with its high carbohydrate content! Fortunately, it is possible to buy concentrated wheat gluten. This high-protein, low-starch flour is absolutely essential to making low-carbohydrate yeast breads.

Buying wheat gluten can be a problem, however, because the nomenclature is not standardized. Some packagers call this "vital wheat gluten" or "pure gluten flour," others simply "wheat gluten." Still others call it "high gluten flour"—this is a real poser, since the same name is frequently used for regular flour that has had extra gluten added to it, something you definitely do not want.

You'll simply have to read the label. The product you want, regardless of what the packager calls it, will have between 75 percent and 80 percent protein—about 24 grams in $1/4$ cup. It will also have a very low carbohydrate count, somewhere in the neighborhood of 6 grams of carbohydrate in that same $1/4$ cup. If your health food store has a bulk bin labeled "high gluten flour" or "gluten flour" with no nutrition label attached, ask to see the bulk manager, and request the information off of the sack the flour came in. (If the label on the bin says "vital wheat gluten" or "pure gluten flour," you can probably trust it.)

At this writing the most widely distributed brand of vital wheat gluten in the United States is Bob's Red Mill. More and more grocery stores are beginning to carry this line of products. If your grocery store doesn't yet, you might request that they get them in.

Wheat Germ

The germ is the part of the wheat kernel that would have become the plant if the grain had sprouted. It is the most nutritious, highest-protein part of the wheat kernel, and is much lower in carbohydrate than the starchy part that becomes white flour. A few recipes in this book call for wheat germ, and raw wheat germ, available at health food stores, is what I use. Raw wheat germ should be refrigerated, as it goes rancid pretty easily.

If you can't get raw wheat germ, toasted wheat germ, such as Kretschmer's, is a usable second best and is widely available in grocery stores.

Wheat Protein Isolate

A few of these recipes, particularly some of the baked goods, call for wheat protein isolate. This is just what it sounds like—it's a protein powder made from wheat, instead of from, say, soybeans. It has a high gluten content but also contains other proteins found in wheat. Wheat protein isolate has very little flavor and very little carbohydrate—just 1.5 grams per cup.

Wheat protein isolate is not widely distributed yet, but it is available through a few online sources. In particular, http://www.locarber.com and http://www.carb-smart.com both carry it.

Whey Protein Powder

Whey is the liquid part of milk—if you've ever seen yogurt that has separated, the clearish liquid is the whey. Whey protein is of extremely good quality, and the protein powder made from it is tops in both flavor and nutritional value. For use in any sweet recipe, the vanilla-flavored whey protein powder—readily available in health food stores—is best. Yes, the kind generally sold for making shakes with. Protein powders vary some in their carbohydrate counts, so find the one with the least carbohydrate! And beware of sugar-sweetened protein powders—the one I use is stevia sweetened and has a little under a gram of carbohydrate per tablespoon.

Natural whey protein powder is just like vanilla whey protein powder, except that it has not been flavored or sweetened. It is bland in flavor, and is used in recipes where a sweet flavor is not desirable. Natural whey protein powder is called for in some of the recipes that other folks have donated to this book—I generally use rice protein powder when a bland protein powder is called for.

Ketatoes

Ketatoes is a low-carb version of instant mashed potatoes. It actually contains some dehydrated potato, diluted with a lot of fiber. You simply mix the powder with equal amounts of water.

Or not. Personally, I find Ketatoes made according to package directions unappealing—they smell good, but the texture is off. However, used in small quantities, Ketatoes mix allows us to give a convincingly potatoey flavor to a variety of dishes. I've used Ketatoes mix in a number of the recipes in this book. Be aware that Ketatoes come in a variety of flavors, but all my recipes call for Ketatoes Classic—that is, plain potato flavor.

If you can't buy Ketatoes in your hometown, there are about a billion online merchants who would be only too happy to ship them to you.

Liquids

Beer

One or two recipes in this book call for beer. The lowest-carbohydrate beer on the market is Michelob Ultra, but I don't much like the stuff. Still, it should be okay for cooking. Miller Lite and Milwaukee's Best Light are better, for my money, and only about 0.5 grams more carb per can.

Broths

Canned or boxed chicken broth and beef broth are very handy items to keep around, and certainly quicker than making your own. However, the quality of most of the canned broth you'll find at your local grocery store is appalling. The chicken broth has all sorts of chemicals in it, and often sugar as well. The "beef" broth is worse—it frequently has no beef in it whatsoever. I refuse to use these products, and you should, too.

However, there are a few canned or boxed broths on the market worth buying. Many grocery stores now carry a brand called Kitchen Basics, which contains no chemicals at all. It is packaged in quart-sized boxes, much like soy milk. Kitchen Basics comes in both chicken and beef. Health food stores also have good-quality canned and boxed broths—both Shelton and Health Valley brands are widely distributed in the United States.

Decent packaged broth will cost you a little more than the stuff that is made of salt and chemicals, but not a whole lot more. If you watch for sales, you can often get it as cheaply as the bad stuff, and stock up—when my health food store runs a sale of good broth for eighty-nine cents a can, I buy piles of the stuff!

One last note—you will also find canned vegetable broth, particularly at health food stores. This is tasty but runs much higher in carbohydrate than the chicken and beef broths do. I'd avoid it.

Carb Countdown Dairy Beverage

A very useful addition to low-carb cuisine is this carbohydrate-reduced milk product, available in full-fat, 1%, and skim, not to mention an exceedingly yummy chocolate variety. To me, Carb Countdown tastes just like milk, and I've used it pretty extensively in these recipes.

I checked with the manufacturer, and Carb Countdown is nationally distributed, so you should be able to find it near you. However, if you cannot, try substituting half-and-half or equal parts of heavy cream and water. For that matter, if you're on the South Beach Diet, low-fat milk is allowed; feel free to use it in place of Carb Countdown wherever I've specified it.

Vinegar

Various recipes in this book call for wine vinegar, cider vinegar, sherry vinegar, rice vinegar, tarragon vinegar, white vinegar, balsamic vinegar, and even raspberry vinegar, for which you'll find a recipe. If you've always thought that vinegar was just vinegar, think again! Each of these vinegars has a distinct flavor all its own, and if you substitute one for the other, you'll change the whole character of the recipe— one splash of cider vinegar in your Asian Chicken Salad (page 383), and you've traded your Chinese accent for an American twang. Vinegar is such a great way to give bright flavors to foods while adding few carbs that I keep *all* of these varieties on hand—it's not like they go bad or anything.

As with everything else, read the labels on your vinegar. I've seen cider vinegar that has 0 grams of carbohydrate per ounce, and I've seen cider vinegar that has 4 grams of carbohydrate per ounce—that's a huge difference! Beware, also, of apple cider *flavored* vinegar—white vinegar with artificial flavors added. I bought this once by mistake, so I thought I'd give you the heads-up. (You'd think the Label Reading Police would be beyond such errors, wouldn't you?)

Wine

There are several recipes in this cookbook calling for either dry red or dry white wine. I find the inexpensive wines that come in a Mylar bag inside a cardboard box to be very convenient to keep on hand for cooking, for the simple reason that they do not go bad, because the contents are never exposed to air. These are not fabulous vintage wines, but they're fine for our modest purposes, and they certainly are handy. I generally have both Burgundy and Chablis wine-in-a-box on hand. Be wary of any wine with "added flavors"—too often, one of those flavors will be sugar. Buy wine with a recognizable name—Burgundy, Rhine, Chablis, Cabernet, and the like, rather than stuff like "Chillable Red."

Nuts, Seeds, and Nut Butters

Flax Seed

Flax seed comes from the same plant that gives us the fabric linen, and it is turning out to be one of the most nutritious seeds there are. Flax seeds have, along with good-quality protein, tons of soluble, cholesterol-reducing fiber and are a rich source of EPAs, the same fats that make fish so heart-healthy.

Most of the recipes in this book that use flax seeds call for them to be ground up into a coarse meal. You can buy preground flax seed meal—Bob's Red Mill puts it out, among others—but I much prefer to grind my own, for the simple reason that the fats in flax seed are very stable so long as the seeds are whole, but go rancid pretty quickly after the seed coat is broken.

In *500 Low-Carb Recipes* I recommended grinding flax seed in your food processor. I have since heard from a few people that a far better tool is an electric coffee grinder, though you'll want to use one you don't use for coffee, or, at the very least, clean it meticulously of coffee residue!

Nut Butters

The only peanut butter called for in this cookbook is "natural" peanut butter, the kind made from ground-up roasted peanuts, peanut oil, salt, and nothing else. Most big grocery stores now carry natural peanut butter; it's the stuff with a layer of oil on top. The oil in standard peanut butter has been hydrogenated to keep it from separating out—that's what gives Skippy and Jif that extremely smooth, plastic consistency—and it's hard to think of anything worse for you than hydrogenated vegetable oil. Except for sugar, of course, which is also added to standard peanut butter. Stick to the natural stuff.

There is now a low-carb version of Skippy peanut butter on the market, under the Carb Options label. It has hydrogenated vegetable oil in it, and I won't touch it.

Health food stores carry not only natural peanut butter, but almond butter, sunflower butter, and sesame butter, generally called tahini. All of these are useful for low carbers.

Keep all natural nut butters in the refrigerator unless you're going to eat them up within a week or two.

Nuts and Seeds

Low in carbohydrates and high in healthy fats, protein, and minerals, nuts and seeds are great foods for us. Not only are they delicious for snacking and for adding crunch to salads and stir-fries, but when ground, they can replace some of the flour in low-carb baked goods—in particular, you'll find quite a few recipes in this book calling for ground hazelnuts, ground almonds, and ground sunflower seeds. Since these ingredients can be pricey, you'll want to shop around. In particular, health food stores often carry nuts and seeds in bulk at better prices than you'll find at the grocery store. I have also found that specialty ethnic groceries often have good prices on nuts; I get my best deal on almonds at my wonderful Middle Eastern grocery, Sahara Mart.

Along with pumpkin and sunflower seeds, you can buy sesame seeds in bulk at health food stores, for a fraction of what they'll cost you in a little shaker jar at the grocery store. Buy them "unhulled" and you'll get more fiber and calcium. You can also get unsweetened shredded coconut at health food stores.

Seasonings

Bouillon or Broth Concentrates

Bouillon or broth concentrate comes in cubes, crystals, and liquids. It is generally full of salt and chemicals and doesn't taste notably like the animal it supposedly came from. It definitely does not make a suitable substitute for good-quality broth if you're making a pot of soup. However, these products can be useful for adding a little kick of flavor here and there—more as seasonings than as soups—and for this use, I keep them on hand. I previously have written that I used chicken bouillon granules but liquid beef bouillon concentrate. I now use a paste bouillon concentrate product called Better Than Bouillon, which comes in both chicken and beef flavors; I do find it preferable to the other kinds. But, hey, use what you have on hand; it should be okay.

Chili Garlic Paste

This is a traditional Asian ingredient, consisting mostly, as the name strongly implies, of hot chilies and garlic. If, like me, you're a chili-head, you'll find endless ways to used the stuff once you have it on hand. Chili garlic paste comes in jars and keeps for months in the refrigerator. Worth seeking out at Asian markets or in the international foods aisle of big grocery stores.

Fish Sauce or *Nuoc Mam*

This is a salty, fermented seasoning widely used in Southeast Asian cooking, available in Asian grocery stores and in the Asian food section of big grocery stores. Grab it when you find it; it keeps nicely without refrigeration. Fish sauce is used in a few (really great) recipes in this book, and adds an authentic flavor. In a pinch, you can substitute soy sauce, although you'll lose some of your Southeast Asian accent.

Garlic

Garlic is a borderline vegetable—one that is fairly high in carbohydrate—but it is very, very good for you. Surely you've heard all about garlic's nutritional prowess by now. Garlic also, of course, is an essential flavoring ingredient in many recipes. However, remember that there is an estimated 1 gram of carbohydrate per clove, and go easy. A "clove," by the way, is one of those little individual bits you get in a whole garlic bulb. If you read "clove" and use a whole bulb (aka a "head") of garlic, you'll get more carbs—and a lot stronger garlic flavor—than you bargained for!

I use only fresh garlic, except for occasional recipes for sprinkle-on seasoning blends. Nothing tastes like the real thing. To my taste buds, even the jarred, chopped garlic in oil doesn't taste like fresh garlic. We won't even *talk* about garlic powder. You may use jarred garlic if you like—half a teaspoon should equal about 1 clove of fresh garlic. If you choose to use powdered garlic, well, I can't stop you, but I'm afraid I can't promise the recipes will taste the same, either. One quarter teaspoon of garlic powder is the rough equivalent of 1 clove of fresh garlic.

By the way, the easiest way to crush a clove or two of garlic is to put the flat side of a big knife on top of it and smash it with your fist. Pick out the papery skin, which will now be easy to do, chop your garlic a bit more, and toss it into your dish. Oh, and keep in mind that the distinctive garlic aroma and flavor only develops after the cell walls are broken—that's why a pile of fresh garlic bulbs in the grocery store doesn't reek—so the more finely you crush or mince your garlic, the more flavor it will release.

Gingerroot

Many recipes in this book call for fresh ginger, sometimes called gingerroot. Fresh ginger is an essential ingredient in Asian cooking, and dried, powdered ginger is *not* a substitute. Fortunately, fresh ginger freezes beautifully—just drop your whole gingerroot (called a "hand" of ginger) into a zipper-lock freezer bag and toss it into the freezer. When the time comes to use it, pull it out, peel enough of the end for your immediate purposes, and grate it—it will grate just fine while still frozen. Throw the remaining root back in the bag, and toss it back into the freezer.

Ground fresh gingerroot in oil is available in jars at some very comprehensive grocery stores. I buy this when I can find it without added sugar, but otherwise, I grate my own.

Low-Sugar Preserves

In particular, I find low-sugar apricot preserves to be a wonderfully versatile ingredient. I buy Smucker's brand and like it very much. This is lower in sugar by *far* than the "all fruit" preserves, which replace sugar with concentrated fruit juice. Folks, sugar from fruit juice is still sugar. I also have been known to use low-sugar orange marmalade and low-sugar raspberry preserves.

Vege-Sal

If you've read my newsletter, *Lowcarbezine!* or my previous cookbooks, you know that I'm a big fan of Vege-Sal. What is Vege-Sal? It's a salt that's been seasoned, but don't think "seasoned salt." Vege-Sal is much milder than traditional seasoned salt. It's simply salt that's been blended with some dried, powdered vegetables; the flavor is quite subtle, but I think it improves all sorts of things. I've given you the choice between using regular salt or Vege-Sal in a wide variety of recipes. Don't worry, they'll come out fine with plain old salt, but I do think Vege-Sal adds a little something extra. Vege-Sal is also excellent sprinkled over chops and steaks in place of regular salt. Vege-Sal is made by Modern Products, and is widely available in health food stores.

Sweeteners

Blackstrap Molasses

What the heck is molasses doing in a low-carb cookbook?! It's practically all carbohydrate, after all. Well, yes, but I've found that combining Splenda with a very small amount of molasses gives a good brown sugar flavor to all sorts of recipes. Always use the darkest molasses you can find—the darker it is, the stronger the flavor and the lower the carb count. That's why I specify blackstrap, the darkest, strongest molasses there is. It's nice to know that blackstrap is also where all the minerals they take out of sugar end up—it may be carb-y, but at least it's not a nutritional wasteland. Still, I use only small amounts.

If you can't get blackstrap molasses—most health food stores carry it—buy the darkest molasses you can find. Most "grocery store" brands come in both light and dark varieties.

Why not use some of the artificial brown sugar–flavored sweeteners out there? Because I've tried them, and I haven't tasted a one I would be willing to buy again. Ick.

Polyols

Polyols, also known as sugar alcohols, are widely used in sugar-free candies and cookies. There are a variety of polyols, and their names all end with "tol": sorbitol, maltitol, mannitol, lactitol, xylitol, and the like. (Okay, there's one exception: isomalt. I don't know what happened there.) Polyols are, indeed, carbohydrates, but they are carbohydrates that are made up of molecules that are too big for the human gut to digest or absorb easily. As a result, polyols don't create much rise in blood sugar, nor much of an insulin release.

This does not, however, mean that polyols are completely unabsorbed. I have seen charts of the relative absorption rates of the various polyols, and I am here to tell you that you do, indeed, absorb carbohydrates from these sweeteners, in varying degrees. Sadly, the highest absorption rate seems to be for maltitol, which is the most widely used of the polyols. You absorb about 2.5 calories for every gram of maltitol you eat. Since you would absorb 4 calories for a gram of sugar, simple arithmetic tells us that you're absorbing more than half of the carbohydrate in the maltitol you eat.

Why do manufacturers use polyols instead of sucralose (Splenda)? Polyols are used in commercial sugar-free sweets because, unlike Splenda and other artificial sweeteners, they will give all of the textures that can be achieved with sugar. Polyols can be used to make crunchy toffee, chewy jelly beans, slick hard candies, moist brownies, and creamy chocolate, just as sugar can.

However, there are one or two problems with polyols. First of all, there is some feeling that different people have differing abilities to digest and absorb these very long chain carbohydrates, which means that for some people, they may cause more of a derangement of blood sugar than for others. Once again, my only advice is to pay attention to your body.

The other problem with polyols is one that is inherent in all indigestible, unabsorbable carbohydrates: they can cause gas and diarrhea. Unabsorbed carbs ferment in your gut, you see, with intestinal gas as a result; it's the exact same thing as happens when people eat beans. I find that even half of a low-carb chocolate bar is enough to cause me social embarrassment several hours later. And I know of a case where eating a dozen and a half sugar-free taffies before bed caused the hapless consumer forty-five minutes of serious gut-cramping intestinal distress at four in the morning.

Don't think, by the way, that you can get around these effects of polyol consumption by taking Beano. It will work, but it will work by making the carbohydrates digestible and absorbable—meaning that any low-carb advantage is gone. I've known folks who have gained weight this way.

What we have here, then, is a sweetener that enforces moderation. Personally, I think this is a wonderful thing!

Since I wrote *500 Low-Carb Recipes*, polyols have become available for the home cook. I have started to use them in my recipes, because they do, indeed, offer a textural advantage. In particular, I got a fair number of complaints about the cookie recipes in *500 Low-Carb Recipes*—people liked the flavor of the cookies but found them too crumbly and sometimes too dry. Polyols solve this problem.

However, I have become increasingly wary of using polyols in any great quantity, because I am convinced we absorb more carbohydrate from them than the food processors want to let on. So here's what I do: When I feel that adding polyol sweetener to a recipe will improve the texture, I use just enough of the sweetener to get the effect I want, and then add Splenda to bring the recipe up to the level of sweetness I'm looking for. This has worked very well for me. It also makes the resulting food easier on both your gut and your blood sugar than it would be if I'd used all polyol.

I use erythritol whenever possible, in preference to maltitol, isomalt, or any of the other granular polyols. Why? Because erythritol has the lowest digestion and absorption rate of all the polyols—you get only 0.3 calories per gram of erythritol, which tells us that we're absorbing very little indeed. Erythritol also seems to be easier on the gut than the other polyols. See Appendix B for mail-order sources of erythritol.

There are, however, recipes where I use other polyols. I use sugar-free dark chocolate not infrequently (and if you haven't tried the sugar-free chocolate yet, you're missing something!). I also use sugar-free pancake syrup and the new sugar-free imitation honey. Obviously, with these products, I'm stuck with whichever polyol the manufacturer used.

I also have found one application in which I can get only maltitol to work: Chocolate sauce. I have tried repeatedly to make a decent no-sugar-added chocolate sauce with erythritol, and it simply isn't happening. The stuff starts out looking all right, but as soon as it cools, it turns grainy on me. Maltitol makes a perfectly textured chocolate sauce. So for that purpose alone, I keep a little maltitol in my pantry.

I confess, I am at a loss as to how to count the carbohydrate grams that polyols add to my recipes, since I can't know which of the polyol sweeteners you'll be using, and they do, indeed, have differing absorption rates. Therefore, I have left them out of the nutritional analyses in this cookbook, which puts me on the same footing as the food processors, I guess. I have mentioned this in the recipe analyses. Be aware that you're probably getting at least a few grams of extra carb per serving in these recipes.

Splenda

If you haven't tried Splenda yet, what are you waiting for? Feed nondieting friends and family Splenda-sweetened desserts and they will never know that you didn't use sugar. It tastes that good.

Splenda has some other advantages. The table sweetener has been bulked so that it measures (in volume, not weight) spoon for spoon, cup for cup like sugar. This makes adapting recipes much easier. Also, Splenda stands up to heat, unlike aspartame, which means you can use it for baked goods and other things that are heated for a while.

Be aware that Splenda granular—the stuff that comes in bulk, in a box or the new "Baker's Bag"—is different than the stuff that comes in the little packets. The stuff in the packets is considerably sweeter—one packet equals 2 teaspoons granular. Whenever the ingredients list says only "Splenda," it means Splenda granular, the stuff you buy in bulk.

It is important to realize that Splenda is not completely carb-free. Because of the maltodextrin used to bulk it, granular Splenda has about a half a gram of carbohydrate per teaspoon, or about one-eighth of the carbohydrate of sugar. So count half a gram per teaspoon, 1 ½ grams per tablespoon, and 24 grams per cup. The stuff in the packets, since it's bulked less, has fewer carbs, so if you want to do the conversion, you can save a few grams. Me, I'd go buggy tearing open all those little packets.

Stevia/FOS Blend

Stevia is short for Stevia rebaudiana, a South American shrub with very sweet leaves. Stevia extract, a white powder from stevia leaves, is growing in popularity with people who don't care to eat sugar, but are nervous about artificial sweeteners.

However, stevia extract has a couple of faults—one, it's so extremely sweet that it's hard to know just how much to use in any given recipe, and two, it often has a bitter taste as well as a sweet one. This is why some smart food packagers have started blending stevia with fructooligosaccharide, also known as FOS. FOS is a sugar, but it's a sugar with a molecule so large that the human gut can neither digest nor absorb it, so it doesn't raise blood sugar or cause an insulin release. FOS has a nice, mild sweetness to it—indeed, it's only half as sweet as table sugar. This makes it the perfect partner for the too-sweet stevia.

This stevia/FOS blend is called for in just a few recipes in this book. It is available in many health food stores, both in packets and in shaker jars. The brand I use is called SteviaPlus, from a company called Sweet Leaf, but any stevia/FOS blend should do for the recipes that call for it.

My favorite use for this stevia/FOS blend, by the way, is to sweeten my yogurt. I think it tastes quite good in yogurt, and FOS actually helps the good bacteria take hold in your gut, improving your health.

Sugar-Free Imitation Honey

This is one of those "I knew low carb had really hit the mainstream when ..." products. I knew we were mainstream when my grocery store started carrying sugar-free imitation honey! This is a polyol syrup with flavoring added to make it taste like honey, and the two I've tried, one by Honey Tree and the other by Steele's, are not bad imitations.

Sugar-free imitation honey is becoming more and more available, and a useful little product it is—in baked goods it adds some extra moisture, while in things like barbecue sauces it adds the familiar syrupy quality. I can get sugar-free imitation honey here in Bloomington at my local Marsh grocery store, and I've heard that Wal-Mart now carries a brand. For that matter, many of the low-carb e-tailers carry Steele's brand of imitation honey. In short, it shouldn't be too hard to get your hands on some.

Remember that sugar-free imitation honey is pretty much pure polyol. Slather it on your low-carb pancakes or biscuits with too free a hand, and you'll pay the price in gastric distress.

Sugar-Free Pancake Syrup

This is actually easy to find; all my local grocery stores carry it—indeed, they have more than one brand. It's usually with the regular pancake syrup, but may be lurking with the diabetic or diet foods. It's just like regular pancake syrup, only it's made from polyols instead of sugar. I use it in small quantities in a few recipes to get a maple flavor.

Vegetables

Avocados

Several recipes in this book call for avocados. Be aware that the little, black, rough-skinned California avocados are lower in carbohydrate (and higher in healthy monounsaturated fat) than the big green Florida avocados. All nutritional analyses were done assuming you used California avocados.

Carrots

Because carrots have a higher glycemic index than many vegetables, a lot of low carbers have started avoiding them with great zeal. But while carrots do have a fairly high blood-sugar impact, you'd have to eat pounds of them to get the quantity that is used to test with. So don't freak when you see a carrot used here and there in these recipes, okay? I've kept the quantities small, just enough to add flavor, color, and a few vitamins, not enough to torpedo your diet.

Frozen Vegetables

You'll notice that many of these recipes call for frozen vegetables, particularly broccoli, green beans, and cauliflower. I use these because I find them very convenient, and I think that the quality is quite good. If you like, you may certainly substitute fresh vegetables in any recipe. You will need to adjust the cooking time, and if the recipe calls for the vegetable to be used thawed, but not cooked, you'll need to blanch your vegetables—boil them for just 3 to 5 minutes.

It's important to know that frozen vegetables are not immortal, no matter how good your freezer is. Don't buy more than you can use up in four to six weeks, even if they're on sale. You'll end up throwing them away.

Onions

Onions are a borderline vegetable; they're certainly higher in carbohydrate than, say, lettuce or cucumbers. However, they're loaded with valuable phytochemicals, so they're very healthful, and, of course, they add an unmatched flavor to all sorts of foods. Therefore I use onions a lot, but I try to use the least quantity that will give the desired flavor. Indeed, one of the most common things I do to cut carb counts on "borrowed" recipes is to cut back on the amount of onion used. If you have serious diabetes, you'll want to watch your quantities of onions pretty carefully, and maybe even cut back further on the amounts I've given.

If you're not an accomplished cook, you need to know that different types of onions are good for different things. There are mild onions, which are best used raw, and there are stronger onions, which are what you want if you're going to be cooking them. My favorite mild onions are sweet red onions; these are widely available, and you'll see I've used them quite a lot in the recipes. However, if you prefer, you can substitute Vidalia onions or Bermuda onions anywhere I've specified sweet red onions. Scallions, also known as green onions, also are mild and best eaten raw or quickly cooked in stir-fries. To me, scallions have their own flavor, and I generally don't substitute for them, but your kitchen won't blow up or anything if you use another sort of sweet onion in their place.

When a recipe simply says "onion," what I'm talking about is good old yellow globe onions, the ones you can buy three or five pounds at a time in net sacks. You'll be doing yourself a favor if you pick a sack with smallish onions in it—that way, when a recipe calls for just a quarter or a half a cup of chopped onion, you're unlikely to be left with half an onion on your hands. For the record, when I say simply "a small onion," I mean one about 1 1/2" (3.75 cm) in diameter, or about 1/4–1/3 cup when chopped. A medium onion would be about 2" (5 cm) in diameter, and would yield between 1/2 and 3/4 cup when chopped. A large onion would be 2 1/2"–3" (6.25–7.5 cm) across, and will yield about a cup when chopped.

Tomatoes and Tomato Products

Tomatoes are another borderline vegetable, but like onions they are so nutritious, so flavorful, and so versatile that I'm reluctant to leave them out of low-carb cuisine entirely. After all, lycopene, the pigment that makes tomatoes red, has been shown to be a potent cancer fighter—who wants to miss something like that?

You'll notice that I call for canned tomatoes in a fair number of recipes, even some where fresh tomatoes might do. This is because fresh tomatoes aren't very good for much of the year, while canned tomatoes are all canned at the height of ripeness. I'd rather have a good canned tomato in my sauce or soup than a mediocre fresh one. Since canned tomatoes are generally used with all the liquid that's in the can, the nutritional content doesn't suffer the way it does with most canned vegetables.

I also use plain canned tomato sauce, canned pizza sauce, canned pasta sauce, and jarred salsa. When choosing these products, you need to be aware that tomatoes, for some reason, inspire food packers to flights of sugar-fancy. They add sugar, corn syrup, and other carb-y sweeteners to all sorts of tomato products. So it is even more important that you *read the labels* on all tomato-based products to find the ones with no added sugar. And keep on reading them! The good, cheap brand of salsa I used for quite a while showed up one day with "New, Improved!" on the label. Guess how they'd improved it? Right. They'd added sugar. I found a new brand!

A small note on ketchup: Commercially-made low-carb ketchup is now available and is often lower carb than my version. All recipes containing ketchup in this book are based on the nutritional analysis of *my* recipes.

Yeast

All of the bread recipes in this book were developed using plain old active dry yeast—not bread-machine yeast and certainly not Rapid Rise yeast. Indeed, one of my testers had some spectacular failures using Rapid Rise yeast in her bread machine with one of my recipes, which worked brilliantly for another tester who used regular yeast.

The best place to buy yeast is at a good health food store, where yeast is generally available in bulk for a fraction of what it would cost you in little packets at the grocery store. Yeast should be stored in the cooler at the health food store, and you should put it in the refrigerator at home.

One last note: don't buy more yeast than you're likely to use up in, oh, four to six weeks. It will eventually die on you, and you'll end up with dough that won't rise. When you're using expensive ingredients, like we do, this is almost more than a body can bear.

Yogurt and Buttermilk

Yogurt and buttermilk both fall into the category of "cultured milks"—milk that has had a particular bacteria added to it and is then kept warm until the bacteria grow. It is these bacteria that give yogurt and buttermilk their characteristic thick texture and tangy flavor.

If you look at the label of either of these cultured milk products, you'll see that the nutrition label claims 12 grams of carbohydrate per cup (and, by the way, 8 grams of protein)—the same carbohydrate count as the milk they're made from. For this reason, many low carbers avoid yogurt and buttermilk.

However, in *The GO-Diet*, Drs. Goldberg and O'Mara explain that, in actuality, most of the lactose—milk sugar—in the milk is converted into lactic acid by the bacteria. This is what gives these foods their sour taste. The labels say "12 grams carbohydrate" largely, they say, because carbohydrate count is determined by "difference." What this means is that the calorie count is first determined. Then the protein and fat fractions are measured, and the number of calories they contribute is calculated. Any calories left over are assumed to come from carbohydrate.

However, Goldberg and O'Mara say, this is inaccurate in the case of yogurt and buttermilk—they say we should count just 4 grams of carbohydrate a cup for these cultured milks. Accordingly, I have added them back to my diet, and I have had no trouble—no weight gain and no triggering of "blood-sugar hunger." I really enjoy yogurt as a snack!

Keep in mind that these numbers *only* apply to *plain* yogurt. The sweetened kind is always higher in carbohydrate. If you like fruit-flavored yogurt, flavor it yourself. You'll find a recipe for making your own plain yogurt, easy as mud pies, in chapter 3, but any plain yogurt is fine.

The carb counts in this book are calculated using that 4 grams of carbohydrate per cup figure.

Miscellaneous Products

As you may have noticed, there are tons of low-carb versions of traditionally high-carb foods now on the market. Two that I frequently use that are certainly worth mentioning are low-carb tortillas and unsweetened shredded or flaked coconut.

chapter two

Snacks, Party Nibbles, and Other Incidental Food

Here, for your entertaining pleasure, is a big bunch of cool stuff to serve at your parties, on family movie night, or when folks are gathered 'round for the big game. You don't have to save them for special occasions, though. A lot of these are great foods to just have hanging around the refrigerator, waiting for that vulnerable moment when you idly open the door.

We start off with a veritable flock of chicken wings. Indeed, I look at this and think the geneticists ought to be working on chickens that look like those six-armed Indian statues....

Chili Lime Wings

1 tablespoon (9g) paprika

1 teaspoon chili powder

1 teaspoon dried oregano, crumbled

1/4 teaspoon salt

1/4 teaspoon pepper

1/2 teaspoon garlic powder

1 1/2 pounds (680 g) chicken wings

3 tablespoons (45 ml) olive oil

1 lime, cut in wedges

In a small bowl, combine all your spices.

If you like individual "drummettes," cut your wings up (or you can buy them that way!). Arrange them in a pan, and brush them with the olive oil. Now sprinkle the spice mixture evenly over your wings.

Roast at 375° F (190° C) for at least 45 minutes, and an hour isn't likely to hurt. You want them crispy! Or, if you have a rotisserie with a basket, that's a great way to cook these as well.

Serve hot, with wedges of lime to squeeze over the wings.

YIELD: About 14 pieces

Each with: 88 calories; 7 g fat; 5 g protein; 1 g carbohydrate; trace dietary fiber; 1 g usable carb.

◎ Chinese Sticky Wings

Mmmmm. Chinese chicken wings...

> 3 pounds (910 g) chicken wings
> ¼ cup dry sherry
> ¼ cup soy sauce
> ¼ cup sugar-free imitation honey
> 1 tablespoon (8 g) grated ginger root
> 1 clove garlic
> ½ teaspoon chili garlic paste

Cut your wings into "drummettes" if you didn't buy them that way (and keep those pointy tips to make chicken broth!). Put your wings in a big zipper-lock bag.

Mix together everything else, and pour it into the bag. Seal the bag, pressing out the air as you go. Turn the bag a few times to coat, and throw it in the fridge for a few hours (and a whole day is brilliant).

Pull out the bag, pour off the marinade into a bowl, and arrange the wings in a shallow baking pan. Give 'em a good hour in an oven preheated to 375° F (190° C), basting every 15 minutes with the marinade.
Serve with plenty of napkins!

YIELD: About 28 pieces

Each with: 62 calories; 4 g fat; 5 g protein; trace carbohydrate; trace dietary fiber; 0 usable carb. Carb count does not include polyols in the sugar-free imitation honey.

Lemon Soy Chicken Wings

These are Chinese-y too, just in a different sort of a way.

    8 whole chicken wings
    3 cloves garlic
    1 tablespoon (8 g) grated ginger root
    2 tablespoons (30 ml) lemon juice
    3 tablespoons (45 ml) soy sauce
    1 tablespoon (15 ml) sugar-free imitation honey
    1 tablespoon (1.5 g) Splenda
    ½ teaspoon chili powder

If you like your wings cut into "drummettes," do that first. (If you keep the pointy tips, they're great for chicken broth.). Put wings in a zipper-lock plastic bag.

Combine everything else, and pour over the wings. Seal the bag, pressing out the air as you go, and turn it a few times to coat. Let wings marinate for at least an hour, and all day won't hurt a bit.

Preheat oven to 375° F (190° C). While the oven's heating, drain the marinade off of the wings, and reserve. Arrange wings in a shallow baking pan, and roast for 1 hour, basting two or three times with the marinade.

YIELD: 16 pieces

Each with: 58 calories; 4 g fat; 5 g protein; 1 g carbohydrate; trace dietary fiber; 1 g usable carb.

Lemon-Mustard Chicken Wings

    10 chicken wings
    3 tablespoons (45 g) brown mustard
    2 tablespoons (3 g) Splenda
    2 tablespoons (30 ml) lemon juice
    ½ teaspoon chili paste
    ¼ teaspoon salt or Vege-Sal

Preheat your oven to 400°F (200°C). Cut wings into drummettes, reserving the pointy tips for broth. Arrange the wings in a baking pan.

Mix together everything else. Brush half of the mixture over the wings, and bake for 20 to 25 minutes. Turn the wings, brush with the rest of the mustard mixture, and bake for another 20 to 25 minutes. Serve.

YIELD: 20 pieces

Each with: 57 calories; 4 g fat; 5 g protein; trace carbohydrate; trace dietary fiber; no usable carb.

Stuffed eggs

Now for the stuffed eggs—so I guess we know which came first, don't we? If you make stuffed eggs to have on hand for snacks, instead of for a party where they'll be eaten up fast, it's good to keep them in a snap-top container. They keep better that way than they do just on a plate.

◉ Southwestern Stuffed Eggs

These spicy eggs were a huge hit at the party I took them to!

6 hard-boiled eggs
2 tablespoons (30 g) mayonnaise
1 tablespoon (15 g) plain yogurt
1 tablespoon (10 g) minced onion
¾ teaspoon chili powder
1 tablespoon (15 ml) cider vinegar
⅛ teaspoon garlic, finely minced

Peel your eggs, and slice each one in half. Remove the yolks to a mixing bowl, and arrange the whites on a platter.

Mash the yolks well with a fork, then mash in the mayonnaise and yogurt. When the mixture is smooth, stir in the seasonings.

Stuff the seasoned yolks into the whites. You may sprinkle a tiny bit of chili powder or paprika on top, to make them look festive, if you like.

YIELD: 12 pieces

Each with: 57 calories; 5 g fat; 3 g protein; 1 g carbohydrate; trace dietary fiber; 1 g usable carb.

◎ Stilton Eggs

For all you blue cheese fans! If you don't have Stilton—the particularly strong English blue cheese—on hand, go ahead and use whatever blue cheese you've got.

    6 hard-boiled eggs
    2 tablespoons (30 g) mayonnaise
    2 tablespoons (30 g) plain yogurt
    2 ounces (60 g) Stilton cheese, crumbled pretty fine
    3 scallions, minced
    1/4 teaspoon salt or Vege-Sal

Peel your eggs and remove the yolks to a mixing bowl. Arrange the whites on a platter.

With a fork, mash the yolks well. Then mash in the mayonnaise and yogurt. When the yolks are smooth and creamy, mash in the Stilton, leaving some small lumps, then stir in the scallions and the salt. Stuff the yolk mixture into the whites.

YIELD: 12 pieces

Each with: 58 calories; 5 g fat; 3 g protein; 1 g carbohydrate; trace dietary fiber; 1 g usable carb.

◎ Tuna Stuffed Eggs

Why does this recipe call for a full dozen boiled eggs, when most of my stuffed egg recipes call for only a half a dozen? Because I didn't want you to be stuck with half a can of leftover tuna, that's why. Use chunk light or even flake tuna—they're cheaper, and it's not as much work to break them up.

    12 hard-boiled eggs
    6 ounces (140 g) canned tuna, drained
    1/2 cup (120 g) mayonnaise
    2/3 cup (110 g) finely minced red onion
    2/3 cup (110 g) finely minced celery
    1 teaspoon chili garlic paste
    2 teaspoons prepared horseradish
    2 tablespoons (20 g) grated Parmesan cheese

Cut the eggs in half, and carefully turn the yolks out into a mixing bowl. Arrange the whites on a plate.

Add the tuna and mayo to the egg yolks, and mash until the tuna is thoroughly broken up.

Now stir in your vegetables. Then add the chili garlic paste and horseradish.

Stuff the yolk-tuna mixture into the whites, piling it high. Sprinkle the Parmesan cheese over the stuffed eggs, and serve.

YIELD: 24 servings

Each with: 84 calories; 7 g fat; 5 g protein; 1 g carbohydrate; trace dietary fiber; 1 g usable carb.

◉ Pâté Eggs

Okay, they're made with liverwurst, not pâté. But they're still tasty and sort of elegant.

> 6 hard-boiled eggs
> 2 ounces (60 g) liverwurst
> 3 tablespoons (45 g) mayonnaise
> 2 teaspoons Worcestershire sauce
> 2 teaspoons brown mustard
> 2 tablespoons (20 g) very finely minced onion
> 2 slices bacon, cooked crisp and drained

Slice each egg in half, and gently turn the yolks out into a mixing bowl. Arrange the whites on a plate.

Add the liverwurst and mayonnaise to the yolks, and mash very thoroughly, till all lumps of liverwurst and yolk disappear. Now stir in the Worcestershire, mustard, and onion, blending well.

Stuff the yolk mixture into the whites, piling it high.

Crumble your bacon fine, and sprinkle a few bacon bits over each stuffed egg, then serve.

YIELD: 12 servings

Each with: 87 calories; 8 g fat; 4 g protein; 1 g carbohydrate; trace dietary fiber; 1 g usable carb.

◉ Guacamole Eggs

The filling of these amazing stuffed eggs is an enchanting spring green! They'll turn color on you as they sit, though, so serve them when they're likely to get eaten up pretty quickly.

> 6 hard-boiled eggs
> 1 California avocado
> 1 tablespoon (15 ml) lime juice
> 1 clove garlic, crushed
> 2 scallions, minced fine
> 1/4 teaspoon Tabasco sauce
> 2 tablespoons (30 g) mayonnaise, or to taste
> 1 tablespoon (15 g) sour cream
> Salt and pepper to taste
> Chili powder

Cut eggs in half, and remove yolks. Put the yolks in a mixing bowl, and set the whites aside on a plate.

Halve the avocado, remove the pit, and scoop the flesh into the bowl with the yolks. Add the lime juice, garlic, scallions, Tabasco, mayo, and sour cream, and mash everything together until quite smooth and creamy. Salt and pepper to taste.

Stuff the yolk mixture into the white, piling it high—you'll have a lot of filling because of that avocado! Sprinkle a little chili powder over them for garnish, and serve immediately!

YIELD: 12 servings

Each with: 84 calories; 7 g fat; 4 g protein; 2 g carbohydrate; 1 g dietary fiber; 1 g usable carb.

Crystal Caskey's Deviled Eggs

Our tester, Kay Winefordner, says to tell you that you could substitute minced ham or shredded barbecue for the bacon, if you like!

6 hard-boiled eggs

4–5 strips bacon, fried until crispy, and drained

½–1 cup (60–120 g) shredded Colby-Jack cheese
(depending on how well you like cheese)

1–2 teaspoons prepared mustard

1–3 tablespoons (15–45 g) mayonnaise, or more to taste

Slice the eggs lengthwise. Put the yolks in a small mixing bowl. Crumble the bacon into the bowl and add the cheese. Put in a squirt of mustard and then mix with mayonnaise until yolks are no longer dry and the mixture can easily be scooped into the whites.

YIELD: 12 servings

Each with: 51 calories; 4 g fat; 4 g protein; trace carbohydrate; 0 g dietary fiber, trace usable carb.

◉ Warm Brie with Sticky Nuts

This is an unusual and delectable party offering. It is also very rich; if you're planning on serving dinner as well, consider sharing this six ways! I think this would also make an elegant dessert.

> 8-ounce (225 g) wheel of Brie (don't buy a slice from a bigger wheel)
> 1/3 cup (40 g) chopped pecans
> 3 tablespoons (45 g) butter
> 1 tablespoon (15 g) polyol
> 1 teaspoon sugar-free imitation honey
> 1 tablespoon (1.5 g) Splenda
> 1/4 teaspoon blackstrap molasses
> 1 pinch salt

Preheat oven to 350°F (180°C). Unwrap cheese, and place it in a shallow baking dish. Put it the oven, and set your timer for 10 minutes.

In the meanwhile, in a saucepan, start sautéing the chopped pecans in the butter—give them about 5 minutes over medium-low heat. Then stir in the four sweeteners, and keep stirring for 3 or 4 minutes. When the cheese is just about ready, stir in the salt.

Fetch the Brie out of the oven, and place it on a serving plate. Scoop the nuts— they'll now be sticky and clumping a bit—out of the butter, and spread them evenly across the top of the cheese. Serve by cutting into 4 wedges, and eat with a fork.

YIELD: 4 servings

Per serving (excluding unknown items): 333 calories; 31 g fat; 13 g protein; 2 g carbohydrate; 1g dietary fiber; 1g usable carb. Carb count does not include polyols.

Tuna Puffs

1 egg
2 tablespoons (20 g) pumpkin seed meal or almond meal
2 tablespoons (20 g) rice protein
1 tablespoon (15 g) butter, melted
2 tablespoons (30 ml) half-and-half
1 1/2 teaspoons lemon juice
1/2 teaspoon chili garlic paste
6 ounces (140 g) canned tuna, drained
4 scallions, sliced thin
Salt and pepper to taste
Easy Orange Salsa (page 440)

Preheat oven to 375°F (190°C), and spray a mini-muffin pan with nonstick cooking spray.

In a mixing bowl, beat the egg for a minute or so. Now stir in the pumpkin seed meal, rice protein, melted butter, half-and-half, lemon juice, and chili garlic paste.

Add the tuna, breaking it up well as you stir it in. Stir in the minced scallions, and salt and pepper to taste.

Spoon into mini-muffin cups, and bake for 12 to 15 minutes.

When Tuna Puffs are done, place on a platter surrounding a bowl of Easy Orange Salsa.

YIELD: 24 puffs

Each with: 25 calories; 1 g fat; 3 g protein; 1 g carbohydrate; trace dietary fiber; 1 g usable carb. Analysis includes the Easy Orange Salsa.

Garlic Cheese Stuffed Mushrooms

These are the easiest stuffed mushrooms you ever made, and really yummy, too.

> 6 small portobello mushrooms, totaling 6 ounces (170 g)
>
> 1 6-ounce (170 g) package garlic and herb spreadable cheese (Boursin or Allouette)
>
> 2 tablespoons (10 g) crushed pork rinds

Wipe the mushrooms clean, and remove the stems (save them to slice and sauté to serve over steaks or in omelets). Divide the cheese between the mushroom caps. Sprinkle each one with a teaspoon of pork rind crumbs.

Arrange your mushrooms in a shallow baking pan. Add just enough water to cover the bottom of the pan. Bake for 30 minutes at 350°F (180°C), and serve hot. These are good with the Mustard-Horseradish Dipping Sauce (page 446), but they're just fine as is.

YIELD: 6 servings

Each with: 27 calories; 2 g fat; 1 g protein; 1 g carbohydrate; trace dietary fiber, 1 g usable carb.

◎ Spinach Stuffed Mushrooms

People scarf these right down!

1 1/2 pounds (680 g) mushrooms, wiped clean

2 tablespoons (30 g) butter

1/2 cup (80 g) chopped onion

4 cloves garlic, crushed

10 ounces (280 g) frozen chopped spinach, thawed

4 ounces (115 g) cream cheese

1/4 teaspoon pepper

1/2 teaspoon salt or Vege-Sal

1 1/2 teaspoons Worcestershire sauce

1/4 cup (40 g) Parmesan cheese, plus a little extra for sprinkling

Preheat oven to 350°F (180°C).

Wipe the mushrooms clean, and remove the stems. Set the caps aside, and chop the stems fairly fine.

In a large, heavy skillet, over medium-low heat, melt the butter. Add the chopped stems, and the onion. Sauté these until the mushroom bits are changing color, and the onion is soft and translucent. Add the garlic, stir it up, and sauté for another couple of minutes.

While that's happening, dump your thawed spinach into a strainer, and press all the water out of it that you can. Now stir it into the mushroom-onion mixture. Next, stir in the cream cheese. When it's melted, add the pepper, salt, Worcestershire, and Parmesan.

Stuff the spinach/mushroom mixture into the mushroom caps. Arrange the stuffed caps in a baking pan as you stuff them.

When they're all stuffed, sprinkle a little Parmesan cheese over them to make them look nice. Add enough water to just barely cover the bottom of the pan.

Bake for 30 minutes. Serve warm.

YIELD: About 40 pieces

Each with: 24 calories; 2 g fat; 1 g protein; 1 g carbohydrate; trace dietary fiber; 1 g usable carb.

◎ Cheese-Pecan Nibbles

These are quite simple to make, and sure to delight your guests. Feel free to use either the regular or the light garlic and herb cheese—they have about the same carb count.

> 2 cups (300 g) pecan halves
> 4 ounces (115 g) garlic and herb spreadable cheese (Boursin or Allouette)

You can make this with canned, roasted, and salted pecans, or, if you prefer, you can roast your own. If you choose the latter, preheat your oven to 350°F (180°C). Spread 2 cups (300 g) of unbroken pecan halves in a shallow baking pan. Stir in 1 teaspoon oil to coat—it will take a fair amount of stirring to get that little oil to coat this many nuts, so keep stirring! Sprinkle with salt, and roast for 8 to 10 minutes. Remove from oven, and let them cool before the next step.

Spread a dollop—between 1/4 and 1/2 a teaspoon—of garlic and herb spreadable cheese on the flat side of a pecan half, and press the flat side of another pecan half against it to make a pecan-and-cheese sandwich! Place on a serving plate, and continue with the rest of the cheese and the rest of the pecans.

YIELD: Enough for about 6 people

Each of whom will get: 300 calories; 30 g fat; 4 g protein; 7 g carbohydrate; 3 g dietary fiber; 4 g usable carbs.

⊚ Cajun Nut Mix

Just a little spicy, and way tasty, this has what we call a "more-ish" flavor.

  1 cup (150 g) dry-roasted peanuts
  1 cup (150 g) cashew pieces, raw
  1 cup (150 g) pecans
  4 tablespoons (60 g) butter
  1 teaspoon paprika
  1/2 teaspoon garlic powder
  1/2 teaspoon onion powder
  1/4 teaspoon cayenne
  1/4 teaspoon dried oregano
  1/4 teaspoon dried thyme
  1/4 teaspoon pepper
  1 teaspoon Worcestershire sauce
  Salt

Combine your nuts in a 9" x 13" (22.5 x 32.5 cm) baking pan.

Melt the butter, and stir all of the seasonings into it. Pour this mixture over the nuts, scraping out any spices that stick to the bottom of the pan you melted the butter in! Stir the nuts to coat.

Roast the nuts at 300°F (150°C) for 45 minutes, stirring every 15 minutes. Salt to taste.

YIELD: 3 cups (450 g), or 9 servings of 1/3 cup (50 g) each

Each with: 306 calories; 28 g fat; 7 g protein; 10 g carbohydrate; 3 g fiber; 7 g usable carbs.

Pepitas Calientes

Hot and sweet and crunchy, these Mexican-style pumpkin seeds will be the hit of any gathering you serve them at. Feel free to double or triple this!

 1 cup (225 g) raw, shelled pumpkin seeds
 2 teaspoons garlic powder
 1/4 teaspoon salt
 2 teaspoons chili garlic paste
 1 teaspoon Splenda
 1 teaspoon lime juice

Heat a medium-sized heavy skillet over medium-high heat. Add the pumpkin seeds, and dry-fry them for a few minutes, stirring constantly. After a little while, you'll see them swell a bit and become a bit plumper. This means they're just about done.

Stir in the garlic, salt, chili garlic paste, Splenda, and lime juice, making sure all the seeds are well coated. Continue to stir over heat until they dry, then serve hot.

YIELD: 4 servings of 1/4 cup (60 g) each

Each with: 78 calories; 3 g fat; 3 g protein; 10 g carbohydrate; 2 g dietary fiber; 8 g usable carbs.

Marilyn Olshansky's Spicy Pecans

Sweet and spicy and good, these pecans will thrill your guests—or just give you something wonderful to snack on.

- 1 tablespoon (9 g) chili powder
- 1 teaspoon cayenne
- 1 tablespoon (20 g) kosher salt
- 1 tablespoon (1.5 g) Splenda
- 2 tablespoons (30 ml) vegetable oil
- 3 cups (450 g) pecan halves
- 1 teaspoon fresh lemon juice (optional)

Combine the chili powder, cayenne, kosher salt, and Splenda in a small bowl.

Heat the oil over medium heat in a large, heavy skillet. Sauté the nuts, stirring, until they are dry and begin to sizzle, about 8 minutes.

Sprinkle the spice mixture over the nuts and stir to coat evenly. Optional: sprinkle the lemon juice over the nuts and cook until it is evaporated.

Turn the nuts out onto layers of paper towels to drain. Serve warm or at room temperature.

YIELD: 9 servings of ⅓ cup (50 g)

Each with: 270 calories; 27 g fat; 3 g protein; 7 g carbohydrate; 3 g dietary fiber; 4 g usable carbs.

Brie and Walnut Quesadillas

⅓ cup (40 g) chopped walnuts
8 ounces (225 g) Brie
6 low-carb tortillas

Preheat your oven to 350°F (180°C). Spread your walnuts in a shallow roasting pan. Put them in the oven, and let them roast for 8 to 10 minutes—set the oven timer!

While that's happening, cut your Brie into quarters, and thinly slice off the rind. Now, slice the Brie, or if it's too soft for that, cut it into little cubes.

Lay a tortilla in a big, heavy skillet over medium-low heat. Cover it with slices or small hunks of Brie, and let it heat until the cheese begins to melt, and the walnuts are done. Scatter ⅓ of the walnuts over the cheese, and top the whole thing with another tortilla. Turn your quesadilla over, and continue to cook till the cheese is good and melty. Transfer to a plate and cover with a lid to keep warm while you make two more!

Cut into wedges, and serve.

YIELD: 6 servings

Each with: 218 calories; 16 g fat; 15 g protein; 12 g carbohydrate; 8 g dietary fiber; 4 g usable carbs.

⊚ Cocktail Ham Tartlets

These hot hors d'oeuvres are a throwback to the 1960s, but they're darned tasty.

Pie Crust (page 132)
2 cans deviled ham, one the 4.25-ounce (120 g) size, the other the
2.25-ounce (60 g) size
3/4 cup (180 g) Simple No-Sugar Pickle Relish (page 441)
2 teaspoons spicy brown mustard

Make your pie crust first, but don't pat it into a pie pan. Instead, you're going to use two 12-cup muffin tins. Spray them with non-stick cooking spray, nip off 1" (2.5 cm) balls of dough with your fingers, and press each one evenly over the bottom of a muffin cup.

Now, preheat your oven to 375°F (190°C). Mix together all the remaining ingredients, and spoon about a teaspoon of the mixture into each muffin cup, spreading it with the back of the spoon.

Bake your Cocktail Ham Tartlets for about 20 minutes, then let them cool just a bit before using the rounded tip of a butter knife to loosen each one and lift it out to a serving plate. Serve warm.

YIELD: 24 servings

Each with: 87 calories; 6 g fat; 6 g protein; 2 g carbohydrate; trace dietary fiber; 2 g usable carbs.

⊙ Curried Chicken Dip

Not only will this mildly spicy dip please your friends and family, but carried in a snap-top container, with a bag of cut-up veggies, it would make a great lunch.

> 5 ounces (140 g) canned chunk chicken, drained
> 3 ounces (85 g) light cream cheese
> 1 tablespoon (15 g) mayonnaise
> 2 tablespoons (20 g) minced red onion
> ³⁄₄ teaspoon curry powder
> 1 teaspoon brown mustard
> ¹⁄₄ teaspoon hot sauce, or to taste
> 2 tablespoons (10 g) minced fresh parsley

Pretty darned easy—just assemble everything in your food processor with the S-blade in place, and pulse till it's smooth. Put your dip in a pretty bowl, and surround it with cucumber slices, celery sticks, and/or pepper strips.

YIELD: 6 servings

Each with: 92 calories; 6 g fat; 7 g protein; 2 g carbohydrate; trace dietary fiber; 2 g usable carbs. Carb count does not include vegetable dippers.

⊙ Sally Waldron's Spicy Blue Cheese Dressing and Dip

A natural with celery sticks, cucumber rounds, or pepper strips.

> ¹⁄₂ cup (120 g) mayonnaise
> ¹⁄₂ cup (120 g) sour cream
> ¹⁄₂ cup (60 g) blue cheese, crumbled
> 1 tablespoon (15 ml) Louisiana-style hot sauce
> Salt and pepper to taste

Simply stir everything together, and it's done!

YIELD: Makes 1 ¹⁄₂ cups (300 g) or 12 servings of 2 tablespoons (25 g)

Each with: 106 calories; 11 g fat; 2 g protein; 1 g carbohydrate; trace dietary fiber;1 g usable carb.

Debbie White's Colorado Chipped Beef Appetizer

16 ounces (455 g) cream cheese, softened

4.5 ounces (125 g) Armour Sliced Dried Beef, chopped

1 cup (150 g) chopped green pepper

¼–⅓ cup (40–50 g) chopped onion

1 teaspoon garlic powder

1 cup (230 g) sour cream

2 tablespoons (30 ml) half-and-half

2 tablespoons (30 ml) water

½ teaspoon pepper

½ cup (60 g) slivered almonds

Mix together all ingredients except almonds and put in a baking dish. Microwave for about 6 to 7 minutes to make it easier to mix and also to warm it up before baking it. Sprinkle with ½ cup slivered almonds and then bake at 350°F (180°C) for 20 minutes, till hot and lightly brown on top. Serve with your favorite low-carb crackers and tons of veggies.

YIELD: Serves at least 12 people.

With 12 servings: 235 calories; 21 g fat; 8 g protein; 5 g carbohydrate; 1 g dietary fiber; 4 g usable carbs.

Sally Miller's Awesome Pimento Cheese

1 pound (455 g) mild cheddar cheese
½ pound (225 g) Muenster cheese
½ pound (225 g) mozzarella cheese
½ pound (225 g) Swiss cheese
½ pound (225 g) Monterey Jack cheese
2 tablespoons (20 g) diced pimento
2 tablespoons (20 g) finely diced green pepper
2 tablespoons (20 g) finely diced green onion
2 cups (470 g) mayonnaise, or to taste—enough to moisten

Shred cheese into a large bowl. Add pimento, green pepper, green onion, and mayonnaise. Mix until well blended. Serve with cut-up veggies and/or low-carb crackers.

Sally's note: "I usually put it in 1/2-pint [235 ml] Mason jars and adorn with curling ribbon and a tag for Christmas giving."

YIELD: Should serve 20 people

Each getting: 413 calories; 39 g fat; 17 g protein; 1 g carbohydrate; trace dietary fiber; 1g usable carb.

☺ Pat Best's Refried Black Soy Beans

Look for those black soy beans at your local health food or natural food grocery—a company called Eden cans them.

2 15-ounce (420 g) cans black soy beans, rinsed, drained, and mashed
1 tablespoon (10 g) finely chopped jalapeno pepper, or to taste
5 ounces (150 ml) chicken broth
2 tablespoons (30 ml) canola oil
2 tablespoons (20 g) finely chopped onion
1/2 teaspoon salt, or to taste
Dash of pepper

In a blender or food processor, puree the black soy beans, jalapeno, and the chicken broth until creamy and smooth. Adjust chicken broth to reach the desired consistency.

In a medium saucepan, warm the oil. Add the onion to the oil and sauté until just tender but not brown or burnt. Carefully add the bean puree to the hot oil and onion mixture, taking care that it does not pop or spit. Heat the bean mixture through, adding the salt and pepper to taste. Keep warm until serving time or prepare ahead and rewarm right before serving.

YIELD: 10 servings

Each has: 106 calories; 7 g fat; 8 g protein; 6 g carbohydrate; 5 g dietary fiber; 1 g usable carb.

Pat Best's Guacamole

Do you have any idea how good for you avocados are?!

4 ripe avocados
1 medium tomato, seeded and coarsely chopped
1/2 cup (80 g) finely chopped onion
1 4-ounce (115 g) can green chili peppers, drained and chopped
1 clove garlic, pressed
2 tablespoons plus 1 teaspoon (35 ml) lime juice
2 tablespoons (5 g) fresh cilantro, chopped
1/2 teaspoon salt
1/4 teaspoon white pepper (optional)

Cut avocados in half lengthwise. Remove pits and scoop flesh into a blender or food processor. Add tomato, onion, peppers, garlic, lime juice, cilantro, salt, and white pepper, if desired. Cover and process until well combined, stopping machine occasionally to scrape down the sides. Transfer to a bowl and cover tightly. Chill several hours before serving.

YIELD: 10 servings (3 cups)

Each has: 140 calories; 12 g fat; 2 g protein; 8 g carbohydrate; 2 g dietary fiber; 6 g usable carbs.

Marcie Vaughn's Sausage Dip

1 pound (455 g) bulk pork sausage
1 14.5-ounce (411 g) can diced tomatoes with green chilies
8 ounces (225 g) cream cheese

Brown and crumble the sausage, but don't drain it. Add the tomatoes and cream cheese. Mix together and enjoy. This can be made in a Crock-Pot, on the stove-top, or in the microwave. Eat with low-carb tortilla chips, pork rinds, or, hey, with a spoon!

YIELD: 15 servings

Each has: 184 calories; 17 g fat; 5 g protein; 2 g carbohydrate; trace dietary fiber; 2 g usable carbs.

Pat Best's Jalapeno Cheese Spread

Our tester suggests that you microwave this gently to bring it up to room temperature if you don't want to wait. He also says this would be great to take to a potluck or pitch-in.

1 ½ cups (180 g) shredded jalapeno Jack cheese
1 3-ounce (85 g) package cream cheese
¼ cup (60 g) butter
⅓ cup (80 ml) heavy cream
1 tablespoon (10 g) chopped green onion
½ teaspoon Dijon-style mustard
¼ teaspoon Worcestershire sauce
Few dashes bottled hot sauce
Assorted high-fiber crackers
Assorted fresh vegetable sticks

Bring cheeses and butter to room temperature. In a small mixer bowl beat cheeses and butter with electric mixer until combined. Add cream, green onion, mustard, Worcestershire sauce, and hot sauce. Beat until smooth. Pack into a 16-ounce (455 g) crock or jar. Refrigerate for at least 6 hours. Serve at room temperature with high-fiber crackers or assorted vegetable sticks.

YIELD: Eight 1/4-cup (60 g) servings

Each has: 205 calories; 20 g fat; 6 g protein; 1 g carbohydrate; trace dietary fiber; 1 g usable carb.

◉ Pat Best's Seven Layer Bean Dip

Our tester, Julie, loved this dip, and says you can use a three-cheese Mexican blend in place of the Monterey Jack, if you prefer.

> 1 1.25-ounce (35 g) packet taco seasoning
>   or 2 tablespoons (12 g) homemade Taco Seasoning (page 531)
> 1 cup (230 g) sour cream
> Refried Black Soy Beans (page 63)
> Pat Best's Guacamole (page 64)
> 1 cup (120 g) shredded Monterey Jack cheese, divided
> ½ 4-ounce (115 g) can sliced black olives
> 1 small tomato, seeded and coarsely chopped
> 2 scallions, chopped, green portion included
> Vegetable sticks for dipping (celery, carrots, peppers, squash, etc.)
> Low-carb chips

Begin by mixing the taco seasoning mix with 1 cup (230 g) sour cream.

To assemble, spread the Refried Black Soybeans on the bottom of your serving dish to start. Then, layer in the following order: guacamole, sour cream mixture, ½ of the cheese, black olives, diced tomato, green onions, and finally the remaining shredded cheese. Cover and chill for several hours. Serve with vegetable sticks or low-carbohydrate chips.

YIELD: Should serve 20 people

Each getting: 176 calories; 14 g fat; 7 g protein; 9 g carbohydrate; 4 g dietary fiber; 5 g usable carbs.

✹ Lorraine Achey's Dilled Almonds

These were inspired by the Sunflower Parmesan Crackers in *500 Low-Carb Recipes*.

>2 cups (300 g) almonds
>3–4 tablespoons (45–60 g) butter, melted
>1 tablespoon Parmesan-Dill Seasoning Mix (page 450)

Preheat oven to 325°F (170°C).

Place nuts in a shallow pan and add butter, mixing to coat well. Spread the nuts out evenly in the pan.

Roast nuts for 15 to 20 minutes.

Remove from oven, sprinkle Parmesan-Dill Seasoning over the almonds and stir to coat.

YIELD: 8 servings

Each has: 262 calories; 24 g fat; 7 g protein; 7 g carbohydrate; 4 g dietary fiber; 3 g usable carbs.

✹ Lynn Avery's Pimiento Cheese

>12 ounces (340 g) American cheese, shredded (Lynn uses Kraft)
>4-ounce (115 g) jar pimientos, drained and chopped or pureed, depending on how you like it
>¼ cup (60 g) Miracle Whip Light salad dressing (you can use mayo; Lynn likes the sweetness of the salad dressing)
>1 tablespoon (15 ml) Worcestershire sauce
>1 tablespoon (15 ml) Tabasco sauce, or to taste
>1 teaspoon celery salt
>1 teaspoon pepper

Mix all ingredients thoroughly. Couldn't be easier! Great stuffed in celery or cherry tomatoes, or spread on low-carb crackers or bread.

Dana's note: You can replace the Miracle Whip Light with mayo with a tiny bit of Splenda added, or Carb Options now has a similar dressing.

YIELD: Makes 8 servings, ¼ cup (60 g) each.

Per serving: 216 calories; 19 g fat; 10 g protein; 2 g carbohydrate; trace dietary fiber; 2g usable carbs.

Barbecued Pumpkin Seeds

2 cups (450 g) pumpkin seeds, roasted

1–2 teaspoons water

2 tablespoons (15 g) Classic Barbecue Rub (page 538)

Put your pumpkin seeds in a dry skillet over medium-high heat, and stir until they start to swell—about 5 minutes. Stir in the water and the barbecue rub, and keep stirring till the seeds are dry again. Serve.

YIELD: 8 servings of $1/4$ cup (60 g) each

Each with: 75 calories; 3 g fat; 3 g protein; 9 g carbohydrate; 2 g dietary fiber; 7 g usable carbs.

Smoked Almonds

These are crunchy with a nice kick!

1 pound almonds

3 tablespoons butter

2 teaspoons barbecue rub (see recipe page 538, or use purchased rub)

2 teaspoons salt

2 teaspoons liquid Barbecue Smoke®

Lay a big flat roasting pan over a burner, and melt the butter in it. Stir in the seasonings, making sure they're blended into the butter. Now add the almonds, and stir until they're well-coated. Roast at 300 for 30-40 minutes. Store in an airtight container.

YIELD: 12 servings

Each with: 248 Calories; 23g Fat; 8g Protein; 8g Carbohydrate; 4g Dietary Fiber; 4 grams usable carbs.

◎ Margaret King's Cheese Crisps

This is so simple, I almost ignored it. I'm really glad I didn't! My tester, Doris, gave this simple recipe a 10. She also said you can fold the cheese in half before it cools, to make something like a taco shell. She filled hers with scrambled eggs for breakfast and tuna salad for lunch—and recommended taco filling for dinner!

Take 1 slice of pasteurized processed American cheese (12, 16, or 24 in a package), put it on a piece of parchment paper on a microwaveable paper plate, and put it in the micro for 50 seconds. It will bubble up and become brown and delish! Take it out, let it cool for a few minutes, and it will be so crisp. Now, this satisfies my need to crunch and is quite tasty!

Each crisp made from one slice of cheese has: 106 calories; 9 g fat; 6 g protein; trace carbohydrate; no fiber; trace usable carbs.

◎ Lynn Avery's Provolone "Chips"

Our tester, Julie, says she likes these better than those high-priced low-carb chips!

Put a slice of provolone on a waxed paper plate and microwave it for about 1:10, or until it starts turning golden brown. When you take it out of the microwave, you can fold it into a "taco shell" as it cools, or just leave it flat. I like to top it with sour cream, guacamole, and salsa for a satisfying and easy Mexican-style lunch.

Each chip made from 1 ounce of cheese has: 100 calories; 8 g fat; 7 g protein; no fiber; 1g usable carb.

⊚ Margaret King's Tortilla Chips

You can buy low-carb tortilla chips, but there's a charm to fresh ones.

> Low-carb tortillas
> Nonstick cooking spray

Spray the tortillas with cooking spray, both sides, and cut them into triangle shapes. Bake on a cookie sheet at 400°F (200°C) for 10 to 15 minutes, until crisp and brown. They make great dippers for all chip and dip needs!

Tester's note: Barbo Gold, who tested these, liked them the way Margaret made them, but thought they were even better baked at 250°F (130°C) for 1 hour and 10 minutes. She also suggests a sprinkle of salt, and even onion powder. Knock yourself out.

Each whole tortilla has: 50 calories; 2 g fat; 5 g protein; 11 g carbohydrate; 8 g dietary fiber; 3 g usable carbs.

⊚ Jill Taylor's Fried Cheese Taco Shells

Who could miss those stale corn ones, out of a box?

> 1 8-ounce (225 g) bag of shredded Mexican 4-Cheese blend
>   Don't use fat-free cheese!

Heat a small nonstick skillet over medium heat until hot. Add ½ cup (30 g) of shredded cheese and fry until brown. Flip over and brown the other side. Do not overcook as it becomes dry and brittle. Light golden brown is good. When cooked, remove from the skillet and place over a rolling pin covered with a kitchen towel. Use another folded piece of kitchen towel to mold the cheese into a taco shape, then put aside to cool. Always wipe the excess fat from the pan before you add more cheese, as it cooks better if it is dry.

If you prefer nachos to tacos, cook the cheese the same way but place flat on a piece of kitchen towel when cooked and cut into "chips" with a pizza cutter before it is cold.

YIELD: Makes 8 tortilla shells or rounds to cut up

Each having: 114 calories; 9 g fat; 7 g protein; trace carbohydrate; no fiber, trace usable carbs.

Mindy Sauve's Low-Carb Nachos Supreme

A fast, teen-friendly dinner!

> 1 pound (455 g) low-fat ground beef
> 1 15-ounce (420 g) can Eden Black Soy Beans, drained
> 1 7 ¾-ounce (220 g) can Mexican Hot-Style Tomato Sauce (if you can't find this, use regular tomato sauce with 3 tablespoons (45 ml) enchilada sauce added!)
> 1 12-ounce (340 g) bag Soy and Flaxseed Tortilla Chips (or make own chips from Margaret King's Tortilla Chips (page 70)
> 2 cups (240 g) grated Mexican Cheese blend (or cheese of choice)
> 1 7 ¾-ounce (220 g) can sliced black olives
> 1 tomato, diced
> Sour cream to taste

Brown and crumble ground beef, and drain fat. Add black soy beans and Mexican tomato sauce. Cook just until all heated through.

Spread the contents of a bag of low-carb chips on a plate; top with ¼ cup (30 g) grated cheese. Spoon ½ cup (60 g) meat/bean mixture on top. Top meat mixture with another ¼ cup (30 g) cheese. Sprinkle with olives. Microwave the whole thing on high for 45 seconds until cheese is melted.

Top with chopped tomato and sour cream to taste.

Dana's note: I might use Pat Best' Refried Black Soy Beans (page 63) instead of the plain black soy beans.

YIELD: Serves 8 or more

Each has: 517 calories; 39 g fat (61.2% calories from fat); 30 g protein; 25 g carbohydrate; 16 g dietary fiber; 9 g usable carbs.

◉ Susan Higgs's Salmon Stuffed Celery

A great party snack or sack lunch.

> 1 15-ounce (420 g) can salmon, drained,
>   or 2 vacuum-packed packages salmon
> 8 ounces (225 g) softened cream cheese
> Juice and zest of one lemon
> 1 teaspoon prepared horseradish
> 1 tablespoon (10 g) dried minced onion flakes
> ¼ teaspoon salt
> 1 tablespoon (15 ml) Worcestershire sauce (you may want to add this
>   1 teaspoon at a time, depending on how well you like the
>   Worcestershire sauce)
> 1 bunch celery, cut in thirds

Mix all ingredients together except celery. Chill for 4 to 8 hours.
Stuff salmon-cheese mixture into celery thirds and serve.

Yield: 20 servings

Each has: 71 calories; 5 g fat; 5 g protein; 1g carbohydrate; trace dietary fiber;
1g usable carbs.

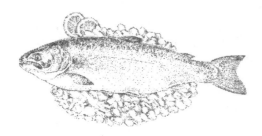

Herbert D. Focken's Sweetened Jalapeno Bites

Our tester, Julie, called this "really interesting, and surprisingly good!" (She also said it really improved low-carb crackers, of which she is not generally fond.)

> 1 12-ounce (340 g) jar sliced jalapeno peppers
> ¾ cup (18 g) Splenda
> Cream cheese—plain or onion-chive flavored
> Pork rinds or low-carb crackers

Dump out the jalapenos, including the liquid, into a bowl, and stir in the Splenda. Pack them back into the jar, put on the lid, and stick it in the fridge for a day or two.

When snack time rolls around, pull out the jar and grab your cream cheese and pork rinds or low-carb crackers. Spread some cream cheese on a pork rind or cracker, top with a slice or two of jalapeno, and stuff it in your face! Repeat.

Your whole jar of sweetened peppers has the following: 94 calories; 2 g fat; 4 g protein; 18 g carbohydrate; 9 g dietary fiber; 9 g usable carbs. Working out the per-piece counts of this was just too darned difficult, so we gave up—but cream cheese is very low carb, and pork rinds are carb-free. If you're using low-carb crackers, read the label.

◉ Linda Guiffre's Pizza Muffin Appetizers

Leftovers—if there are any—can be eaten cold the next day for lunch.

1–2 tablespoons (15–30 ml) olive oil
1 clove garlic, minced
½ cup (75 g) chopped green pepper
½ cup (75 g) chopped red pepper
½ small onion, chopped
1 cup (100 g) chopped mushrooms
¼ cup (25 g) chopped olives
¼–½ teaspoon red pepper flakes, or to taste
½ teaspoon Italian seasoning
Dash black pepper
2 eggs
⅔ cup (100 g) grated Parmesan cheese
1 ½ cups (180 g) shredded mozzarella
8 ounces (225 g) cream cheese, softened
Approximately 30 slices of deli-sized pepperoni
½ cup (120 g) pizza sauce (optional)

In the olive oil sauté the garlic, peppers, and onion until almost soft. Add the mushrooms and sauté a minute or two more. Turn off the heat and add the olives, red pepper flakes, Italian seasoning, and pepper.

In a bowl, lightly beat your eggs, then add the Parmesan, mozzarella, and cream cheese. Add your sautéed vegetables and mix all ingredients until blended.

Line each mini-muffin cup with a slice of pepperoni (forming a basket). Use a teaspoon to drop the vegetable-cheese mixture into the pepperoni cup.

Bake for 25 minutes at 325°F (170°C) or until very lightly browned.

If desired, serve with a bit of pizza sauce on top (may top each muffin with sauce 10 minutes prior to end of baking time, then return to oven to finish baking—or simply top muffins with sauce when done), but they're good plain, too.

Yield: Makes about 30 mini-muffin-sized bites

Each with: 98 calories; 8 g fat; 4 g protein; 2 g carbohydrate; trace dietary fiber; 2g usable carbs.

◎ Nancy Harrigan's Spinach Balls

Our tester, Patty Mishler, rated this a 10!

> 3 boxes, 10 ounces (280 g) each, frozen chopped spinach, thawed and squeezed dry
> 2 cups (250 g) almond meal
> 1 1/2 cups (185 g) chopped macadamia nuts
> 1 teaspoon salt
> 1/4 teaspoon garlic powder
> 2 tablespoons (20 g) dried minced onion
> 1/2 cup (80 g) grated Parmesan cheese
> 2 eggs or 4 egg whites
> 1 stick butter, melted

Mix together and form into 1" (2.5 cm) balls.

Bake ats 350°F (180°C) for 20 min.

These may be baked dry and served with hollandaise sauce or a mustard sauce as an hors d'oeuvres. The balls should be bite-sized for this. Or you can bake these in Nancy Harrigan's Coconut Ginger Sauce (page 445).

Nancy's note: "I like to bake these in the Coconut Ginger Sauce (page 445). Mix the sauce and pour over balls before baking. This sauce will need to be doubled for the whole batch of Spinach Balls. I bake them in this sauce (using butter) with raw shrimp. Add a salad and you've got a fabulous dinner!

"I also like to make up the whole batch, put the balls on a cookie sheet, and freeze them, then put them in a freezer bag and take them out as needed."

Yield: About 8 servings (6 balls each)

Each with: 464 calories; 38 g fat; 20 g protein; 17 g carbohydrate; 6 g dietary fiber; 11 g usable carbs. Analysis does not include any sauce or dip.

Audra Olsen's Asparagus/Salami Roll-Ups

    1 pound (455 g) fresh or frozen asparagus
    1 pound (455 g) hard salami, the smaller round ones
    4 ounces (115 g) cream cheese

If you're using fresh asparagus, snap the end off each spear where it breaks naturally, then plunge into boiling water for just 20 to 30 seconds; drain. If using frozen asparagus, just thaw it.

Preheat oven to 375°F (190°C) degrees.

Lay out a slice of salami, spread with cream cheese, and place an asparagus spear on one end, rolling it up. Seal with a dab of cream cheese and lay on a cookie sheet. Once all processed, bake for 20 minutes. Serve.

Yield: Serves 4

Each serving will have: 397 calories; 33 g fat; 19 g protein; 6 g carbohydrate; 1 g dietary fiber; 5 g usable carbs.

chapter three

Eggs, Cheese, and the Like

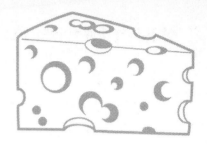

I've said it before, I'll say it again: eggs are not just for breakfast! They're one of the most versatile foods we have in our low-carb diet, and for the protein they offer—with almost no waste—they're a heckuva bargain. Better yet, many egg recipes are fast! So have a dozen eggs—or more—in the fridge at all times.

We're also including recipes that get their protein from cheese in this chapter, just because it seemed like a good idea. One of the best things about cheese is that it keeps well. Further, it doesn't need defrosting. And all you have to do is heat it up to make it seem like a meal, instead of a snack.

Of course, if you're a low-carb vegetarian, eggs and cheese will be among the staples of your diet. But everyone can enjoy meals centered around eggs and cheese!

There are also some recipes in this chapter that involve substantial quantities of things like sausage, ham, or bacon, along with the eggs and cheese. It was sort of a judgment call, you know?

Here, repeated from two previous books, is the single skill I'm determined to teach every low carber:

Dana's Easy Omelet Method

If I had to choose just one skill to teach to every new low carber, it would be how to make an omelet. They're fast, they're easy, and they make a wide variety of simple ingredients seem like a meal!

First, have your filling ready. If you're using vegetables, you'll want to sauté them first. If you're using cheese, have it grated or sliced and ready to go. If you're making an omelet to use up leftovers—a great idea, by the way—warm them through in the microwave and have them standing by.

Spray your omelet pan well with cooking spray if it doesn't have a good nonstick surface, and put it over medium-high heat. While the skillet's heating, grab your eggs—2 is the perfect number for this size pan, but 1 or 3 will work—and a bowl, crack the eggs, and beat them with a fork. Don't add any water or milk or anything, just mix them up.

The pan is hot enough when a drop of water thrown in sizzles right away. Add a tablespoon of oil or butter, slosh it around to cover the bottom, then pour in the eggs, all at once. They should sizzle, too, and immediately start to set. When the bottom layer of egg is set around the edges—this should happen quite quickly—lift the edge using a spatula and tip the pan to let the raw egg flow underneath. Do this all around the edges, until there's not enough raw egg to run.

Now, turn your burner to the lowest heat if you have a gas stove. If you have an electric stove, you'll have to have a "warm" burner standing by; electric elements don't cool off fast enough for this job. Put your filling on one-half of the omelet, cover it, and let it sit over very low heat for a minute or two, no more. Peek and see if the raw, shiny egg is gone from the top surface (although you can serve it that way if you like—that's how the French prefer their omelets), and the cheese, if you've used it, is melted. If not, re-cover the pan and let it go another minute or two.

When your omelet is done, slip a spatula under the half without the filling and fold it over; then lift the whole thing onto a plate. Or you can get fancy and tip the pan, letting the filling side of the omelet slide onto the plate, folding the top over as you go, but this takes some practice.

This makes a single-serving omelet. I think it's a lot easier to make several individual omelets than to make one big one, and omelets are so fast to make that it's not that big a deal. Anyway, that way you can customize your omelets to each individual's taste. If you're making more than 2 or 3 omelets, just keep them warm in your oven, set to its very lowest heat.

Now here are some ideas for what to put in your omelets!

◎ Club Omelet

One of the few high-carb meals I miss is the turkey club sandwich—so here's the omelet equivalent!

2 slices bacon, cooked and drained
2 ounces (55 g) turkey breast slices
1/2 small tomato, sliced
1 scallion, sliced
2 eggs
1 tablespoon (15 g) mayonnaise

Have your bacon cooked and drained—I like to microwave mine and crumble it up. Cut the turkey into small squares, and have the tomato and scallion sliced and at hand.

Beat the eggs, and make your omelet according to Dana's Easy Omelet Method (page 77), adding just the bacon and turkey while it's still cooking. Then add the tomato and scallion, spread the mayo on the other side, fold, and serve.

Yield: 1 serving

Each with: 383 calories; 28 g fat; 29 g protein; 5 g carbohydrate; 1 g dietary fiber; 4 g usable carbs.

Mexican Avocado and Ham Omelet

This is actually a fairly traditional combination in Mexico.

> 1 pinch paprika
> 1/4 teaspoon salt
> 2 tablespoons (30 g) sour cream
> 2 eggs
> 1/4 cup (30 g) ham, minced
> 2 tablespoons (25 g) diced tomato
> 1/2 avocado, sliced

Have everything cut up before you start cooking. Stir the paprika and salt into the sour cream.

Now, make your omelet according to Dana's Easy Omelet Method (page 77). When bottom is set, add ham and tomato, cover the skillet, and set the burner to low. Let it cook for a minute or two until top is set. Arrange avocado slices on the ham and tomato, fold omelet, and top with seasoned sour cream to serve.

Yield: 1 serving

Each with: 509 calories; 42 g fat; 23 g protein; 12 g carbohydrate; 3 g dietary fiber; 9 g usable carbs.

Roman Mushroom Omelet

Believe it or not, this is classical Italian food, with no pasta in sight.

> 2 cups (200 g) sliced mushrooms
> 1/4 small onion, sliced thin
> 1 stalk celery, diced fine
> 2 tablespoons (30 ml) olive oil
> 1 clove garlic
> 1/2 teaspoon chicken bouillon concentrate
> 1/2 teaspoon Splenda
> Salt and pepper
> 4 eggs
> 1/2 cup (80 g) shredded Romano cheese

In your big skillet, start sautéing the mushrooms, onion, and celery in the olive oil. When the mushrooms have changed color and the onion is translucent, add the garlic, chicken bouillon granules, and Splenda, stirring till the bouillon dissolves. Let cook for another minute or so. Salt and pepper the mushroom mixture to taste, and remove from skillet.

Now, in your omelet pan, make 2 omelets, one after the other, according to Dana's Easy Omelet Method (page 77), using the mushrooms as filling, with ¼ cup (40 g) of shredded Romano cheese on top. Cover and cook till cheese melts, fold, and serve. (You can keep the first omelet warm long enough to make the second omelet by simply covering the plate with a spare pot lid. For that matter, you can halve this recipe to make one omelet!)

Yield: 2 omelets

Each with: 388 calories; 30 g fat; 22 g protein; 8 g carbohydrate; 1 g dietary fiber; 7 g usable carbs.

◎ Sloppy Tom Omelet

I like this omelet as a quick lunch. Indeed, I've been known to make Sloppy Toms just to have them on hand for this purpose. If you have a favorite low-carb Sloppy Joe recipe, feel free to use it instead.

> 2 eggs
> ¼ cup (50 g) Sloppy Toms (page 259)
> 1 ounce (30 g) cheddar cheese or Monterey Jack, sliced or shredded

If your Sloppy Toms are left over, straight out of the fridge, warm them a bit in the microwave before you start cooking the eggs. Then make your omelet according to Dana's Easy Omelet Method (page 77), adding the cheese first, then the Sloppy Toms on top of the cheese. Cover, turn burner to low, and finish cooking, then fold and serve.

Yield: 1 serving

Each with: 346 calories; 23 g fat; 27 g protein; 7 g carbohydrate; 1 g dietary fiber; 6 g usable carbs.

Ropa Vieja Omelet

Here's another way to use your Ropa Vieja (page 319)

1/3 cup (70 g) Ropa Vieja
1 ounce (30 g) Monterey Jack cheese
1/4 California avocado, sliced
2 eggs

Warm your Ropa Vieja in the microwave, slice or shred your cheese, and slice your avocado; have everything standing by!

Now heat your omelet pan, and add a little oil. Beat up your eggs, and when the skillet's hot, pour them in and make your omelet according to Dana's Easy Omelet Method (page 77).

When it's time to add the filling, put the cheese in first, then the Ropa Vieja, then the avocado. Cover, turn burner to low, and finish cooking, then fold and serve.

Yield: 1 serving

Each with: 445 calories; 34 g fat; 29 g protein; 5 g carbohydrate; 2 g dietary fiber; 3 g usable carbs.

Inauthentic Machaca Eggs

True Machaca is made with beef that you've salted and dried, then rehydrated in boiling water, and pounded into shreds. It's very tasty, but I don't know a lot of people who want to do that much work. The beef shreds from the Ropa Vieja work beautifully in this scramble!

2 tablespoons (30 ml) olive oil
1 cup (200 g) Ropa Vieja (page 319)
½ green bell pepper, diced
½ onion, chopped
1 clove garlic, crushed
1 cup (225 g) canned tomatoes with green chilies, drained
5 eggs
¼ cup (20 g) chopped fresh cilantro

Heat the olive oil in a large, heavy skillet, and add the Ropa Vieja, diced pepper and onion, and the garlic. Sauté them together, stirring often, until the onion and pepper are becoming a little soft. In the meanwhile, measure your tomatoes and scramble up your eggs.

Okay, your onion is translucent, and your pepper's starting to soften. Add the tomato, stir it up, then pour in the beaten eggs. Scramble until the eggs are set. Divide evenly between two plates, top each serving with half the cilantro, and serve.

Feel free to add some chopped jalapenos or more green chilies to this, if you'd like it spicy. Or you could use a pasilla or Anaheim chili in place of the green pepper.

Yield: 2 to3 servings

Assuming 2 servings, each will have: 520 calories; 39 g fat; 30 g protein; 12 g carbohydrate; 2 g dietary fiber; 10 g usable carbs.

Italian Sausage and Mushroom Scramble

2 ounces (55 g) Italian sausage link
1 tablespoon (15 ml) olive oil
¾ cup (75 g) chopped mushrooms
2 tablespoons (16 g) grated carrot
1 scallion
3 eggs
2 tablespoons (20 g) grated Parmesan cheese

Slice the sausage down the middle the long way, then lay flat side down and slice into half-rounds, about ¼" (6.25 mm) thick. Heat the olive oil in a large skillet, over medium-low heat, and start browning the sausage.

In the meanwhile, cut up your mushrooms, grate your carrot, and slice your scallion. When the sausage is browned on the first side, turn it over, and add the veggies. Cook, stirring now and then, until the mushrooms soften a bit.

Beat the eggs with the Parmesan, and pour over the sausage and vegetables. Scramble till set, and serve.

Yield: 1 to 2 servings

Assuming 1 serving, it will have: 582 calories; 48 g fat; 30 g protein; 7 g carbohydrate; 1 g dietary fiber; 6 g usable carbs.

Spring Ham and Mushroom Scramble

Ham and eggs scrambled together are nothing new—it's the seasoning that makes this taste fresh as springtime!

½ cup (50 g) sliced mushrooms
½ cup (55 g) ham cubes
1 teaspoon butter
4 eggs
¾ teaspoon dried dill weed
½ teaspoon lemon juice
4 scallions, sliced ¼" (6.25 mm) thick

In a small-to-medium–sized nonstick skillet, start sautéing the mushrooms and ham cubes in the butter. While that's happening, scramble your eggs with the dill and lemon.

When the mushrooms are limp and have changed color, add the eggs and sliced scallions to the skillet. Scramble till eggs are set, and serve.

Yield: 2 servings

Each with: 225 calories; 14 g fat; 18 g protein; 5 g carbohydrate; 1 g dietary fiber; 4 g usable carbs.

◎ Springtime Scramble

4 stalks asparagus
8 fresh snow pea pods
1 scallion
3 eggs
1 teaspoon olive oil

Snap the bottoms off your asparagus where they break naturally, then cut the stalks into ½" (1.25 cm) pieces, on the diagonal. Pinch the ends off the snow peas, and pull off the strings, then cut them into ½" (1.25 cm) pieces, too. Put the two in a microwaveable bowl, add just a couple of teaspoons of water, cover, and microwave on high for just 3 minutes. Uncover as soon as the microwave beeps! While this is happening, slice your scallion, including the crisp part of the green, and beat up your eggs.

Okay, pull your asparagus and snow peas out of the microwave. Spray a medium skillet with nonstick cooking spray, and place over medium heat. Add the olive oil, and let it start heating. Drain the asparagus and snow peas, and throw 'em in the skillet, along with the scallion. Now pour in the eggs, and scramble till set. That's it!

Yield: 1 serving

Each with: 267 calories; 18 g fat; 19 g protein; 8 g carbohydrate; 2 g dietary fiber; 6 g usable carbs.

Marilee Wellersdick's Bean Sprout Scramble

Like bean sprouts? They're very low carb and quite good for you.

> 2 tablespoons (30 g) butter
> 1 tablespoon (10 g) minced onion
> 1/2 cup (25 g) bean sprouts
> 3 eggs
> Salt and pepper
> 1 tablespoon (15 g) sour cream (optional)

Melt the butter in a nonstick skillet. Add the onion and sprouts and stir until the sprouts are tender crisp (onions should be translucent by then). Scramble the eggs, add salt and pepper, and add them to the skillet, stirring the mixture until the eggs are set. To serve, top with a dollop of sour cream, if desired.

Yield: This recipe is for 1 serving

Assuming 1 serving, each will have: 550 calories; 40 g fat; 18 g protein; 6 g carbohydrate; 2 g dietary fiber; 4 g usable carbs.

◎ Quiche Lorraine

Quiche has somehow acquired a reputation for being foofy, girly food—but it's entirely made of stuff men love! So tell your husband this is "Bacon, Egg, and Cheese Pie," and watch him yum it down.

1 Pie Crust, unbaked (page 132)

8 ounces (225 g) Gruyere cheese

12 slices bacon

5 eggs

1/2 cup (120 ml) Carb Countdown Dairy Beverage

1/2 cup (120 ml) heavy cream or you can use 1 cup (240 ml)
  half-and-half in place of the Carb Countdown and the cream

1 pinch ground nutmeg

1 tablespoon (15 ml) dry vermouth

1/2 teaspoon salt or Vege-Sal

1/4 teaspoon pepper

Have your crust ready in the pan and standing by.

Preheat oven to 350°F (180°C).

Shred your cheese, and cook and drain your bacon—I microwave my bacon, and I find that 1 minute per slice on high is about right, but your microwave may be a little different.

First put the cheese in the pie shell, covering the bottom evenly. Crumble the bacon evenly over the cheese.

Now whisk together the eggs, Carb Countdown Dairy Beverage, cream, nutmeg, vermouth, salt, and pepper. Pour this over the cheese and bacon. Bake for 45 minutes, then cool. It's actually traditional to serve Quiche Lorraine at room temperature, but you certainly may warm it if you like.

Yield: 8 servings

Each with: 470 calories; 37 g fat; 32 g protein; 4 g carbohydrate; 1 g dietary fiber; 3 g usable carbs.

Spinach Mushroom Quiche

1 Almond-Parmesan Crust, prebaked (page 132)

8 ounces (225 g) sliced mushrooms

1/2 cup (80 g) chopped onion

2 tablespoons (30 g) butter

10 ounces (280 g) frozen chopped spinach, thawed

3 eggs

3/4 cup (175 ml) heavy cream

3/4 cup (175 ml) Carb Countdown Dairy Beverage

2 tablespoons (30 ml) dry vermouth

1/2 teaspoon salt

1/4 teaspoon pepper

1 1/2 cups (180 g) shredded Monterey Jack cheese

Have your crust ready first.

In a large, heavy skillet, over medium-high heat, sauté the mushrooms and onion in the butter until the onion is translucent and the mushrooms are limp. Transfer into a large mixing bowl, preferably one with a pouring lip.

Dump your thawed spinach into a strainer, and using clean hands, squeeze all the moisture out of it you can. Add it to the mushrooms and onions.

Now add the eggs, cream, and Carb Countdown Dairy Beverage. Whisk the whole thing up until well combined. Whisk in the vermouth, salt, and pepper.

Cover the bottom of the Almond-Parmesan Crust with the Monterey Jack, and put it in the oven at 325°F (170°C) for just a couple of minutes, or until the cheese just starts to melt. Take it out of the oven, and pour in the egg-vegetable mixture—your quiche will be very full! Very carefully place it back in the oven. It's a good idea to place a flat pan under it, on the floor of the oven, to catch any drips.

Bake for 50 to 60 minutes, or until just set in the center. Let cool. Quiche is traditionally served at room temperature, but if you like it warm, it's better to make this ahead, let it cool, and even chill it, then cut slices and warm them for a minute or two on 70 percent power in your microwave, rather than serving it right out of the oven.

Yield: 8 servings

Each with: 480 calories; 43 g fat; 17 g protein; 10 g carbohydrate; 4 g dietary fiber; 6 g usable carbs.

Deb Gajewski's Zucchini Quiche

Our tester, Linda, thought this was a very tasty recipe—even her husband, no big fan of vegetables, liked this.

> 2 cups (240 g) zucchini, cut in thin half-rounds
> 2 tablespoons (30 g) butter
> 12 cherry tomatoes
> 2 tablespoons (15 g) low-carb bake mix
> 2 extra large eggs
> ¾ cup (180 g) yogurt
> 1 teaspoon oregano
> 8 ounces (225 g) cream cheese, Kraft ⅓ less fat
> ⅓ cup (50 g) Parmesan cheese

Preheat oven to 375°F (190°C). Spray a 9" (22.5 cm) pie plate with nonstick cooking spray.

In your big, heavy skillet, sauté the zucchini in the butter until it's limp. Add the tomatoes. Cook for 3 more minutes. Cool for 5 to 10 minutes. Stir in the low-carb bake mix and spoon the whole thing into buttered 9" (22.5 cm) pie plate.

In a separate bowl, lightly beat your eggs. Add the yogurt and oregano, then whisk in the cream cheese in small bits. Mix together lightly. Spoon on top of the vegetables, and sprinkle the Parmesan on top.

Bake for 30 minutes at 375°F (190°C) or until firm in center. Serve.

Yield: Makes 4 servings

Each with: 333 calories; 25 g fat; 17 g protein; 9 g carbohydrate; 2 g dietary fiber; 7 g usable carbs.

◉ Jan Carmichael's Sausage Mushroom Quiche

Serve this with a salad on the side, and warm up any leftovers for breakfast.

    1 pound (445 g) bulk sausage, hot or mild as you prefer
    1 cup (160 g) chopped white onions
    1 cup (100 g) sliced fresh mushrooms
    4 eggs plus 1 egg yolk, lightly beaten
    ½ teaspoon Dijon mustard
    ½ teaspoon dry mustard
    ⅛ teaspoon cayenne pepper
    ⅛ teaspoon nutmeg
    1 cup (120 g) shredded Monterey Jack cheese
    1 cup (150 g) grated Parmesan
    2 cups (480 ml) heavy cream
    1 teaspoon chopped parsley

Preheat your oven to 300°F (150°C).

First, cook sausage, onions, and mushrooms together, crumbling the sausage, until sausage is brown and vegetables cooked through. Drain, drain, drain. (Jan usually pours off excess grease, then drains it further by placing mixture on paper towels.) Press this mixture into the bottom of 10" (25 cm) pie plate you've sprayed with nonstick spray. (Alternatively, our tester suggests a 9" x 13" (22.5 x 32.5 cm) rectangular baking dish.)

Next, whisk together the 4 eggs and 1 yolk with the Dijon mustard, dry mustard, cayenne pepper, nutmeg, Jack cheese, and ⅔ cup (100 g) of the Parmesan cheese. Mix well.

Pour your cream into a heavy-bottomed saucepan, and put it over low heat. Heat just to the boiling point (do not boil!). Then pour this scalded cream into the egg mixture. Mix and pour custard over sausage crust in pie plate. Bake at 300°F (150°C) for around 35 minutes or until set. Sprinkle with remaining Parmesan cheese and parsley. Let cool for 15 minutes before cutting.

Note: Jan says, "I've also used leftover chicken and broccoli in place of the sausage and mushrooms. It's all good!"

Yield: 8 servings

Each will have: 591 calories; 55 g fat; 19 g protein; 5 g carbohydrate; trace dietary fiber; 5 g usable carbs.

◎ Tracie Jansen's Cheesy Spinach Pie

This would make a great brunch dish, or light supper, and could be a real ace in the hole if you have vegetarians coming to dinner.

>3 large eggs
>1/2 cup (120 ml) heavy cream
>1/4 teaspoon garlic powder
>1/4 teaspoon Tabasco sauce
>2 tablespoons (15 g) low-carb baking mix
>Salt and pepper
>1 1/2 cups (180 g) shredded Cheddar cheese
>1/4 cup (50 g) shredded Parmesan cheese
>1 10-ounce (280 g) box frozen chopped spinach, thawed and well drained

Preheat oven to 350°F (180°C). Grease a 9" (22.5 cm) pie plate.

Whisk together the eggs, cream, garlic powder, Tabasco, baking mix, and salt and pepper.

Stir in cheeses and spinach until well combined. Pour mixture into prepared pie plate.

Bake for approximately 35 minutes, or until set and starting to brown on top. Let cool slightly, then cut into 8 wedges.

Tracie's note: "This recipe can be adapted many ways. For a Greek Spinach Pie, add oregano and substitute feta cheese. I will use whatever cheese I have in the fridge … Swiss, blue, mozzarella … or a combination of any of those."

Yield: About 8 servings

Each with: 188 calories; 15 g fat; 11 g protein; 3 g carbohydrate; 1 g dietary fiber; 2 g usable carbs.

⌾ UnPotato Tortilla

Don't think Mexican flatbread, think eggs. In Spain, a "tortilla" is much like an Italian frittata—a substantial egg dish, cooked in a skillet and served in wedges. This one is my version of a traditional dish served in tapas bars all over Spain. As bar food goes, it's a heckuva step up from beer nuts and stale popcorn!

¼ head cauliflower
1 medium turnip
1 medium onion, sliced thin
3 tablespoons (45 ml) olive oil
6 eggs
Salt and pepper

Thinly slice your cauliflower—include the stem—and peel and thinly slice your turnip. Put them in a microwaveable casserole with a lid, add a couple of tablespoons of water, and microwave on high for 6 to 7 minutes.

In the meanwhile, start the onion sautéing in 2 tablespoons (30 ml) of the olive oil in an 8" (20 cm) to 9" (22.5 cm) skillet—a nonstick skillet is ideal, but not essential. If your skillet isn't nonstick, give it a good squirt of nonstick cooking spray first. Use medium heat.

When your microwave goes beep, pull out the veggies, drain them, and throw them in the skillet with the onion. Continue sautéing everything, adding a bit more oil if things start to stick, until the veggies are getting golden around the edges—about 10 to 15 minutes. Turn the burner to low, and spread the vegetables in an even layer on the bottom of the skillet.

Scramble up the eggs with a little salt and pepper, and pour over the vegetables. Cook on low for 5 to 7 minutes, lifting the edges frequently to let uncooked egg run underneath. When it's all set except for the top, slide the skillet under a low broiler for 4 to 5 minutes, or until the top of your tortilla is golden. (If your skillet doesn't have a flameproof handle, wrap it in foil first.) Cut in wedges to serve. A little chopped parsley is nice on this, but not essential.

Yield: 6 servings

Each with: 139 calories; 11 g fat; 6 g protein; 4 g carbohydrate; 1 g dietary fiber; 3 g usable carbs.

◎ Eliot Sohmer's Bacon Cheese Frittata

Y'know, it strikes me that this one is the epitome of the stereotype of low-carb food—eggs, bacon, cheese. And a beautiful thing it is, too.

> 6 eggs
> 1 cup (240 ml) whole milk or Carb Countdown Dairy Beverage
> 2 tablespoons (30 g) butter, melted
> 1/2 teaspoon salt
> 1/4 teaspoon pepper
> 1/4 cup (25 g) chopped green onion
> 5 bacon strips, cooked and crumbled
> 1 cup (120 g) cheddar cheese, shredded

Preheat oven to 350°F (180°C). Spray an 7"–11" (27.5x17.5 cm) baking dish with nonstick cooking spray.

In a mixing bowl, whisk together the eggs, milk or Carb Countdown Dairy Beverage, butter, salt, and pepper. Stir in the green onion, crumbled bacon, and cheese. Pour into prepared dish, and bake, uncovered, for 25 to 30 minutes, or until a knife inserted in center comes out clean.

Yield: Serves 6

Each with: 232 calories; 18 g fat; 13 g protein; 3 g carbohydrate; trace dietary fiber; 3 g usable carbs.

Artichoke and Friends Frittata

>
> 3 tablespoons (45 ml) olive oil
>
> 1/4 pound (115 g) zucchini (about 1 really little zucchini), diced small
>
> 3 tablespoons (30 g) chopped onion
>
> 1 clove garlic, crushed
>
> 1/2 small green pepper, diced
>
> 1/2 small red pepper, diced
>
> 1 cup (300 g) canned artichoke hearts, drained and chopped
>
> 1 cup (110 g) 1/4" (6.25 mm) ham cubes
>
> 1/4 cup (15 g) chopped fresh parsley
>
> 10 eggs
>
> 1 tablespoon (5 g) oregano
>
> 1/3 cup (50 g) grated Parmesan cheese

For this you need an oven-safe skillet—a big cast-iron skillet works great. Spray the skillet with nonstick cooking spray, and put it over medium-high heat. Add the olive oil, and start sautéing the zucchini, onion, garlic, and peppers. When the vegetables are starting to soften, stir in the artichoke hearts, ham cubes, and fresh parsley. Let the whole thing continue cooking while you . . .

Scramble up the eggs with the oregano and Parmesan.

Arrange the stuff in the skillet in an even layer, and pour in the eggs. Cover the pan, turn the burner to low, and let the whole thing cook for 15 to 20 minutes, or until all but the top is set.

Run the skillet under the broiler for 3 or 4 minutes until it starts to brown a little, then cut frittata in wedges to serve.

Yield: 4 to 5 servings

Assuming 5 servings, each will have: 308 calories; 21 g fat; 20 g protein; 8 g carbohydrate; 1 g dietary fiber; 7 g usable carbs.

Diane Lyon's
Savory Cheese and Ham Torte

This is great for any meal, both hot and cold. It even looks great! Our tester, Kim Pulley, says this was "one of the best of the bunch."

1 10-ounce (280 g) package frozen chopped spinach
3 8-ounce (225 g) packages cream cheese, softened
1/2 cup (120 ml) heavy cream
1 tablespoon (15 g) Dijon mustard
1/2 tablespoon (10 g) salt
1 teaspoon (10 g) dried oregano
4 eggs
1 1/2 cups (180 g) shredded Swiss or Gruyere cheese
1/2–3/4 cup (55–80 g) diced ham
2 tablespoons (10 g) chopped fresh parsley

Preheat oven to 325°F (170°C). Grease a 9" (22.5 cm) springform pan.

Place your box of frozen spinach in the microwave on a paper towel and cook on high for 4 to 5 minutes. Carefully remove and drain, squeezing out most of the moisture—it's good to dump it in a sieve and press it hard with the back of a spoon. Set aside to cool.

In a large bowl, beat cream cheese and next 5 ingredients until smooth. Fold in cheese, ham, parsley, and cooked spinach. Pour mixture into prepared pan. Bake about 1 1/4 hours or until knife inserted in center of torte comes out clean. Cool torte slightly in pan on wire rack. Cover and refrigerate until cold, about 3 hours. To serve, run a thin knife blade around the edge, then carefully remove side of pan. Cut torte into wedges.

Diane's note: I cut it into 12 wedges and heat in the microwave as needed when I want it warm, but it is equally delicious cold.

Yield: 12 wedges

Each will have: 327 calories; 30 g fat; 12 g protein; 3 g carbohydrate; trace dietary fiber; 3 g usable carbs.

◎ Eliot Sohmer's Spinach Soufflé

This simple but great dish would be a fine side dish, but also would serve well as a vegetarian entree. Our tester, Kay Winefordner, emphasizes the need to drain the spinach very well!

 2 cups (450 g) cottage cheese
 3 eggs, beaten
 3 10-ounce (280 g) packages frozen chopped spinach, thawed
 2 cups (240 g) grated cheddar cheese
 Salt to taste

Spray a 9" x 11" (22.5 x 27.5 cm) baking pan with nonstick cooking spray. Preheat your oven to 350°F (180°C).

Mix cottage cheese and eggs with spoon in mixing bowl. Drain your spinach very well—it's best to dump it into a colander and press it hard with your hands or the back of a spoon, or even actually pick it up in handfuls and squeeze it hard! Stir the spinach, 1 ½ cups (180 g) of the cheddar, and salt if you like, into the egg mixture. Pour into your prepared pan. Sprinkle the reserved cheddar cheese on top. Bake 30 to 45 minutes at 350°F (180°C) until set.

Yield: Serves 6

Each getting: 276 calories; 16 g fat; 26 g protein; 9 g carbohydrate; 4 g dietary fiber; 5 g usable carbs.

⊚ Betsy Calvin's Breakfast Casserole

This easy, crowd-pleasing brunch dish would also make a filling supper. Our tester, Ray, who liked this a lot, suggested halving this recipe for smaller groups.

> 1 pound (455 g) bulk Italian sausage (Betsy uses Bob Evan's brand)
> 5 cups (600 g) shredded sharp cheddar
> 12 eggs
> 1 cup (240 ml) heavy cream

Preheat oven to 325°F (170°C). Spray an 9" X12" (22.5 x 30 cm) pan with nonstick cooking spray.

First, cook and crumble your sausage, and drain it.

Spread 2 ½ cups (300 g) of cheese in the prepared pan. Whisk your eggs in a bowl, then pour on top of the cheese. Add the sausage, then the cream, and top with the remaining cheese. Bake at 325°F (170°C) for 45 minutes. Delicious!!!!

Yield: 8 servings

Each with: 683 calories; 59 g fat; 35 g protein; 3 g carbohydrate; 0 g dietary fiber; 3 g usable carbs.

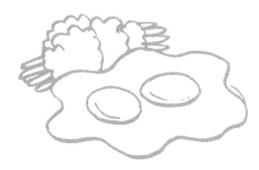

Stephanie H.'s French Toasty Eggs

This quick and easy microwave recipe makes eggs taste like a Danish. Our tester, Ray, called this "fast and great"—a real treat you can make on a busy morning!

2 ounces (55 g) cream cheese

2 eggs, lightly beaten

2 tablespoons (30 ml) sugar-free pancake syrup, divided
(do not use aspartame-sweetened syrup)

Ground cinnamon, to taste (careful, cinnamon is one of those
carb-y spices)

Soften the cream cheese in a microwave safe bowl, about 20 to 30 seconds on high. Then add the eggs and 1 tablespoon (15 ml) of the syrup, stirring to mix. This shouldn't mix completely; you'll have little bits of cream cheese remaining. Microwave for about a minute, then stir to break up any lumps. Microwave until you have a large puffy pancakelike result; in my microwave this takes another minute. Drizzle with remaining syrup and top with a few sprinkles of cinnamon.

Yield: Single serving

Each with: 331 calories; 29 g fat; 15 g protein; 3 g carbohydrate; trace dietary fiber; 3 g usable carbs.

◉ Cheese "Danish"

A contributor identified only as "Hihopeso1" writes, "This is my version of a Weight Watchers Danish with an English muffin, which of course has way too many carbs. I used to fix this for my kids as breakfast before school but never really appreciated just how good it probably was for them" Our tester, Ray, says this is, "very quick, very easy, very good." What more could you want? Oh, yes—it's a good source of calcium, too!

>   1 slice low-carb bread, toasted and buttered
>   Up to ¼ cup (60 g) cottage cheese, or as much as your toast will hold
>   Cinnamon to taste
>   Splenda to taste

Toast the bread, butter is optional; spread on the cottage cheese and sprinkle with cinnamon and Splenda. Put under the broiler until the cheese starts to bubble.

Yield: 1 "Danish"

Carb count will depend on what brand of low-carb bread you use. To that, add: 53 calories; 1 g fat; 8 g protein; 3 g carbohydrate; trace dietary fiber; 3 g usable carbs.

◎ Jill Boelsma's Scottish Eggs

This is a decarbed version of what is actually a classic recipe. Our tester, Ray, called this "fabulous!" and when asked if he'd make it again, answered with a hearty "Oh, yeah!"

    4 hard-boiled eggs
    1 pound (455 g) Jimmy Dean or other bulk breakfast sausage
    Spicy pork rinds, crushed

Preheat oven to 350°F (180°C).

Peel your hard-boiled eggs.

Divide the sausage into 4 equal portions and flatten each into a thin patty between your palms. Encase each hard-boiled egg in sausage by slowly wrapping a patty around it; then roll in pork rind crumbs. Place on a cookie sheet you've sprayed with nonstick cooking spray, and bake for 20 to 25 minutes.

Yield: 4 servings

Each with: 577 calories; 52 g fat; 23 g protein; 2 g carbohydrate; 0 g dietary fiber; 2 g usable carbs.

◉ Jody's Breakfast Wrap

Our tester, Julie, now calls this recipe "a low-carb staple."

> 1 or 2 strips bacon
> 1–2 eggs
> 1 low-carb tortilla
> 2–3 tablespoons (20–30 g) shredded cheese—cheddar or Monterey Jack are good

First, you need to deal with the bacon and the scrambled eggs. I'd microwave the bacon—lay it on a microwave bacon rack or in a glass pie plate, and nuke it on high (a minute per slice is about right in my microwave, but microwaves vary). Keep an eye on it the first couple of times, and you'll get the timing down. Drain your bacon on a paper towel while you scramble the eggs.

You can scramble your egg or eggs plain or add a splash of cream if you like. Just beat 'em up in a bowl. Spray a medium skillet with nonstick cooking spray, and add a little butter if you want to. Heat over medium-high flame, pour in the eggs, and scramble till set.

Lay your low-carb tortilla on a microwaveable plate. Sprinkle the cheese on it, and microwave on high for 10 to 20 seconds—you just want to melt the cheese. Add the scrambled egg and bacon, roll it up, and enjoy!

Tester's note: Julie says the eggs and bacon can even be made ahead and put into a plastic snap-top container, and then used for a couple of days in a row for a fast and easy breakfast on the go. Just nuke the bacon and egg separately (it needs more nuke time than the tortilla), nuke the tortilla with the cheese, combine, and go. Breakfast made in less than a minute, and totally portable for the commute to work!

Yield: 1 serving

Made with 2 eggs and 3 tablespoons (30 g) of cheese, this has: 254 calories; 17 g fat; 20 g protein; 12 g carbohydrate; 8 g dietary fiber; 4 g usable carbs.

Sharon Walsh's Mushroom-Spinach-Egg-Muffin Thing or Something Like That

That's the name my husband gave this recipe, and I liked it so much, I kept it! Whatever you call it, it's a great breakfast or supper!

> 4 eggs and 1/2 cup (120 ml) egg whites or 6 eggs
> 1/2 10-ounce (280 g) package frozen chopped spinach, thawed and well drained
> 1/2 cup (50 g) finely chopped fresh mushrooms
> 1/2 cup (60 g) shredded cheddar
> 1/2 cup (60 g) shredded mozzarella
> 1/2 cup (115 g) ricotta cheese
> 1 tablespoon (10 g) minced onion
> 1 tablespoon (5 g) Mrs. Dash (or other seasoning mix)
> 1 tablespoon (10 g) chopped garlic
> 1 teaspoon salt or Vege-Sal
> 1/4 teaspoon pepper

Preheat your oven to 350°F (180°C). Spray a 12-cup muffin tin with nonstick cooking spray.

Whisk up your eggs in a mixing bowl. Add the vegetables, cheeses, and seasonings, and mix thoroughly. Spoon into the prepared muffin cups and bake for 20 to 25 minutes or until brown, puffy, and set.

Note: Sharon says these can be made ahead and reheated in your microwave for a quick breakfast or lunch. She likes turkey bacon on the side!

Yield: 4 servings, 3 muffins each.

Each serving has: 269 calories; 19 g fat; 20 g protein; 5 g carbohydrate; 1 g dietary fiber, 4 g usable carbs.

◎ Swiss Puff

This is a great comfort-food-type supper.

> 4 eggs
> 3/4 teaspoon salt or Vege-Sal
> 1/2 teaspoon pepper
> 1 tablespoon (15 g) butter
> 1 batch Ultimate Fauxtatoes (page 136)
> 2 cups (240 g) shredded Swiss cheese
> 4 scallions, sliced, including the crisp part of the green shoot
> 2 tablespoons (10 g) chopped parsley
> 4 drops hot sauce

Separate your eggs. (Since whites with even a tiny speck of yolk in them will stubbornly refuse to whip up, do yourself a favor and separate each egg into a small cup or bowl.) Dump the yolks into the Fauxtatoes and beat them in; add the salt, pepper, and butter. Dump your (presumably yolkless) egg whites into a deep mixing bowl and set aside.

Stir the shredded Swiss cheese into the Fauxtatoes, then stir in the scallions, parsley, and hot sauce.

Now, using an electric mixer, beat the whites until they stand in soft peaks. Fold gently into the Fauxtatoes. Spoon the whole thing into a 6-cup (1.4 L) casserole you've sprayed with nonstick cooking spray. Bake for 40 to 45 minutes at 375°F (190°C).

Yield: 4 to 5 servings

Assuming 4 servings, each will have: 422 calories; 25 g fat; 32 g protein; 18 g carbohydrate; 8 g dietary fiber; 10 g usable carbs.

Jill Taylor's Chili Relleno Casserole

Love Mexican food? I do! Here's a great Mexican-style casserole. Since traditional Chilies Rellenos is delicious but labor-intensive, this is a really great alternative.

> 2–3 roasted green chilies
> ½ pound (225 g) sharp cheddar, finely shredded
> 8 ounces (225 g) salsa
> ½ pound (225 g) Monterey Jack, finely shredded
> 5 eggs
> 1 cup (240 ml) whipping cream

Preheat oven to 350°F (180°C).

Chop your green chilies and spread half of them in the bottom of a 9" x 13" (22.5 x 32.5 cm) casserole dish you've sprayed with nonstick cooking spray. Spread the cheddar evenly over the chilies, then pour the salsa over the top. Add the Monterey Jack, then top with the remaining green chilies.

In a mixing bowl, beat the eggs and cream until combined and pour over the chilies and cheese. Bake at 350°F (180°C) for approximately 1 hour or until set. Serve with green salad as a light lunch or as a side with your favorite entrée.

Jill's note: "Do not use a dish that is smaller but deeper. The result is better when the casserole rises to about 2" (5 cm) in height."

Yield: 10 servings

Each will have: 301 calories; 25 g fat (75.6% calories from fat); 15 g protein; 4 g carbohydrate; trace dietary fiber; 4 g usable carbs.

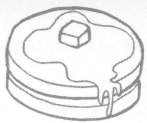

chapter four

Breads, Muffins, Cereals, Crackers, and Other Grainy Things

Baking is the most complicated, fluky kind of cooking, involving, as it does, stuff like chemistry. And of course, "regular" baked goods are made with flour and sugar and things like that! Substituting for the various ingredients is a complex task, full of trial and error. More than any other chapter, the recipes in this one made my dogs, Jed and Molly, happy—because they're the ones who get to eat the failures. Hey, I find this stuff out the hard way so you won't have to.

With more and more low-carb baked goods entering the market, you may decide not to bother with making your own. However, I will warn you to *read the labels* of those low-carb baked goods. Many of them are higher carb than I would care to use on a regular basis, and a distressing number use ingredients I won't put in my body, including white flour and hydrogenated vegetable oil. Eat this sort of thing on a regular basis, and you run the risk of compromising the health benefits of your low-carb diet.

Yet low-carb baking is very possible, and for many people it's the thing that lets them be comfortable with the idea of staying low carb forever. Once you know you can have a slice of bread or a muffin or a cracker if you really want one, a lot of that "This diet is so *weird*!" feeling evaporates. Too, if you're one of those many people I hear from who simply can't face another plate of fried eggs, having recipes for muffins, pancakes, waffles, and other familiar breakfast-y foods with enough protein to keep you full and energetic is a real boon.

And anyway, baking is *fun*! Memories of baking with my mother are some of the brightest of my childhood. And nothing makes your house smell better.

So try some low-carb baking! It'll take a modest stock of specialty ingredients, since that white-flour thing just ain't happenin'. Give chapter 1, "Ingredients," a read, then tie on an apron and give it a shot.

◉ Zucchini Bread

Many low carbers tell me they miss having "a little something" with a cup of coffee or tea for breakfast, and express a profound weariness with eggs. Here's something for you! This Zucchini Bread is moist, sweet, cinnamon-y, and delicious—not to mention being low carb and having as much protein per slice as a couple of eggs!

> 1/2 cup (120 ml) canola oil
>
> 1/4 cup (85 g) sugar-free imitation honey
>
> 2 eggs
>
> 1/3 cup (80 g) plain yogurt
>
> 1 cup (125 g) pumpkin seed meal (see page 24)
>
> 1 cup (125 g) vanilla whey protein powder
>
> 1 1/2 teaspoons baking soda
>
> 1/2 teaspoon salt
>
> 1 teaspoon cinnamon
>
> 1/3 cup (18 g) Splenda granular
>
> 1 cup (125 g) chopped walnuts
>
> 1 1/2 cups (180 g) shredded zucchini (about one 6" [15 cm] zucchini)

Preheat the oven to 350°F (180°C).

In a good-sized mixing bowl, combine the oil, imitation honey, eggs, and yogurt. Whisk these together. Now, in a second bowl, measure the dry ingredients: the ground pumpkin seeds, vanilla whey protein powder, baking soda, salt, cinnamon, and Splenda. Stir them together, making sure any little lumps of baking soda get broken up. Now whisk the dry ingredients into the wet ingredients. Stir just until everything is well combined; no need for prolonged beating. Finally, stir in the walnuts and the shredded zucchini, mixing well.

Pour into a loaf pan you've sprayed well with nonstick cooking spray—my loaf pan is large, 5" x 9" (13 x 22.5 cm). Bake for about 50 minutes, or until a toothpick inserted into the center comes out clean. Turn out onto a wire rack for cooling.

Yield: About 16 slices

Each with: 194 calories; 14 g fat, 14 g protein; 5 g carbohydrate; 2 g dietary fiber—for a usable carb count of just 3 g a slice. Carb count does not include polyols in the sugar-free imitation honey.

◉ Cranberry Nut Muffins

I tried Cranberry Nut Bread, and it was a failure—all the cranberries rose, so the top of the bread was soggy. But muffins worked out fine!

$\frac{1}{2}$ cup (60 g) pecans

$\frac{1}{2}$ cup (50 g) cranberries

$\frac{3}{4}$ cup plus 2 tablespoons (110 g) almond meal

$\frac{3}{4}$ cup (90 g) vanilla whey protein powder

2 tablespoons (30 g) gluten

2 tablespoons (30 g) polyol

$\frac{1}{4}$ cup (6 g) Splenda

2 $\frac{1}{2}$ teaspoons baking powder

2 eggs

$\frac{3}{4}$ cup (180 ml) carb Countdown Dairy Beverage

3 tablespoons (45 g) butter, melted

$\frac{1}{4}$ teaspoon orange extract

Preheat your oven to 400°F (200°C). Spray a 12-cup muffin tin with nonstick cooking spray, or line it with paper muffin cups if you prefer.

Chop your pecans, then your cranberries—I do them by pulsing the S-blade of my food processor, and if you do them in this order, you won't have pecans sticking to the moisture left behind by the cranberries. Set aside.

In a mixing bowl, combine all of the dry ingredients. Stir together, to make sure everything is distributed evenly.

Whisk together the eggs, Carb Countdown Dairy Beverage, melted butter, and orange extract.

Make sure your oven is up to temperature before you add the wet ingredients to the dry ingredients. When it is, pour the wet ingredients into the dry ingredients, and stir the two together with a few swift strokes of your whisk or a spoon. Do not overmix! A few lumps are fine. Now add the pecans and cranberries, and stir just enough to incorporate into the batter. Spoon into muffin cups, and bake for 20 minutes. Remove from pan to a wire rack to cool.

Yield: 12 muffins

Each with: 202 calories; 13 g fat; 18 g protein; 5 g carbohydrate; 2 g dietary fiber; 3 g usable carb. Carb count does not include polyol sweetener.

☺ Pumpkin Muffins

Just as with the Cranberry Nut Muffins, these Pumpkin Muffins happened because I couldn't get Pumpkin Bread to work out!

⅓ cup (50 g) almond meal
¼ cup (25 g) gluten
¼ cup (30 g) vanilla whey protein powder
¼ teaspoon salt
¼ cup (6 g) Splenda
1 teaspoon baking powder
½ teaspoon ground cinnamon
½ teaspoon ground nutmeg
½ cup (120 g) canned pumpkin
1 egg
2 tablespoons (30 g) butter, melted
¼ teaspoon orange extract
⅓ cup (80 ml) Carb Countdown Dairy Beverage
½ cup (60 g) chopped pecans

Preheat oven to 400°F (200°C). Spray a 12-cup muffin tin with nonstick cooking spray, or, if you prefer, line it with paper muffin cups.

In a mixing bowl, measure all your dry ingredients. Stir them together, to evenly distribute ingredients.

Combine the canned pumpkin, egg, melted butter, orange extract, and Carb Countdown Dairy Beverage and whisk together. Make sure your oven is up to temperature before you take the next step!

Pour the wet ingredients into the dry ingredients and, with a few swift strokes, combine them. Stir just enough to make sure there are no big pockets of dry stuff; a few lumps are fine. Stir in the pecans quickly, and spoon into prepared muffin tin. Bake for 20 minutes; remove from pan to a wire rack to cool.

Yield: 12 muffins

Each with: 119 calories; 8 g fat; 9 g protein; 3 g carbohydrate; 6 g usable carbs.

Libby Sinback's Peach Sour Cream Muffins

Julie tested these muffins and said her whole family liked them!

1 cup (125 g) soy flour

1 cup (120 g) Designer Whey French vanilla protein powder

1 teaspoon baking powder

½ teaspoon salt

½ teaspoon baking soda

2 tablespoons (15 g) of stevia-FOS blend

1 cup (240 g) sour cream

½ cup (120 g) butter, melted

2 tablespoons (30 ml) cream

3 eggs

2 teaspoon orange peel

1 ½ cups (300 g) frozen peaches, slightly thawed, then diced

Preheat oven to 350°F (180°C).

Combine all dry ingredients, including the stevia-FOS blend, in a small bowl. Combine sour cream, butter, cream, eggs, and orange peel in a larger mixing bowl. Mix peaches in with dry ingredients, then fold into larger bowl with wet ingredients. Mix all ingredients until everything's wet, then pour into paper-lined muffin tins, filling almost to the top.

Bake for 20 to 25 minutes at 350°F (180°C) degrees.

Yield: Makes 12 large muffins

Each with: 266 calories; 16 g fat; 19 g protein; 13 g carbohydrate; 2 g dietary fiber; 11 g usable carbs.

⊚ Gingerbread Waffles

Really make Sunday breakfast something special! Double or triple this recipe, and you'll have extra waffles to freeze and reheat on busy mornings. Tip—they'll be a lot crispier and tastier if you reheat them in the toaster than if you microwave them.

> 1 cup almond meal
> 1 cup (120 g) vanilla whey protein powder
> 1/2 teaspoon salt
> 1/4 cup (6 g) Splenda
> 1 tablespoon (5 g) baking powder
> 2 teaspoons ground ginger
> 1 1/2 cups (360 ml) Carb Countdown Dairy Beverage or 3/4 cup (180 ml)
>   heavy cream and 3/4 cup (180 ml) water
> 2 eggs
> 4 tablespoons (60 g) butter, melted

Start waffle iron heating.

Combine dry ingredients. In a glass measuring cup, whisk together the carb-counting milk or cream and water and the eggs, then stir the butter into them. Pour this into the dry ingredients, with a few quick strokes.

Ladle the batter into the waffle iron, and bake until done—my waffle iron has a light that goes out when the waffle is ready, but follow the instructions for your unit.

Serve with whipped cream.

Yield: 6 servings

Each with: 448 calories; 32 g fat; 35 g protein; 9 g carbohydrate; 3 g dietary fiber, 6 g usable carbs.

⊚ Exceedingly Crisp Waffles

You have to separate eggs and all, but these waffles are worth it!

> 1/2 cup (60 g) almond meal
> 1/3 cup (40 g) vanilla whey protein powder
> 1/4 cup (30 g) oat flour
> 1/2 teaspoon baking powder
> 1 tablespoon (1.5 g) Splenda
> 1/4 teaspoon baking soda
> 3/4 cup (180 ml) buttermilk
> 1/4 cup (60 ml) Carb Countdown Dairy Beverage or half-and-half
> 6 tablespoons (90 ml) canola oil
> 1 egg

In one mixing bowl, combine the almond meal, vanilla whey, oat flour, baking powder, Splenda, and baking soda. Stir the dry ingredients together.

Measure the buttermilk and Carb Countdown Dairy Beverage into a glass measuring cup. Add the canola oil.

Now's the time to plug in your waffle iron and get it heating; you want it to be ready as soon as your batter is!

Separate that egg, making sure you don't get even a tiny speck of yolk in the white. Add the yolk to the liquid ingredients. Put the white in a small, deep bowl, and beat until stiff. Set aside.

Whisk all the liquid ingredients together, and pour them into the dry ingredients. Mix everything quickly with a few quick strokes of your whisk. Mix only enough to be sure all the dry ingredients are moistened.

Add about 1/3 of the beaten egg white to the batter, and fold in gently, using a rubber scraper. Then fold in the rest of the egg white.

Bake immediately, according to the directions that come with your waffle iron. Serve with butter and sugar-free pancake syrup, cinnamon and Splenda, or low-sugar preserves.

Yield: How many waffles you get will depend on the size of your waffle iron; I got 6.

Each with: 282 calories; 21 g fat; 15 g protein; 9 g carbohydrate; 2 g dietary fiber, 7 g usable carbs.

⚙ Mary Lou Theisen's Best Low-Carb Waffle

Our tester agrees these waffles are great.

>   4 ounces (115 g) cream cheese, softened
>   2 tablespoons vanilla whey protein powder
>   2 medium eggs (not large!)
>   1 teaspoon Splenda
>   1 teaspoon vanilla extract
>   1/2 teaspoon baking powder

Heat up waffle iron while mixing ingredients. Soften cream cheese in the microwave for about 45 seconds. (You want the cream cheese nice and smooth.) Add the whey protein powder, eggs, Splenda, vanilla extract, and baking powder. Mix until smooth. Pour mixture into hot waffle iron (I do not grease the waffle iron, as the waffles come out crispier without it). I heat the waffle for 2 minutes (this, of course, depends on what kind of waffle maker you have). Take the waffle out; top with low-carb whipped cream and cinnamon or butter and sugar-free syrup.

Note: Our tester, Barbo Gold, who loved this recipe, suggests making these with chocolate whey protein powder for a chocolate treat.

Yield: 2 servings

Each with: 326 calories; 25 g fat; 21 g protein; 4 g carbohydrate; trace dietary fiber; 4 g usable carbs.

⚙ Julie Sandell's Low-Carb Blueberry Pancakes

Our tester, Ray Stevens, says these are not only quick and easy, but good-looking enough for company.

>   2 eggs
>   1/2 cup (115 g) whole-milk cottage cheese
>   1 scoop (1/4 cup [30 g]) vanilla flavored whey protein
>   2 tablespoons (15 g) low-carb bake mix
>   1/2 teaspoon baking powder
>   Pinch of salt
>   1/2 cup (80 g) frozen blueberries

Mix all ingredients in order given. Drop by large spoonfuls onto well-greased pan. Cook until bubbly on top. Flip and cook a minute longer.

Note: Julie says you can substitute a chopped-up sugar-free chocolate bar for the blueberries, and that sure sounds good to me!

Yield: Makes 3 servings of about 5 pancakes each.

Per serving: 183 calories; 5 g fat; 26 g protein; 8 g carbohydrate; 2 g dietary fiber; 6 g usable carbs.

⊚ Jill Taylor's Soy Pancakes

Our tester, Julie, says even her seven-year-old son Austin will eat these pancakes!

$\frac{1}{2}$ cup (60 g) soy flour
$\frac{1}{2}$ teaspoon baking powder
$\frac{1}{2}$ teaspoon Salt
$\frac{1}{2}$ teaspoon cinnamon
2 packets of artificial sweetener
1 teaspoon vanilla essence
$\frac{1}{2}$ cup (180 ml) water
2 eggs
Oil for cooking, or use a nonstick pan

Put all ingredients except the oil in a blender and mix until smooth. Let the batter rest for 5 minutes. Heat a small skillet over medium to low heat until hot. Add 1 to 2 tablespoons (15–30 ml) of the batter and cook until small bubbles appear. Flip over and cook for a further 30 to 45 seconds.

Serve with fresh fruit, whipped cream, and sugar-free maple syrup.

Yield: Batter makes between 8 and 12 pancakes, depending on how big you make them, so carb count per pancake will vary.

Each will have: 58 calories; 4 g fat; 3 g protein; 2 g carbohydrate; trace dietary fiber; 2 g usable carbs.

Jeanette Wiese's Best Pancakes I've Ever Had!

Our tester, Ray, calls these "hard to tell from the real thing."

> 1 scoop Designer Whey vanilla protein powder
> 1 scoop Designer Whey plain protein powder
> 1/3 cup (40 g) almond meal
> 2 teaspoons baking powder
> Dash of cinnamon
> 1 ounce (30 g) cream cheese
> 2 eggs
> 2–4 teaspoons Splenda
> 1/4 cup (60 ml) oil
> 1/2 teaspoon vanilla extract

In one bowl, stir together protein powders, almond flour, baking powder, and cinnamon. Soften cream cheese in microwave. In second bowl, whisk the eggs into the cream cheese until well combined. Add sweetener, oil, and vanilla; whisk well.

Add egg mixture to dry ingredients, whisking until well combined.

Cook pancakes in a heavy skillet—it's best to use a nonstick skillet, but if you don't have one, at least give it a good squirt of nonstick cooking spray. Then heat it over medium-low heat. Use a 1/4 cup (60 ml) measuring cup, almost full, for each pancake. The mixture will be pretty thick, so use a small spatula to help drop the batter in a pan and spread it slightly to make round. Turn them carefully. These will cook faster than regular pancakes, so keep an eye on them. Our tester, Ray, points out that unlike "regular" pancakes, where you tell when the first side is done by the bubbles around the edges, these have few bubbles. Instead, he says, a "visible skin" forms on top of the pancake, and this is your signal to flip it.

Yield: Makes about 7 pancakes

Each with: 194 calories; 13 g fat; 17 g protein; 4 g carbohydrate; trace dietary fiber; 4 g usable carbs.

◎ Oat Bran Pancakes

I like these for their grainy-cinnamony flavor. I eat 'em with butter and a little cinnamon and Splenda.

1/2 cup (50 g) oat bran
1 cup (120 g) vanilla whey protein powder
1 1/4 cups (155 g) almond meal
1/4 cup (6 g) Splenda
1 teaspoon baking powder
1/2 teaspoon baking soda
1/8 teaspoon salt
1/2 teaspoon cinnamon
2 cups (480 ml) buttermilk
2 eggs

In a medium-sized mixing bowl, combine all the dry ingredients, and stir to distribute evenly. Measure the buttermilk in a glass measuring cup, and break the eggs into it. Whisk the two together. Dump the buttermilk-and-egg mixture into the dry ingredients. Mix with a few quick strokes of the whisk, just enough to make sure all the dry ingredients are incorporated.

Heat a heavy skillet or griddle over a medium-high flame until a single drop of water skitters around when dripped on the surface. Using a hot-pot holder, remove from the heat just long enough to spray with nonstick cooking spray, then return to the heat (the spray is flammable, so you don't want to be spraying it at a hot burner!).

Pour about 2 to 3 tablespoons (30–45 ml) of batter at a time onto the hot griddle. Cook until bubbles around the edges start to break and leave little holes, then flip and cook other side.

Serve with butter and your choice of sugar-free pancake syrup, sugar-free jelly or preserves, or cinnamon and Splenda.

Yield: 8 servings

Each with: 287 calories; 14 g fat; 32 g protein; 12 g carbohydrate; 3 g dietary fiber; 9 g usable carbs.

"Whole Wheat" Buttermilk Pancakes

½ cup (60 g) almond meal
½ cup (60 g) vanilla whey protein powder
¼ cup (25 g) gluten
2 tablespoons (15 g) wheat germ
1 tablespoon (15 g) wheat bran
1 teaspoon baking powder
½ teaspoon baking soda
1 cup (240 ml) buttermilk
1 egg
2 tablespoons (30 g) butter, melted

In a mixing bowl, combine the dry ingredients. Stir together so everything is evenly distributed.

In a 2-cup (475 ml) glass measure, combine the buttermilk, egg, and melted butter; stir together.

Take a moment to set your big skillet or griddle over medium heat, so it's ready when you are.

Now, pour the wet ingredients into the dry ingredients, and stir together with a few swift strokes of your whisk.

When your skillet is hot enough that a single drop of water sizzles and dances around when dripped on the surface, you're ready to cook. If your skillet doesn't have a good nonstick surface, spray it with nonstick cooking spray. (Turn off the burner first, or remove the skillet from the burner and turn away from the flame—that spray is flammable!) Now you're ready to fry your pancakes—I like to use 2 tablespoons (30 ml) of batter per pancake. Fry the first side until the bubbles around the edges leave little holes when they break, then flip and cook the other side. Repeat until all the batter is used up!

Serve with butter and your choice of low-sugar preserves, cinnamon and Splenda, or sugar-free syrup—and don't think you're limited to maple-flavored pancake syrup! Consider your favorite sugar-free coffee-flavoring syrup.

Yield: 5 servings (about 15 pancakes)

Each with: 233 calories; 13 g fat; 23 g protein; 7 g carbohydrate; 2 g dietary fiber; 5 g usable carbs.

⊚ John Smolinski's Low-Carb Dutch Baby

A very popular puffy, oven-baked pancake.

> 3 ounces (85 g) cream cheese, softened
> 2 eggs
> ½ cup (120 ml) heavy cream
> 1 teaspoon vanilla
> 2 tablespoons (16 g) vanilla whey protein powder
> ½ teaspoon baking powder
> 1 teaspoon Splenda
> 1–2 tablespoons (30 g) butter

Preheat your oven to 425°F (220°C) degrees. While the oven is heating up, put your cream cheese in a microwaveable mixing bowl, and microwave for 30 to 45 seconds to soften. Using an electric mixer or a whisk, beat the eggs, heavy cream, vanilla, whey protein powder, baking powder, and Splenda in with the cream cheese—incorporating plenty of air is a good thing here. Spray a 9" (22.5 cm) cake pan with nonstick cooking spray, then put 1 to 2 tablespoons (15–30 g) of butter in the pan, and put it in your oven. Let the butter melt, and then tilt the pan to make sure the entire pan is coated with the melted butter.

Pour the cream cheese mixture into the hot cake pan (make sure you use oven gloves to do this step and to put the cake pan back into the oven). Bake for 10 to 12 minutes. You will have a fluffy, big Dutch baby. Use a spatula to carefully work it out of the pan. (You can flip the Dutch baby out on one plate, then use another plate to flip it back so that it faces up.) Top with sour cream and warm sugar-free maple syrup, butter and cinnamon-Splenda, or a squeeze of lemon juice and a sprinkle of Splenda.

Yield: 2 servings

Each with: 583 calories; 54 g fat; 21 g protein; 6 g carbohydrate; trace dietary fiber; 6 g usable carbs.

◎ Graham Crackers

These are wonderful! Eat them as is, with some milk or reduced-carb dairy beverage, or spread them with a little cream cheese.

> ⅔ cup (80 g) vanilla whey protein powder
> ⅔ cup (80 g) almond meal
> ⅓ cup (35 g) oat bran
> ¼ (25 g) wheat gluten
> ½ cup (50 g) wheat bran
> ½ cup (50 g) wheat germ
> 1 teaspoon baking powder
> ½ teaspoon baking soda
> ½ teaspoon salt
> ½ cup (120 ml) coconut oil
> ¼ cup (50 g) granular polyol sweetener
> ¼ cup (6 g) Splenda
> 1 ½ teaspoons blackstrap molasses
> ½ cup (120 ml) Carb Countdown Dairy Beverage

In a mixing bowl, combine the vanilla whey protein powder, almond meal, oat bran, wheat gluten, wheat bran, wheat germ, baking powder, baking soda, and salt. Stir to evenly distribute ingredients. Set aside.

Using an electric mixer, beat the coconut oil with the granular polyol sweetener, Splenda, and blackstrap until the mixture is fluffy. Now beat in the dry ingredients and the carb-reduced milk gradually, alternating which you add.

When all the dry ingredients and milk are beaten in, scrape the dough into a ball, and refrigerate overnight. (This does something magical to the texture. I don't understand it myself.)

Okay, next day you can pull your dough out of the fridge. Let it warm up for 15 or 20 minutes—while that's happening, you can preheat your oven to 350°F (180°C).

Divide the dough into two equal parts. Cover a cookie sheet with baking parchment or a Teflon pan liner, and place one of the dough balls on it. Cover it with another sheet of baking parchment, or another pan liner. Using a rolling pin, roll out the dough between the two layers of parchment or liner, just a little thinner than a commercial graham cracker. Peel off the top sheet, and use a pizza cutter or a sharp, thin-bladed knife to score into squares. Prick each cracker 3 or 4 times with a fork.

Repeat this with the second dough ball, with a second set of parchment or pan liners (you can use the same top sheet for both).

Bake for about 15 to 20 minutes, or until browning a bit around the edges. Let cool, rescore, and break apart. Store in an airtight container.

Yield: 36 crackers

Each with: 68 calories; 4 g fat; 6 g protein; 3 g carbohydrate; 1 g dietary fiber, 2 g usable carbs. Carb count does not include polyol sweetener.

⊚ Parmesan Garlic Crackers

These are a variation on a cracker in *500 Low-Carb Recipes*—for you garlic fans, and I know your name is Legion!

>   1 cup (225 g) sunflower seeds
>   ½ cup (80 g) grated Parmesan cheese
>   1 ½ teaspoons garlic powder
>   1 ½ teaspoons onion powder
>   ¼ cup (60 ml) water

Preheat oven to 325°F (170°C).

Dump the sunflower seeds into your food processor, with the S-blade in place. Run the food processor until the seeds are ground fine.

Add the Parmesan and the garlic and onion powders, and pulse to combine. Now turn on the processor, and pour in the water. As soon as a soft dough forms, turn it off.

Cover a baking sheet with baking parchment, and turn the dough out onto it. Cover the dough with another sheet of baking parchment. Using a rolling pin, roll the dough out between the two layers of parchment, taking the time to get the dough seriously thin—so long as there are no holes, the thinner, the better.

Peel off the top sheet of parchment, and, using a thin-bladed sharp knife or a pizza cutter, score dough into diamonds or squares. Bake for about 30 minutes, or until evenly browned. Peel off the parchment, break along scored lines, and cool. Store in a tightly lidded container.

Yield: will depend on what size you make your crackers, of course. I make mine small, about the size of Wheat Thins, and get 6 dozen.

Each with: 14 calories; 1 g fat; 1 g protein; trace carbohydrate; trace dietary fiber; no usable carbs. Heck, the whole batch has 34 g of carbs and 15 g of fiber, or a usable carb count of 19 g!

Sunflower Wheat Crackers

These taste a bit like Wheat Thins, and would be wonderful with dips—or just by themselves!

> 1 cup (225 g) sunflower seeds
> 1/2 cup (50 g) wheat germ
> 1/4 cup (25 g) wheat bran
> 1/4 cup (25 g) oat bran
> 1/2 teaspoon salt
> 4 tablespoons (60 ml) canola oil
> 1/4 cup (60 ml) water
> 1 tablespoon (1.5 g) Splenda

In your food processor, using the S-blade, grind the sunflower seeds until they're a fine meal. Add the wheat germ, wheat bran, oat bran, salt, and Splenda, and pulse to mix.

Now pour in the oil, and pulse to mix that in. Finally, add the water, and pulse to make an evenly blended dough.

Cover a cookie sheet with baking parchment or a Teflon pan liner. Turn the dough out onto this. Cover with another sheet of parchment or another pan liner. Now roll the dough out through the top sheet, making it as thin as you can without making holes in it. It's really worth the time to make this seriously thin.

Using a knife with a thin, straight, sharp blade, or a pizza cutter, score the dough into squares or diamonds. I make mine about the size of Wheat Thins.

Bake for about 30 minutes, or until evenly golden. Rescore to help you separate the crackers without breaking them. Store in a tightly lidded container.

Yield: About 6 dozen small crackers.

Each with: 22 calories; 2 g fat; 1 g protein; 1 g carbohydrate; trace dietary fiber; 1 g usable carb.

◎ Ruth Green's Cinnamon Crackers

A sweet, cinnamony, crunchy treat.

> 1 cup (150 g) whole roasted almonds
> 1/3 cup (40 g) vanilla-flavored whey protein powder
> 1 teaspoon cinnamon
> 2 tablespoons (3 g) Splenda
> A scant 1/2 cup (60 ml) water (take out 1 tablespoon water)

Preheat oven to 325°F (170°C).

Process the almonds in your food processor until finely ground. Then add all of the dry ingredients and pulse the processor to blend. Now add the water; process to mix. Using a rubber spatula, scrape bowl once.

Cover a cookie sheet with baking parchment. Turn the dough out onto this, and cover with another sheet of parchment. Flatten with your hands or a rolling pin until quite thin. Peel off top sheet of parchment, and score into squares or diamonds using your pizza cutter. (If the dough sticks to the top parchment as you take it off and your crackers do not have a smooth top, reduce your water slightly.)

Bake for about 25 minutes, until a cracker in the center feels firm when you tap on it. It kind of makes a thumping sound.

Yield: The number of crackers per batch depends on how thin you like your crackers and how big you cut them—I roll my batch out to be about 11" x 11" (27.5 x 27.5 cm). Assuming you get 4 dozen crackers …

Each cracker will have: 25 calories; 2 g fat; 2 g protein; 1 g carbohydrate; trace dietary fiber; 1 g usable carb.

⊚ Ruth Green's Coconut Crackers

3/4 cup (115 g) whole roasted almonds
1/3 cup (40 g) vanilla-flavored whey protein powder
1/3 cup (25 g) unsweetened coconut flakes
2 tablespoons (3 g) Splenda
Scant 1/2 cup (60 ml) water

Process the almonds in your food processor until finely ground. Then add all of the dry ingredients and pulse the processor to blend. Now add the water; process to mix. Using a rubber spatula scrape bowl once.

Cover a cookie sheet with baking parchment. Turn the dough out onto this, and cover with another sheet of parchment. Flatten with your hands or a rolling pin until quite thin. Peel off top sheet of parchment, and score into squares or diamonds using your pizza cutter. (If the dough sticks to the top parchment as you take it off and your crackers do not have a smooth top, reduce your water slightly.)

Bake for about 25 minutes, until a cracker in the center feels firm when you tap on it. It kind of makes a thumping sound. Ruth's note: "For a cool variation, use lemon juice in place of the water."

Yield: The number of crackers per batch depends on how thin you like your crackers and how big you cut them—I roll my batch out to be about 11" x 11" (27.5 x 27.5 cm). Assuming you get 4 dozen crackers . . .

Each cracker will have: 25 calories; 2 g fat; 2 g protein; 1 g carbohydrate; trace dietary fiber; 1 g usable carb.

Buttermilk Drop Biscuits

You wouldn't believe how much trouble I had coming up with a decent low-carb biscuit! Everything I made either ran all over the baking sheet or was unpleasantly heavy. And I couldn't get a dough that could be rolled out and cut without sticking! Finally, I hit on the idea of drop biscuits baked in a muffin tin, and sure enough, it worked out great.

1 cup (125 g) almond meal
1/2 cup (125 g) rice protein
1/4 cup (25 g) gluten
2 tablespoons (30 g) butter
2 tablespoons (30 ml) coconut oil
1/2 teaspoon salt
2 teaspoons baking powder
1/2 teaspoon soda
3/4 cup (180 ml) buttermilk

Preheat oven to 475°F (240°C)—the oven must be up to temperature before you add the buttermilk to the dry ingredients, so do this first!

Put everything but the buttermilk into your food processor, with the S-blade in place. Pulse food processor to cut in shortening—you want it evenly distributed in the dry ingredients. Dump this mixture—it should have a mealy texture—into a mixing bowl.

Spray a 12-cup muffin tin with nonstick cooking spray. Don't use paper muffin cups; you want the browning you'll get from direct contact with the hot metal.

Check to make sure your oven is up to temperature—if it isn't, have a quick cup of tea until it's hot. Now measure the buttermilk and pour it into your dry ingredients, and stir it in with a few swift strokes—don't overmix; you just want to make sure everything's evenly damp. This will make a soft dough. Spoon it into your prepared muffin tin, smoothing the tops with the back of the spoon. Put in the oven immediately, and bake for 10 to 12 minutes, or until golden on top. Serve hot with butter, and, if you like, low-sugar preserves or sugar-free imitation honey.

Yield: 12 biscuits

Each with: 153 calories; 10 g fat; 14 g protein; 4 g carbohydrate; 1g dietary fiber; 3 g usable carbs.

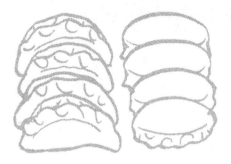

Yeast Breads

Now we come to a few yeast-raised items. I offer these with a certain trepidation. Of all the recipes in *500 Low-Carb Recipes*, the yeast bread recipes have turned out to be the most problematic. They all work beautifully for me, or I wouldn't have included them. Many readers love them, but many others have written me complaining that they can't get them to rise for love nor money. It's impossible to troubleshoot, because there are so many variables involved—the problem could be a different brand of ingredients, the particular bread machine, hard versus soft water, dead yeast, the weather—all sorts of things. For what it's worth, some people have had success using an extra teaspoon of yeast, while others find that making sure that the yeast doesn't touch the liquid ingredients until the kneading starts makes a difference.

So there are just a few yeast-raised recipes here: dinner rolls and two loaf breads. All call for a bread machine, and the quantities are for a 1-pound (455 g) loaf, which is what my machine makes. If you have a bigger machine, you'll just have to multiply.

◎ Dinner Rolls

These have a more elastic texture than carb-y dinner rolls; it comes from the high protein content. (They're so high in protein, you could have a leftover roll in the morning and call it breakfast.) But they come out wonderfully crusty and have a good yeasty flavor. We had them for a holiday meal, and everyone liked them, texture and all.

> 5 1/2 ounces (155 ml) water
> 3 tablespoons (25 g) instant dry milk
> 3/4 cup (75 g) wheat gluten
> 3/4 cup (75 g) wheat protein isolate
> 1/2 cup (60 g) oat flour
> 2 tablespoons (30 g) butter
> 1/2 teaspoon salt
> 2 teaspoons active baker's yeast (one packet)

Put everything in your bread machine, in the order specified with your unit. Put dough through two knead-and-rise cycles. Remove from machine.

Spray a 12-cup muffin tin with nonstick cooking spray.

Nip off bits of dough, and roll them into balls about 1" (2.5 cm) in diameter. Place three dough balls in a clover-leaf configuration in each muffin tin. Dough will be extremely elastic! Don't worry about trying to make each ball completely smooth.

Let rolls rise for 60 to 90 minutes in a warm place. Preheat oven to 350°F (180°C), and bake rolls for 10 to 15 minutes, or until golden.

Serve with plenty of butter!

Yield: 12 rolls

Each with: 172 calories; 4 g fat; 26 g protein; 8 g carbohydrate; 1 g dietary fiber; 7 g usable carbs.

Maple Oat Bread

Sugar-free pancake syrup gives this bread a very special flavor.

7 ounces (205 ml) water
2 teaspoons sugar-free pancake syrup
¾ cup (75 g) wheat gluten
½ cup (60 g) wheat protein isolate
¼ cup (25 g) rolled oats
2 tablespoons wheat bran
¼ cup (25 g) wheat germ
2 tablespoons (8 g) flax seed meal
1 tablespoon (8 g) oat flour
¼ teaspoon salt
1 tablespoon (15 g) butter, softened
2 teaspoons active baker's yeast (one packet)

Put ingredients in bread machine in order given, unless the instructions with your unit call for something quite different—then do it according to instructions!

Run bread machine through two knead-and-rise cycles. In my cheapie, low-tech, twelve-year-old bread machine, this means unplugging the machine when the first knead-and-rise cycle is through, plugging it back in, and hitting start again—but if your machine will automatically run two knead-and-rise cycles before baking, go with it. After the second rise, let the bread bake. Remove promptly from bread case when done, and cool before slicing and/or wrapping.

Yield: 12 slices

Each with: 133 calories; 3 g fat; 21 g protein; 5 g carbohydrate; 2 g dietary fiber; 3 g usable carbs. Carb count does not include the polyols in the sugar-free pancake syrup.

◎ Poppy Seed Bread

This bread has a firm, close-grained texture that lends itself to thin slicing. It also doesn't rise more than about 4" (10 cm), but I liked the flavor and texture so much, I thought I'd include it anyway. Don't eat poppy seeds if you're facing a drug test! You run the risk of testing positive for opiates.

⅔ cup (160 ml) water
⅔ cup (70 g) gluten
3 tablespoons (20 g) wheat bran
3 tablespoons (25 g) oat flour
⅔ cup (80 g) almond meal
⅓ cup (35 g) wheat protein isolate
2 tablespoons (15 g) poppy seeds
3 tablespoons (25 g) powdered milk
1 tablespoon (15 g) butter, softened
2 teaspoons active baker's yeast
½ teaspoon salt
1 tablespoon (1.5 g) Splenda

Put everything in a bread machine in the order specified in the instructions that come with your unit. Run the dough through two knead-and-rise cycles, then bake. Remove from bread case immediately, and cool before slicing thin to serve.

Yield: About 12 slices

Each with: 154 calories; 7 g fat; 19 g protein; 6 g carbohydrate; 2 g dietary fiber; 4 g usable carbs.

Elizabeth Dean's Next Best Thing to Cornbread

A decarbed version of Southern-style cornbread.

> Butter for greasing pan
> 1 cup (125 g) almond meal
> 1/2 cup (60 g) soy flour
> 1/2 cup (60 g) natural-flavor whey protein powder
> 1 teaspoon stevia/FOS
> 1 tablespoon (5 g) baking powder
> 1/2 teaspoon salt
> 4 tablespoons (60 g) butter, melted
> 1 egg
> 1/2 cup (120 g) cream
> 1/2 cup (120 ml) water
> 1/2 teaspoon butter flavoring

Preheat oven to 400°F (200°C). Put a little butter in an ovenproof skillet or 8" x 8" (20 x 20 cm) pan and place in oven until butter is melted. Swirl melted butter around to grease pan.

Combine dry ingredients in a large mixing bowl and mix well. In another bowl, combine the remaining ingredients and mix well. Pour the liquid mixture all at once into the dry mixture. Stir until combined, but do not overmix.

Pour the batter into the prepared pan and bake until top is golden and a toothpick inserted tests clean, about 15 to 20 minutes.

Yield: About 16 servings

Each will have: 120 calories; 7 g fat; 10 g protein; 5 g carbohydrate; trace dietary fiber; 5 g usable carbs.

Sharyn Taylor's Granny's Spoon Bread

A decarbed version of this old-time favorite. Our tester, Ray, said, "I remember my granny's homemade bread like this, and this tastes just like it."

- 2 cups (480 ml) soy milk (or substitute Carb Countdown Dairy Beverage)
- 3 tablespoons (45 g) butter, melted
- 2 heaping tablespoons (12 g) Atkins Bake Mix (or other low-carb bake mix)
- 2 heaping tablespoons (20 g) corn meal
- 1 ½ teaspoons salt
- 2 teaspoons baking powder
- 4 slices stale low-carb bread, crumbled (Sharyn uses Nature's Own Wheat and Fiber, with 5 g per slice, but use the lowest-carb bread at your store.)
- 2 eggs, slightly beaten

Preheat oven to 425°F (220°C).

Grease an 8″ (20 cm) cast-iron skillet, or a baking pan of about the same size. Heat milk and butter together (do not boil). Sift together the dry ingredients. Now stir in the heated milk and butter mixture, and pour it over crumbled bread. Stir in the eggs—mixture will be very soft.

Pour into pan and bake until brown.

Sharyn's Note: You can put 3 or 4 slices of bacon on top for added flavor. You could also add grated cheddar cheese to mixture before baking, if you want, but I like it just the way it is with butter on top.

Yield: Makes 8 servings

Each with: 112 calories; 8 g fat; 6 g protein; 6 g carbohydrate; 1 g dietary fiber; 5 g usable carbs.

◎ Dean's Granola

Donna Hodach-Price writes, "When I announced my intent to begin cooking low carb, my husband, Dean (who is really an 'old hippie') was very sad to hear that my homemade, traditional granola was no longer on the 'acceptable' list. He moped for months until I became more comfortable with low-carb cooking. After a while, I went to work on developing my own low-carb version of his favorite. While this pared-down version does *not* contain the 6 cups of rolled oats or the full cup of honey, it is very tasty and relatively low carb! The first time he tasted it, he gave it 'two thumbs up.'"

2 cups (100 g) All-Bran Extra Fiber Cereal

3 cups (210 g) shredded unsweetened coconut

2 cups (200 g) rolled oats

1 cup (125 g) pecan pieces

1 cup (225 g) raw pumpkin seeds (shelled)

1 cup (225 g) raw sunflower seeds (shelled)

1 cup (95 g) sliced almonds

1/2 cup (60 g) sesame seeds

1 cup (125 g) ground flax seeds

3 tablespoons (25 g) ground cinnamon

1/2 cup (60 g) vanilla whey protein powder

1 teaspoon salt

1 cup (240 g) butter (2 sticks), melted

1 1/2 cups (38 g) Splenda

Preheat oven to 350°F (180°C).

In very large bowl, combine all dry ingredients. Add Splenda to melted butter and stir to combine. Pour butter mixture over dry ingredients and mix well.

Place mixture into two large, shallow baking pans and bake approximately 45 minutes, stirring every 15 minutes or until lightly toasted. *Do not allow to overbake!*

Cool completely at room temperature before storing in tightly covered storage container.

Yield: 13 servings of 1 cup

Each with: 631 calories; 56 g fat; 15 g protein; 27 g carbohydrate; 12 g dietary fiber; 15 g usable carbs.

Almond-Parmesan Crust

This is a good "crumb crust" for savory dishes, like quiche.

> 1 ⅓ cups (200 g) almonds
> ½ cup (75 g) grated Parmesan cheese
> 6 tablespoons (90 g) butter, melted
> 1 tablespoon water

In your food processor, using the S-blade, grind the almonds until they're the texture of cornmeal. Add the Parmesan cheese, and pulse to combine. Pour in the butter and the water, and run the processor until a uniform dough is formed— you may need to stop the processor and run a butter knife around the bottom edge of the processor bowl halfway through.

Turn out into a 10" (25 cm) pie plate you've sprayed with nonstick cooking spray. Bake at 350°F (180°C) for about 10 to 12 minutes. Cool before filling.

Yield: 8 servings

Each with: 238 calories; 22 g fat; 7 g protein; 5 g carbohydrate; 3 g dietary fiber, 2 g usable carbs.

Pie Crust

Because rolling this pie crust out doesn't work well, you'll have to settle for one-crust pies. But that's lots better than no-crust pies! I'm very pleased with how the texture of this crust worked out; it's brittle and flaky, just like a pie crust should be.

> ½ cup (60 g) almond meal
> ⅓ cup (40 g) rice protein
> ¼ cup (25 g) gluten, wheat
> 1 pinch baking powder
> ½ teaspoon salt
> ⅓ cup (80 ml) coconut oil, chilled
> 1 tablespoon (15 g) butter, chilled
> 3 tablespoons (45 ml) ice water

Put the almond meal, rice protein, gluten, baking powder, and salt in your food processor, with the S-blade in place. Add the coconut oil and the butter, and pulse the food processor until the shortening is cut into the dry ingredients—it should be sort of mealy in texture.

Do use ice water, not just cold water—I put an ice cube in a cup and cover it with water, and let the water sit for a minute. Now add 1 tablespoon of this water, pulse the food processor briefly, then repeat 2 more times, with the other 2 tablespoons of water.

I find that pressing this crust into place works better than rolling it out. Dump out the dough into a 9" (22.5 cm) pie plate, and press it into place evenly across the bottom and up the sides; then crimp the top rim, if you want to be spiffy about it.

You can now bake your pie shell empty and use it for any recipe that calls for a prebaked pie shell, or you can fill and bake it according to any recipe that calls for an unbaked pie shell. If you want to prebake your pie shell, preheat your oven to 450°F (230°C). Prick the bottom of the pie shell all over with a fork, then add a layer of dried beans, marbles, or clean, round pebbles—this is to keep your pie shell from buckling. Bake for 10 minutes, take it out of the oven, and remove the beans, marbles, or pebbles, dealing gingerly with any that may have embedded themselves a bit. Return the crust to the oven for another 3 to 5 minutes, then cool and fill.

Yield: 8 servings

Each with: 194 calories; 15 g fat; 15 g protein; 3 g carbohydrate; 1 g dietary fiber; 2 g usable carbs.

chapter five

Hot Vegetables and Other Sides

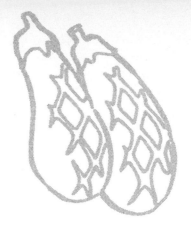

Perhaps the hardest adjustment new low-carb cooks have is that third of the plate that used to be filled by potatoes or rice. What goes there now?

Vegetables! Wonderful, delicious, nutritious vegetables. Here you'll find a mind-boggling selection of utterly fabulous hot vegetable dishes to mix and match with any main dish, or even serve alone. Have fun trying them—you're going to find a lot of new favorites, and I bet you get your family to eat vegetables they never knew they liked.

We kick this chapter off with a slew of cauliflower recipes. As all long-time low carbers know, cauliflower is the Great Fooler, substituting for potatoes and rice in many a dish. Heck, I never go to the grocery store without picking up another head. Sounds strange to you? No stranger than buying potatoes by the ten-pound sack, and a whole lot better for you.

For the basic recipes for Fauxtatoes (page 529) and Cauliflower Rice (page 530), see chapter 15. Here we're going to start right in with the cool variations!

◎ The Ultimate Fauxtatoes

I'm not crazy about Ketatoes by themselves, but added to pureed-cauliflower Fauxtatoes, they add a potato-y flavor and texture that is remarkably convincing!

> 1/2 head cauliflower
> 1/2 cup (25 g) Ketatoes mix
> 1/2 cup (120 ml) boiling water
> 1 tablespoon (15 g) butter
> Salt and pepper

Trim the bottom of the stem of your cauliflower, and whack the rest of the head into chunks. Put them in a microwaveable casserole with a lid. Add a couple of tablespoons of water, cover, and microwave on high for 8 to 9 minutes.

While that's happening, measure your Ketatoes mix and boiling water into a mixing bowl, and whisk together.

When the microwave beeps, pull out your cauliflower—it should be tender. Drain it well, and put it in either your food processor, with the S-blade in place, or in your blender. Either way, puree the cauliflower until it's smooth. Transfer the pureed cauliflower to the mixing bowl, and stir the cauliflower and Ketatoes together well. Add the butter, and stir till it melts. Salt and pepper to taste, and serve.

Yield: 4 servings

Each with: 140 calories; 5 g fat; 10 g protein; 14 g carbohydrate; 8 g dietary fiber; 6 g usable carbs.

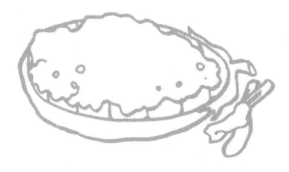

Chipotle-Cheese Fauxtatoes

 1 large chipotle chile canned in adobo, minced; reserve 1 teaspoon sauce
 ½ cup (60 g) shredded Monterey Jack cheese
 1 batch The Ultimate Fauxtatoes (page 136)

Stir the minced chipotle, a teaspoon of the adobo sauce it was canned in, and the shredded cheese into the Ultimate Fauxtatoes. Serve immediately!

Yield: 4 servings

Each with: 193 calories; 10 g fat; 14 g protein; 14 g carbohydrate; 8 g dietary fiber; 6 g usable carbs.

Nancy O'Connor's Creamy Garlic-Chive Fauxtatoes

Miss baked potatoes with sour cream and chives? Try this.

 4 cups (600 g) fresh cauliflower
 ½ cup (115 g) cream cheese with chives
 2 tablespoons (30 g) butter
 1 clove garlic, crushed
 Salt and pepper to taste

Put your cauliflower in a microwaveable casserole with a lid. Add a couple of tablespoons water, cover, and nuke it on high for 8 minutes or so, until tender.

Blend cooked cauliflower in food processor with the cream cheese, butter, and garlic. Salt and pepper to taste, then serve.

Yield: 3 servings

Each with: 236 calories; 20 g fat; 5 g protein; 10 g carbohydrate; 3 g dietary fiber; 7 g usable carbs.

Bubble and Squeak

This is my decarbed version of a tradition Irish dish—and very tasty, too!

> 1 tablespoon (15 g) butter
> 2 cups (150 g) shredded cabbage
> 1 medium carrot, shredded
> ¾ cup (120 g) chopped onion
> 1 batch The Ultimate Fauxtatoes (page 136)
> ½ cup (60 g) shredded cheddar cheese

Melt the butter in your big, heavy skillet and sauté the veggies until the onion is turning translucent and the cabbage has softened a bit.

Spray a 6-cup (1.4 L) casserole dish with nonstick cooking spray. Spread ⅓ of the Fauxtatoes on the bottom, then make a layer of ½ the cabbage mixture. Repeat the layers, then finish with a layer of Fauxtatoes. Top with the cheese. Bake at 350°F (180°C) for 45 minutes, then serve, scooping down through all the layers.

Yield: 6 servings

Each with: 167 calories; 9 g fat; 10 g protein; 14 g carbohydrate; 6 g dietary fiber; 8 g usable carbs.

Trish Z.'s Pork Rind Stuffing

This is remarkably like cornbread stuffing! By the way, Trish runs a website that carries a few hard to find specialty products—www.lowcarber.com

> 1 cup (120 g) chopped celery
> ¼ cup (40 g) chopped onion
> Salt and pepper, to taste
> Poultry seasoning, to taste
> 1 packet Splenda or other sweetener
> 2 tbsp (30 g) butter
> ¼ cup (60 ml) cream
> 3 ½ ounces (105 ml) chicken broth (about ¼ can)
> 10 ounces (280 g) pork rinds, crushed
> 4 eggs

Sauté celery, onion, salt, pepper, poultry seasoning, sweetener, and butter in a frying pan until transparent and tender. Add other ingredients and mix together until the pork rinds are coated and moist. Put into baking dish and bake for 35 to 50 minutes until set like regular bread stuffing. Feel free to add more eggs or cream to get the texture you are used to. Some people also add mushrooms, sage, sausage, or oysters.

Yield: 8 servings

Each will have: 276 calories; 18 g fat; 25 g protein; 2 g carbohydrate; trace dietary fiber; 2 g usable carbs.

◉ Hellzapoppin Cheese "Rice"

Another recipe I've adapted from the funniest cookbook ever written, *The I Hate To Cook Book,* by Peg Bracken. And truly fabulous it is, too.

> 1/3 cup (55 g) cooked wild rice
> 4 eggs
> 1 cup (240 ml) Carb Countdown Dairy Beverage
> 1/4 cup (60 g) minced onion
> 1 tablespoon (15 ml) Worcestershire sauce
> 1 teaspoon salt
> 1/2 teaspoon dried thyme
> 1/2 teaspoon dried marjoram
> 3 1/3 cups (500 g) shredded cauliflower (about 1/2 head)
> 1 pound (455 g) grated sharp cheddar cheese
> 1 10-ounce (280 g) box frozen chopped spinach, thawed

You need to have your wild rice cooked before you start. Make more than you need for this recipe and stash it in a snap-top container in the freezer; next time you'll have it on hand!

Beat the eggs till they're foamy, then whisk in the Carb Countdown Dairy Beverage, onion, Worcestershire, salt, thyme, and marjoram. Now, stir in the raw cauli-rice, the wild rice, the cheese, and the spinach. Stir till everything is well combined.

Pour the whole thing into a casserole dish you've sprayed with nonstick cooking spray, and bake it at 375°F (190°C) for 35 to 40 minutes.

Yield: 6 servings

Each with: 409 calories; 30 g fat; 27 g protein; 10 g carbohydrate; 3 g dietary fiber; 7 g usable carbs.

Japanese Fried "Rice"

½ head cauliflower, shredded
2 eggs
1 cup (75 g) snow pea pods, fresh
2 tablespoons (30 g) butter
½ cup (80 g) diced onion
2 tablespoons (16 g) shredded carrot
3 tablespoons (45 ml) soy sauce
Salt and pepper

Put the shredded cauliflower in a microwaveable casserole with a lid, add a couple of tablespoons of water, cover, and microwave on high for 6 minutes.

While that's happening, scramble the eggs and pour them into a skillet you've sprayed with nonstick cooking spray, over medium-high heat. As you cook the eggs, use your spatula to break them up into pea-sized bits. Remove from skillet and set aside.

Remove the tips and strings from the snow peas, and snip into ¼" (6.25 mm) lengths. (By now the microwave has beeped—take the lid off your cauliflower or it will turn into a mush that bears not the slightest resemblance to rice!) Melt the butter in the skillet, and sauté the pea pods, onion, and carrot for 2 to 3 minutes.

Add the cauliflower, and stir everything together well. Stir in the soy sauce, and cook the whole thing, stirring often, for another 5 to 6 minutes. Salt and pepper a bit, and serve.

Yield: 5 servings

Each with: 91 calories; 6 g fat; 4 g protein; 5 g carbohydrate; 1 g dietary fiber; 4 g usable carbs.

Lonestar "Rice"

1/2 head cauliflower, shredded

1/4 cup (40 g) chopped onion

1 cup (100 g) sliced mushrooms

1/2 cup (40 g) snow pea pods, fresh, cut in 1/2" (1.25 g) pieces

1 tablespoon (15 ml) olive oil

1 tablespoon (15 g) butter

1/4 teaspoon chili powder

2 teaspoons beef bouillon granules or concentrate

Put the cauliflower in a microwaveable casserole with a lid. Add a couple of tablespoons of water, cover, and microwave on high for 6 minutes.

While that's cooking, sauté your onions, mushrooms, and snow peas in the olive oil and butter, in your big skillet. I like to use the edge of my spatula to break up the mushrooms into smaller pieces, but leave the slices whole if you like them better that way—up to you. When the mushrooms have changed color and the snow peas are tender-crisp, drain your cooked cauli-rice, and stir it in. Add the chili powder and beef bouillon, and stir to distribute the seasonings well, then serve.

Yield: 3 servings

Each with: 99 calories; 9 g fat; 2 g protein; 5 g carbohydrate; 1 g dietary fiber; 4 g usable carbs.

◎ Venetian "Rice"

This is rich tasting and slightly piquant.

> ½ head cauliflower
> 1 tablespoon (15 ml) olive oil
> 2 tablespoons (30 g) butter
> 1 cup (100 g) sliced mushrooms
> 3 anchovy fillets, minced
> 1 clove garlic, crushed
> 3 tablespoons (30 g) grated Parmesan cheese

Run the cauliflower through the shredding blade of your food processor. Put it in a microwaveable casserole with a lid, add a couple of tablespoons of water, cover, and nuke on high for 5 to 6 minutes. When it's done, uncover immediately!

Combine the olive oil and butter in your big heavy skillet over medium heat, swirling together as the butter melts. Add the mushrooms and sauté until they're soft and changing color. If your mushroom slices are quite large, you may want to break them up a bit with the edge of your spatula as you stir.

When the mushrooms are soft, stir in the minced anchovies and garlic. Add the cauli-rice, undrained—that little bit of water is going to help the flavors blend. Stir well to distribute all the flavors.

Stir in the Parmesan, and serve.

Yield: 3 to 4 servings

Each will have: 148 calories; 10 g fat; 4 g protein; 2 g carbohydrate; 1 g dietary fiber; 1 g usable carb.

Cheesy Cauliflower

4 cups (600 g) cauliflower florets, cut $\frac{1}{2}$" (1.25 cm) thick
$\frac{1}{3}$ cup (50 g) chopped onion
$\frac{1}{2}$ green bell pepper, diced
2 tablespoons (30 ml) olive oil
4 cloves garlic, crushed
$\frac{1}{2}$ teaspoon dried basil
$\frac{1}{2}$ cup (120 ml) half-and-half
1 cup (120 g) shredded Monterey Jack cheese

Put your cauliflower in a microwaveable casserole with a lid. Add a tablespoon or two of water, cover, and nuke on high for 7 minutes.

While that's happening, start the onion and pepper sautéing in the olive oil, in a large heavy skillet over medium-high heat.

By the time the microwave goes beep, your pepper and onion should be getting soft. Drain the cauliflower, and dump it into the skillet. Stir everything around together. Stir in the garlic, and sauté for another minute or two.

Now stir in the basil, half-and-half, and shredded cheese. Keep stirring till the cheese is melted. Let the whole thing cook for another minute or two, then serve.

Yield: 5 servings

Each with: 195 calories; 15 g fat; 8 g protein; 8 g carbohydrate; 2 g dietary fiber; 6 g usable carbs.

Gratin of Cauliflower and Turnips

2 1/2 cups (375 g) turnip slices
2 1/2 cups (375 g) sliced cauliflower
1 1/2 cups (360 ml) carb-counting milk
1/4 cup (60 ml) heavy cream
3/4 cup (90 g) blue cheese, crumbled
1/2 teaspoon pepper
1/2 teaspoon salt
1 teaspoon dried thyme
Guar or xanthan (optional)
1/4 cup (40 g) Parmesan cheese

Combine the turnips and cauliflower in a bowl, making sure they're pretty evenly interspersed.

In a saucepan, over lowest heat, warm the carb-counting milk and heavy cream. When it's hot, add the blue cheese, pepper, salt, and thyme. Stir with a whisk until the cheese is melted. It's good to thicken this sauce just slightly with your guar or xanthan shaker.

Spray a casserole dish with nonstick cooking spray. Put about 1/3 of the cauliflower and turnip slices in the dish, and pour 1/3 of the sauce evenly over them. Make two more layers of vegetables and sauce. Sprinkle the Parmesan cheese over the top. Bake at 375°F (190°C) for 30 minutes.

Yield: 6 servings

Each with: 142 calories; 10 g fat; 7 g protein; 8 g carbohydrate; 3 g dietary fiber; 5 g usable carbs.

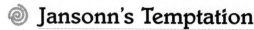 Jansonn's Temptation

This Swedish favorite is traditionally made with potatoes. I have no idea how this decarbed version compares, but it's utterly delicious in its own right. This is the natural side dish to serve with Swedish Meatballs (page 317).

2 turnips
1/2 head cauliflower
1 onion
2 tablespoons (30 g) butter
1 tablespoon (15 g) anchovy paste
1/4 teaspoon salt, or Vege-Sal
1/4 teaspoon pepper
1/2 cup (120 ml) heavy cream

Preheat oven to 400°F (200°C).

Peel your turnips and cut them into smallish strips—about the size of fast food French fries. Cut up your cauliflower, too—cut it in strips as much as possible (include the stem), but of course, being cauliflower, it'll crumble some. No biggie. Combine the turnips and cauliflower.

Slice your onion quite thin. Melt the butter in your heavy skillet, over medium heat, and sauté your onion slices until they're limp and turning translucent.

Spray an 8" x 8" (20 x 20 cm) baking dish with nonstick cooking spray. Layer the turnip/cauliflower mixture and the onions in the baking dish.

Stir the anchovy paste, salt, and pepper into the cream until the anchovy paste is dissolved. Pour this mixture over the vegetables.

Bake for 45 minutes, then serve.

Yield: 5 servings

Each with: 155 calories; 14 g fat; 2 g protein; 6 g carbohydrate; 2 g dietary fiber; 4 g usable carbs.

Melissa Wright's Two-Cheese Cauliflower

1 head of cauliflower (or 1 1/2 pounds frozen cauliflower)

1 large egg

1 cup (225 g) small curd whole-milk cottage cheese

1 cup (230 g) sour cream

1/2 teaspoon salt

1/8 teaspoon black pepper

8 ounces (225 g) sharp cheddar cheese, shredded

2 tablespoons (10 g) chopped parsley, optional

Preheat the oven to 350°F (180°C). Lightly spray a 2-quart baking dish with nonstick cooking spray.

Put the cauliflower florets in a microwaveable casserole, add two tablespoons of water, and cover. Microwave it for about 10 to 11 minutes, or until very tender (see package directions if using frozen).

Whisk egg in a large bowl. Add cottage cheese, sour cream, salt and pepper; mix well. Stir in cheddar cheese.

Remove the cauliflower from the microwave and drain thoroughly. Fold the cauliflower into the cheese mixture and gently mix well. Spoon the cauliflower mixture into the prepared baking dish. Sprinkle with chopped parsley, if desired. Bake for 30 minutes. Serve immediately.

As a variation of this, you can stir in two tablespoons of poppy seeds. This gives it a kind of polka-dot look and adds a subtle sophistication to the flavor.

Yield: 8 servings

Each with: 213 calories; 17 g fat; 13 g protein; 3 g carbohydrate; trace dietary fiber; 3 g usable carbs.

Stephanie Hill's Creamy Cauliflower and Bacon Casserole

1 medium head cauliflower

12 ounces bacon, cut in 1" (2.5 cm) pieces

1/2 cup (80 g) diced onion

1 1/2 teaspoons minced garlic, optional

6 ounces (170 g) cream cheese, softened

2 tablespoons (20 g) grated Parmesan cheese

2 tablespoons (30 ml) heavy cream, or as needed

Salt and pepper to taste

3 ounces (85 g) sharp cheddar cheese, grated

Preheat oven to 325°F (170°C). (If you're cooking something else in the oven, this can probably cook alongside it with no problems.) Spray a large casserole dish with nonstick cooking spray and set aside.

Chop the cauliflower into bite-sized pieces and cook until tender, either by steaming or in salted, boiling water. Drain and set aside.

In a Dutch oven or large, heavy saucepan, sauté the bacon pieces over medium to medium-high heat until half done. (You can drain off a portion of the bacon fat if desired.) Add the onion and cook until the onion is soft. Then add the garlic and sauté for a few moments, but do not burn. Add the cream cheese and Parmesan cheese, stirring until melted and creamy. Add the cream if necessary. Remove from heat and stir in the drained cauliflower and mix thoroughly. Add salt and pepper to taste. Pour cauliflower mixture into prepared casserole dish, and top with shredded cheddar. Bake until cheddar is melted and bubbly, about 10 minutes. Let casserole sit for five minutes before serving.

Note: Once you add the onion, the bacon will not crisp. If you want crispy bacon, cook it until crisp, remove to drain, and return it to the pan.

Tester's note: Ray, our tester, calls this "an easy, nifty dish" but warns that he lost a fair quantity of the chopped cauliflower through the holes in his bamboo steamer. If you have a steamer with fairly large holes, consider steaming your cauliflower whole, then chopping it. Ray also says he likes to add more shredded cheddar!

Dana's note: Me, I'd microwave that chopped cauliflower for about 7 minutes on high.

Yield: 6 servings

Per serving: 518 calories; 45 g fat; 24 g protein; 4 g carbohydrate; 1 g dietary fiber; 3 g usable carbs.

Leslie's Broccoli and Cauliflower Casserole

1 large onion, chopped

1 stick butter

1 pound (455 g) bag frozen chopped broccoli, cooked until soft

1 pound (455 g) bag frozen cauliflower, cooked until soft,
  and lightly mashed

2 large eggs, beaten

3 packets Splenda

1 teaspoon chicken base or bouillon concentrate, dissolved in
  two tablespoons (30 ml) water

1 cup (50 g) pork rind crumbs

1 1/2 cups (180 g) shredded cheddar cheese

4 slices provolone cheese

Preheat your oven to 350°F (180°C).

Sauté your onion in the butter until softened. Add to broccoli and cauliflower. Stir in the rest of your ingredients except the provolone. Pour everything into a 9" x 13" (22.5 x 32.5 cm) pan you've sprayed with nonstick cooking spray.

Bake for 30 minutes. Top with provolone and bake for another 5 to 10 minutes until cheese the melts.

Yield: 8 to 10 servings

Assuming 10 servings, each will have: 350 calories; 26 g fat; 24 g protein; 4 g carbohydrate; 2 g dietary fiber; 2 g usable carbs.

Tee's Cajun Dirty UnRice

1 bag broccoslaw (or any bagged coleslaw would work)

1/2 pound bulk breakfast sausage (or finely ground Italian sausage
  or beef if desired)

1–2 teaspoons Tee's Cajun Seasoning Mix (page 451), or to taste

1 tablespoon (15 ml) olive oil

Dash cream

Finely shred the broccoslaw with a hand chopper or in a food processor to size of rice grains (or you could use grated cauliflower). Sauté sausage until no longer pink. Add broccoslaw, cajun seasoning, and olive oil and sauté til broccoslaw is tender-crisp. When done, top with a dash of cream and mix in completely. Serve immediately.

Yield: Serves 6

Each having: 197 calories; 18 g fat; 6 g protein; 4 g carbohydrate; 2 g dietary fiber; 2 g usable carbs.

◎ Anne Logston's Cheesy Broccoli Casserole

Broccoli and cheese are a classic combination, dressed up here with some almonds for crunch.

> 8 ounces (225 g) cream cheese
> 1 pound (455 g) bag frozen broccoli florets
> 1/4 cup (60 ml) heavy whipping cream
> 1/2 cup (75 g) Parmesan cheese
> 1/2 cup (60 g) shredded cheddar cheese
> 1/4 cup (25 g) sliced almonds

Preheat oven to 350°F (180°C). Microwave cream cheese briefly to soften. Thaw and drain broccoli and lay in baking pan you've sprayed with non-stick cooking spray.

In a small saucepan, melt your cream cheese, then thin it with the cream and pour the whole thing over the broccoli. Sprinkle with the Parmesan and stir to coat the broccoli evenly. Sprinkle the cheddar cheese over the top.

Bake at 350°F (180°C) for 30 minutes. Ten minutes before casserole is done, sprinkle almonds over the top.

Yield: 4 servings

Each with: 425 calories; 38 g fat; 16 g protein; 8 g carbohydrate; 3 g dietary fiber; 5 g usable carbs.

Broccoli Dijon

For the work involved—practically none—this is really great.

>   1 pound (455 g) frozen broccoli cuts or spears
>   ¼ cup (60 ml) vinaigrette dressing (I use Paul Newman's Olive Oil
>   and Vinegar)
>   1 tablespoon (15 g) Dijon mustard
>   3 scallions, sliced thin

I like to use broccoli cuts for this, but use spears or florets if that's what you have on hand; it'll be fine. If your broccoli is frozen in a clump, throw the bag on the floor, hard, a few times to break it up, or, if it's a box, slam all sides of it against the counter. This will make sure it's separated, and cooks evenly. Put your smashed-apart broccoli, still frozen, in a microwaveable casserole with a lid. Add a couple of tablespoons of water, cover, and nuke on high for 7 minutes. It should be tender-crisp by then, but if there are still cold spots, stir it and give it another minute or two. Don't overcook!

While the broccoli is cooking, measure the dressing and the mustard into a bowl, and whisk together.

Okay, broccoli's done! Drain it, then pour the dressing over it and toss. Add the scallions, toss again, and serve immediately.

Yield: 3 to 4 servings

Assuming 3 servings, each will have: 141 calories; 11 g fat; 5 g protein; 9 g carbohydrate; 5 g dietary fiber; 4 g usable carbs.

Leslie's Low-Carb Broccoli Cornbread

If you can't find La Tiara brand or other low-carb corn taco shells locally, you can easily order them online. Or you can use low-carb tortilla chips, instead—our tester, Ray, did this and said they worked fine.

1 ½ cups (185 g) almond meal

6 La Tiara Low Carb Taco Shells, ground, about ½ cup

1 teaspoon baking powder

1 cup (250 g) butter, softened

2 packets Splenda or 4 teaspoons Splenda granular

5 eggs

¾ cup (175 g) ricotta cheese or cottage cheese

10 ounces (280 g) frozen chopped broccoli, thawed and drained

1 cup (160 g) onion chopped

Preheat your oven to 350°F (180°C). Spray a rectangular baking dish with nonstick cooking spray.

In a mixing bowl, stir together the almond meal, ground taco shells, and baking powder, and set aside.

With your electric mixer, whip the butter with the Splenda until well combined. Add the eggs, one at a time, beating after each addition. Beat in dry ingredients a little at a time until well combined. Stir in ricotta, then add broccoli and chopped onion. Spread in the prepared baking dish, and bake for 55 minutes.

Yield: Serves 8 to 10

Assuming 10 servings, each will have: 356 calories; 28 g fat; 17 g protein; 16 g carbohydrate; 6 g dietary fiber; 10 g usable carbs.

Michele Holbrook's Broccoli Bake

If you can't find those Keto Crumbs locally, you can order them online.

> 24-ounce (680 g) bag frozen broccoli
> 1 16-ounce (455 g) block Velveeta cheese, cubed (or 3 cups [360 g] shredded cheddar cheese)
> ½ cup (120 ml) heavy cream (or light cream)

Topping

> ½ 3-ounce (85 g) can French's fried onions, crushed
> ½ 2–3 ounce (55–85 g) bag fried pork skins, crushed
> ¼ cup (30 g) Keto Soy Crumbs
> ½ teaspoon each salt, pepper, garlic powder, and onion powder

Preheat oven to 350°F (180°C).

Grease a 2-quart baking dish. Put in broccoli (still frozen), cheese, and cream, and stir the three together. Mix topping ingredients together and spread over broccoli. Bake for 1 to 1 ½ hours, then serve.

Dana's note: Velveeta has considerably more carbohydrate in it than regular cheddar cheese does—if you get 12 servings from this casserole, the Velveeta alone will contribute 7 g of carbs per serving, while the cheddar will contribute less than 1 gram per serving. Personally, I'd go with the cheddar, but I know some folks like the meltability of Velveeta better.

Yield: 12 servings

Each with: 312 calories; 20 g fat; 20 g protein; 13 g carbohydrate; 3 g dietary fiber; 10 g usable carbs.

Holiday Green Bean Casserole

You know that green bean casserole that mom serves every holiday? The one with the mushroom soup and the onion rings? It's pretty high carb. I'd rather have beans amandine, myself. But for you green bean casserole diehards—and I know that there are more than a few of you out there!—here's the new, decarbed version.

> 1 medium onion
> ¼ cup (30 g) low-carb bake mix or rice protein powder
> ¼ teaspoon salt or Vege-Sal

$^{1}/_{4}$ teaspoon paprika

Oil for frying

4 cups (600 g) frozen green beans, cut style

1 4-ounce (115 g) can mushrooms

2 tablespoons (20 g) minced onion

1 tablespoon (15 g) butter

1 cup (240 ml) heavy cream

$^{1}/_{2}$ teaspoon Worcestershire sauce

$^{1}/_{2}$ teaspoon chicken or beef bouillon concentrate

1 teaspoon soy sauce

Salt and pepper to taste

$^{1}/_{2}$ teaspoon guar or xanthan gum

Slice the onion thin, and separate into rings. Mix together the bake mix or protein powder, salt or Vege-Sal, and paprika. "Flour" the onion rings—the easiest way is to put the "flouring" mixture in a small paper sack, and shake a few onion rings at a time. Heat about $^{1}/_{4}$" (6.25 mm) of oil in a heavy skillet, over medium heat, and fry the "floured" onion rings, turning once, until golden brown and crisp. Drain on absorbent paper. You can do this part well in advance, if you like.

When you're ready to make your casserole, start your green beans cooking—I like to microwave mine on high for about 7 or 8 minutes, but you can steam them if you prefer. While that's happening, drain the liquid off the mushrooms, and reserve it. Sauté the mushrooms and the minced onion in the butter until the onion is limp and translucent. Now add the cream, the reserved mushroom liquid, the Worcestershire sauce, the bouillon concentrate, and the soy sauce, and stir, then salt and pepper to taste.

Now you have a choice: you can either pour this mixture into a blender or use a hand blender. Either way, sprinkle the guar or xanthan over the top, and run the blender just long enough to blend in the thickener, and to chop the mushrooms a bit—but not to totally puree them; you want some bits of mushroom.

Okay, we're on the home stretch. Drain your cooked green beans, and put them in a 1$^{1}/_{2}$-quart (1.4 L) casserole dish that you've sprayed with nonstick cooking spray. Stir in the mushroom mixture and half of those fried onions. Bake it in a 350°F (180°C) oven for 25 to 30 minutes, then top it with the rest of the fried onions, and bake for another 5 minutes.

Yield: 6 servings

Each with: 254 calories; 11 g carbohydrate and 4 g of fiber, for a usable carb count of 7 g; 6 g protein. For the record, this comes to just over half of the carb content of the original recipe—and just about the same calorie count.

Stir-Fried Green Beans and Water Chestnuts

2 tablespoons (30 ml) oil
2 cups (300 g) frozen green beans, thawed
1/2 cup (100 g) canned water chestnuts, sliced or diced, drained
1 clove garlic, crushed
1/4 cup (60 ml) chicken broth
1 1/2 teaspoons soy sauce
Guar or xanthan

Heat the oil in a skillet or wok, over high heat. Add the green beans and water chestnuts, and stir-fry until the green beans are tender-crisp. Stir in the garlic, chicken broth, and soy sauce, and let simmer for a couple of minutes; thicken the pan juices just a little with your guar or xanthan shaker, and serve.

Yield: 3 servings

Each with: 126 calories; 9 g fat; 2 g protein; 10 g carbohydrate; 3 g dietary fiber; 7 g usable carbs.

Janet Hoy's Twice-Fried Green Beans

Here's an unusual Chinese-style vegetable dish. Be aware that cooking hot pepper at high temperature can make you cough, so turn on the vent fan or open a window or two!

Good-quality cooking oil for deep- and stir-frying
1 ½" (3.75 cm) fresh gingerroot, or to taste
2 chopped garlic cloves, or to taste
1 pound (455 g) fresh green beans, washed, dried, and trimmed
1 teaspoon red pepper flakes or Thai pepper sauce (without added sugar), optional
1 teaspoon sesame oil (or pepper oil, if you like)
1–2 tablespoons (15–30 ml) soy sauce (I like tamari)
1 tablespoon (1.5 g) Splenda

Heat oil to 375°F (190°C) degrees in a deep-fat fryer or deep, heavy saucepan. While oil is heating, peel and coarsely chop ginger and garlic. Fry green beans a batch at a time 2 to 3 minutes or until skin crinkles. Drain on a clean towel.

In a wok or frying pan, over high heat, sauté ginger, garlic, and red pepper flakes in oil. Add sesame oil, soy sauce, and Splenda. When these are lightly cooked, add the cooked green beans and stir-fry for a couple of minutes until ingredients are thoroughly mixed.

Janet's note: "This is my own version of a Chinese restaurant favorite. It's especially good with chunks of precooked chicken breast meat added to the stir fry."

Tester's note: Ray Stevens says a wok really is better for this recipe than a skillet, so if you have a wok, use it.

Yield: Makes 4 servings

Each with: 116 calories; 8 g fat; 3 g protein; 10 g carbohydrate; 4 g dietary fiber; 6 g usable carbs.

Stephanie H.'s Green Beans Old Roman Style

Here's a simple but very cool way of dressing up green beans.

> 1 pound (455 g) green beans, fresh or frozen
> 6 ounces (170 g) bacon, cut into 1" (2.5 cm) slices
> 2 teaspoons coarse ground mustard with horseradish

Cook the green beans by your preferred method until just tender, then drain and set aside.

Sauté the bacon in a big skillet to the desired degree of doneness (I typically don't need it to be very crisp at all). Add the drained green beans to the pan along with the mustard and stir well over medium-high heat until everything is heated through. (If your bacon is particularly fatty, or you're watching fat intake, you could always drain off a bit of the bacon fat before adding the green beans and mustard, but do leave some for flavoring.)

Stephanie's note: "This works with other mustards, but the horseradish mustard adds a nice presence. You can also dress this up with other additions, like onion, garlic, slivered almonds, thinly sliced red onion, and so forth, but I prefer it straight or with a little minced garlic."

Dana's note: My preferred method, as no doubt you've gathered by now, would be to put those beans in a microwaveable casserole with a lid, add a couple of tablespoons of water, cover, and nuke 'em on high for about 6 or 7 minutes. Then I'd check for doneness, and if I thought they needed another couple of minutes, I'd stir them, re-cover them, and nuke 'em a little longer.

Yield: About 4 servings

Each with: 278 calories; 21 g fat; 15 g protein; 8 g carbohydrate; 3 g dietary fiber; 5 g usable carbs.

Debra Rodriguez's Green Bean Casserole

Our tester, Doris Courtney, gave this a 10. This recipe has the added convenience of not calling for you to thaw your frozen green beans.

1 1-pound (455 g) bag frozen French-cut green beans
1 cup (225 g) Bertolli portobello mushroom pasta sauce
¼ medium onion, sliced very thin
Soy sauce
Salt and pepper to taste

Preheat oven to 350°F (180°C).

Open green beans and dump the entire bag (still frozen) into a greased 2-quart (1.9 L) casserole dish. Add the pasta sauce, the thinly sliced onions, and a few dashes of soy sauce. Mix this all together. Add salt and pepper if desired. Bake for approximately 25 to 30 minutes.

Dana's note: If you can't get Bertolli sauce where you live, you can use any jarred spaghetti sauce with mushrooms. Look for one with no added corn syrup or sugar.

Yield: Serves 4 to 6

Assuming 6, each will have: 42 calories; trace fat; 2 g protein; 9 g carbohydrate; 3 g dietary fiber; 6 g usable carbs.

◉ Cindy Shields's BBQ Green Bean Casserole

4 cups (400 g) green beans
8 slices bacon, cooked and crumbled
½–1 cup (80–160 g) diced onion
1 tablespoon (10 g) minced garlic
1 cup (250 g) low-carb barbecue sauce
    (purchased or homemade from the recipe on page 525)
1 cup (120 g) shredded cheddar

Preheat oven to 350°F (180°C).

Combine green beans, bacon, onion, garlic, and half of the barbecue sauce in a casserole dish. Bake for 20 minutes, remove, top with cheese and remaining barbecue sauce and bake an additional 10 minutes or until cheese has melted.

Yield: 8 to 10 servings

Assuming 8 servings, each will have: 156 calories; 10 g fat; 7 g protein; 12 g carbohydrate; 3 g dietary fiber; 9 g usable carbs.

Marco Polo Stir-Fried Vegetables

2 cups (450 g) frozen broccoli florets, thawed
1 cup (100 g) sliced mushrooms
2 tablespoons (30 ml) peanut oil, or other oil for sautéing
1/4 cup (60 ml) reserved Marco Polo Marinade (page 445)

In a heavy skillet or wok, over high heat, stir-fry the vegetables in the oil until the broccoli is just tender-crisp. Stir in the reserved marinade, and let the whole thing cook for another couple of minutes—this will kill any raw steak germs still in the marinade. Serve with your Marco Polo Steak (page 446)!

Yield: 4 servings

Each with: 132 calories; 13 g fat; 4 g carbohydrate and 1 g fiber, for a usable carb count of 3 g; 2 g protein.

Asparagus with Curried Walnut Butter

1 pound (455 g) asparagus
4 tablespoons (60 g) butter
2 tablespoons (16 g) chopped walnuts
1 teaspoon curry powder
1/2 teaspoon cumin
1 1/2 teaspoons Splenda

Snap the ends off of the asparagus where they want to break naturally. Put in a microwaveable container with a lid, or use a glass pie plate covered with plastic wrap. Either way, add a tablespoon or two of water, and cover. Microwave on high for 5 minutes. Don't forget to uncover as soon as the microwave goes beep, or your asparagus will keep cooking and be limp and sad!

While that's cooking, put the butter in a medium skillet over medium heat. When it's melted, add the walnuts. Stir them around for 2 to 3 minutes, until they're getting toasty. Now stir in the curry powder, cumin, and Splenda, and stir for another 2 minutes or so.

Your asparagus is done by now! Fish it out of the container with tongs, put it on your serving plates, and divide the Curried Walnut Butter between the three servings.

Yield: 3 servings

Each with: 189 calories; 19 g fat; 3 g protein; 5 g carbohydrate; 2 g dietary fiber; 3 g usable carbs.

◎ Grilled Asparagus with Balsamic Vinegar

1 pound (455 g) asparagus
2 tablespoons (30 ml) olive oil
2 tablespoons (30 ml) balsamic vinegar
3 tablespoons (30 g) grated Parmesan cheese

Start your electric tabletop grill heating (or you can do this over your backyard grill!). Snap the ends off the asparagus where they break naturally. Put them on a plate and drizzle with the olive oil. Toss the asparagus a bit, to make sure it's all coated with the oil.

Place the asparagus on your grill—you'll probably have to do it in two batches, unless your grill is a lot bigger than mine. Set a timer for 10 minutes. (If grilling out of doors, just keep an eye on it, and grill until it's tender, with brown spots.)

If you've had to do two batches, put the first batch on a plate and cover it with a pot lid to keep it warm while the second batch cooks. When all the asparagus is done, and all on the plate, drizzle with the balsamic vinegar. Roll it about to coat it, then top it with the Parmesan and serve.

Yield: 3 servings

Each with: 184 calories; 16 g fat (74.2% calories from fat); 6 g protein; 7 g carbohydrate; 2 g dietary fiber; 5 g usable carbs.

Asparagus with Sun-Dried Tomatoes

1 pound (455 g) asparagus

1 tablespoon (15 ml) olive oil

2 tablespoons (30 g) butter

2 tablespoons (20 g) minced red onion

1/2 clove garlic, crushed

2 tablespoons (10 g) sun-dried tomato halves, minced

2 teaspoons lemon juice

Snap the ends off of the asparagus where they want to break naturally. Put them in a microwaveable casserole with a lid, add a couple of tablespoons of water, and cover—but don't nuke it yet. Make your sauce, first.

In a medium skillet, heat the olive oil and the butter, swirling them together as the butter melts. Add the onion, garlic, and sun-dried tomatoes to the oil and butter, and sauté until the onion is soft, being careful not to brown the onions or garlic. Stir in the lemon juice. Turn off the heat.

Okay, back to your asparagus. Microwave it on high for just 5 minutes. Uncover it the second it's done! Divide it between 3 or 4 serving plates, spoon the sauce over it, and serve.

Yield: 3 to 4 servings

Assuming 3 servings, each will have: 156 calories; 13 g fat; 3 g protein; 10 g carbohydrate; 3 g dietary fiber; 7 g usable carbs.

Barbo Gold's To-Die-For Asparagus Skillet

1 1/2–2 pounds (680 g–1 kg) asparagus, cut rather short
1 tablespoon (15 ml) extra-virgin olive oil
2 tablespoons (30 ml) good balsamic vinegar
Water
Salt and pepper

Place asparagus in a large nonstick skillet. Add oil and vinegar and enough water to not quite cover the asparagus. Cover the skillet, and cook on medium-high. Peek now and then to see when you need to add a bit more water. Then go ahead and cook it down till it's almost, but not quite, dry. Test the asparagus with a fork; it should be crisp-tender. (Well, okay, keep the tender part in your mind rather than the crisp part.) They will be perfect! Salt and pepper to taste. Eat hot or cold and betcha can't eat just one.

Yield: 4 servings

Each with: 59 calories; 4 g fat (48.3% calories from fat); 3 g protein; 6 g carbohydrate; 3 g dietary fiber; 3 g usable carbs.

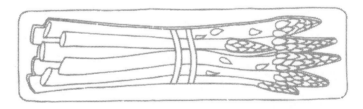

◎ Karen Sonderman's Roasted Asparagus

Our tester, Julie, says, "My seven-year-old son scarfed down almost the whole batch. I had to fight him for a sample for myself! He's never liked asparagus before, but he begged me to buy more asparagus and make this again tomorrow night! This was amazing."

> 3 pounds (1.4 kg) fresh asparagus, all about the same thickness
> 1–3 tablespoons (15–45 ml) olive oil
> Fresh ground pepper to taste
> Salt to taste

Preheat oven to 450°F (230°) degrees.

Gently bend each asparagus stalk until it snaps. Toss the part that was below the break.

Pour 1 tablespoon (15 ml) olive oil into an ovenproof dish or shallow baking pan large enough to accommodate the asparagus. Add fresh ground black pepper and salt to taste.

Place the asparagus in the olive oil and roll it in the oil and seasonings until it is well coated.

Place in preheated oven and roast until just tender—5 to 7 minutes for thin spears, 8 to 10 for medium, 10 to 12 for thick.

Remove and serve immediately.

You can easily top the asparagus with favorite sauces or melt butter until golden brown and pour over top, but it is delicious just as is! Adjust the amount of oil and seasonings for larger or smaller quantities of asparagus.

Tester's note: Julie very much recommends that along with fresh ground pepper, you use fresh ground coarse sea salt, or kosher salt, instead of regular table salt.

Yield: About 10 servings

Each with: 29 calories; 1 g fat; 2 g protein; 3 g carbohydrate; 1 g dietary fiber; 2 g usable carbs.

◎ Chili Lime Pumpkin

It's such a shame fresh pumpkin is available for only a couple of months in the autumn; it's so wonderful. This side dish is a tad high in carbs, but it's so unusual and so good I had to include it. Don't try shelling the seeds from the pumpkin you're cooking to complete the recipe—it's a tedious task! Just roast them and salt them as is, and snack on them later.

> 1 little pumpkin, about 2 pounds (1 kg)
> 2 tablespoons (30 g) butter
> 1 tablespoon (15 ml) oil
> 1/2 cup (120 g) shelled pumpkin seeds (pepitas)
> 1 teaspoon chili garlic paste
> 2 teaspoons lime juice

Whack your pumpkin in half and scoop out the seeds. Peel off the hard rind, then cut the flesh into slices about 1/4" (6.25 mm) thick.

Put the butter and the oil in your big, heavy skillet over medium heat. Swirl them together as the butter melts. Now, lay the slices of pumpkin flat in the butter/oil mixture, and sauté until lightly golden on both sides, and tender, yet still al dente. You'll need to do this in more than one batch; keep the stuff that's done warm on a plate under a pot lid.

While this is happening, toast your pepitas by stirring them in a dry skillet over medium-high heat until they swell a bit—about 4 to 5 minutes. Remove from the heat when they're done.

When the pumpkin's all cooked, put it all back in the skillet. Mix together the chili garlic paste and the lime juice, and gently mix it in, coating all of the pumpkin slices.

Lay the pumpkin slices on serving plates, top each serving with a tablespoon of toasted pumpkin seeds, and serve.

Yield: 8 servings

Each with: 89 calories; 5 g fat; 2 g protein; 10 g carbohydrate; 1 g dietary fiber; 9 g usable carbs.

Donna Barton's
Pumpkin Mousse Casserole

½ cup (120 ml) half-and-half

1 tablespoon (15 g) butter

1 29-ounce (810 g) can pumpkin

2 eggs, slightly beaten

1 cup (25 g) Splenda

½ teaspoon each salt, cinnamon, ginger, nutmeg

1 teaspoon vanilla

3 tablespoons (45 ml) exactly, Jack Daniels whiskey

Topping

½ cup (60 g) chopped pecans

⅓ cup (25 g) unsweetened coconut flakes

3 tablespoons (45 g) butter, melted

Preheat oven to 350°F (180°C).

Heat half-and-half and butter in the microwave just until warm. Combine the pumpkin with the butter and half-and-half in a large mixing bowl. Mix well. Add all remaining ingredients except toppings. (Be sure to measure the whiskey exactly. Too much will ruin it.)

Mix thoroughly. Transfer to an ungreased casserole dish.

Combine pecans and coconut flakes. Use fingertips to sprinkle all over the top. Drizzle melted butter over the topping ingredients. (Coconut flakes can be omitted, if desired.) Bake 30 to 35 minutes, or until the center is firm.

Let stand at least 15 minutes. This doesn't have to be served piping hot. It's just as good at room temp.

Yield: 8 to 10 servings

Assuming 10 servings, each will have: 167 calories; 13 g fat; 3 g protein; 9 g carbohydrate; 3 g dietary fiber; 6 g usable carbs.

◉ Dragon's Teeth

This hot stir-fried cabbage is fabulous. If you didn't think cabbage could be exciting, try this! Have the exhaust fan on or a window open when you cook this—when the chili garlic paste hits that hot oil, it may make you cough. Worth it!

> 1 head Napa cabbage
> ¼ cup (60 g) chili garlic paste
> 1 teaspoon salt
> 2 teaspoons Splenda
> 2 teaspoons toasted sesame oil
> 2 tablespoons (30 ml) soy sauce
> 2 tablespoons (30 ml) peanut or canola oil
> 2 teaspoons rice vinegar

I like to cut my head of Napa cabbage in half lengthwise, then lay it flat-side down on the cutting board and slice it about ½" (1.25 cm) thick. Cut it one more time, lengthwise, down the middle, and then do the other half head.

Mix together the chili garlic paste, salt, Splenda, toasted sesame oil, and soy sauce in a small dish, and set by the stove.

In a wok or huge skillet, over highest heat, heat the peanut or canola oil. Add the cabbage and start stir-frying. After about a minute, add the seasoning mixture, and keep stir-frying until the cabbage is just starting to wilt—you want it still crispy in most places. Sprinkle in the rice vinegar, stir once more, and serve.

Yield: 4 servings

Each with: 98 calories; 10 g fat; 1g protein; 3 g carbohydrate; trace dietary fiber; 3 g usable carbs.

◎ Roasted Cabbage with Balsamic Vinegar

This is a simple way to cook a lot of cabbage!

1/2 head red cabbage
1/2 head cabbage
3 tablespoons (45 ml) olive oil
Salt and pepper
2 tablespoons (30 ml) balsamic vinegar

Preheat oven to 450°F (230°C).

Coarsely chop the two kinds of cabbage, and separate the leaves. Put it in a good-sized roasting pan, and toss it with the olive oil until it's coated all over. Salt and pepper, and toss again.

Put cabbage in oven, and roast for 15 to 20 minutes, stirring once or twice, until it's just browning around the edges, but still not entirely limp. Sprinkle with the balsamic vinegar, toss again, and serve.

Yield: 5 to 6 servings

Assuming 5 servings, each will have: 77 calories; 8 g fat; trace protein; 1 g carbohydrate; trace dietary fiber; 1 g usable carb.

Linda Carroll-King's Red Cabbage Recipe

Even non-low-carbers will love this quick and easy cabbage dish.

> 8 ounces (225 g) shredded red cabbage
> 1–2 tablespoons (15–30 ml) extra-light olive oil
> ½ cup (60 ml) rice vinegar
> Splenda to taste

Sauté cabbage in the olive oil in your big frying pan, covered, over medium-low heat. Every few minutes, remove the lid, and stir. Cook until softened but not mushy. Stir in the rice vinegar and Splenda and cook for another 2 minutes.

Linda's note: "You can use bagged shredded cabbage for this and save a bunch of time and effort." Our tester, Julie, agrees this is a great idea.

Yield: Serves 2

Each with: 154 calories; 14 g fat; 2 g protein; 9 g carbohydrate; 2 g dietary fiber; 7 g usable carbs.

Susan Higgs's Skillet Cabbage

Our tester, Julie, calls this "Good stuff."

> 6 slices bacon
> 1 medium onion, chopped
> 3 stalks of celery, finely chopped or sliced
> 1 head green cabbage, finely chopped, sliced, or shredded
>   (my family likes it sliced)
> 2 tablespoons (30 g) butter, optional
> Salt and pepper to taste

In your big, heavy skillet, fry the 6 slices of bacon up crisp, then remove from pan to cool. Add the onions and celery to the hot bacon grease in the pan. Cook these until almost caramelized—certainly till they're a bit browned.

Add the cabbage and give it a good stir, and add the 2 tablespoons (30 g) of butter if you think you need it. Cover the pan and let the cabbage cook down until crisp-tender (or whatever doneness your family likes). Taste for seasonings and add salt and pepper to your desired taste. Crumble bacon and add back to the cabbage mixture, giving it a good stir. Serve.

Susan's notes: "Optionally, you can add apple cider vinegar or soy sauce to change the flavor of this dish depending on what you are serving it with. For example, I'll do the apple cider vinegar add-in if I'm using this as a side dish for ribs or pulled bbq pork, or the soy sauce if it's an accompaniment to an Asian main dish. Sometimes when I'm making this as a main dish, I'll include chopped green pepper with the celery and onions as well as a 15-ounce (420 g) can of diced tomatoes with their juice with the cabbage. During the winter, I occasionally also add garlic, a quart of chicken stock, and some bouillon to turn it all into a soup (including the green pepper and tomatoes). I think its versatility is what makes this an awesome recipe for folks who cook for their families."

Yield: 4 main dishes or 6 side dishes

Each of 6 servings will have: 82 calories; 7 g fat; 2 g protein; 3 g carbohydrate; 1 g dietary fiber; 2 g usable carbs.

◎ Spinach Mushroom Kugel

I came up with this for a Passover column I wrote, but it's a great side dish for anyone, any time of year!

> 8 ounces (225 g) sliced mushrooms
> 1 medium onion, chopped
> 2 tablespoons (30 ml) olive oil
> 3 10-ounce (280 g) boxes frozen chopped spinach, thawed and drained
> 2 eggs
> ¾ cup (180 g) mayonnaise
> 1 teaspoon beef bouillon concentrate
> 2 tablespoons (20 g) almond meal
> ½ teaspoon guar or xanthan

Preheat oven to 350°F (180°C).

Sauté mushrooms and onion in the oil until the onion is translucent and the mushrooms soften. Transfer to a mixing bowl, reserving 9 mushroom slices for garnish, and add spinach; mix well.

Stir together eggs, mayo, and bouillon concentrate till the concentrate dissolves. Stir into vegetables. Stir in the almond meal. Sprinkle ¼ teaspoon of the guar or xanthan over mixture and stir in well; repeat with the second ¼ teaspoon.

Spread evenly in a greased 8" x 8" (20 x 20 cm) baking dish. Decorate with reserved mushrooms. Bake for 1 hour. Cut in squares to serve.

Yield: 9 servings

Each with: 214 calories; 20 g fat; 6 g protein; 7 g carbohydrate; 3 g dietary fiber; 4 g usable carbs.

Mary Lou Theisen's
Three Cheese Spinach Bake

Our tester, Julie, loved this recipe—and so did her seven-year-old son and two-year-old daughter! She said it was easy and "tasted like a million bucks."

> 2 10-ounce (280 g) packages frozen chopped spinach
> ½ cup plus 2 tablespoons (150 g) unsalted butter, divided
> 1 medium onion, chopped
> 2 cloves garlic, minced
> 1 cup (240 ml) heavy cream
> 8 ounces (225 g) cream cheese
> ¾ cup (120 g) fresh grated Parmesan cheese
> Salt and pepper to taste
> ½ cup (60 g) thinly shredded Monterey Jack cheese
>   (you can also use mild cheddar cheese instead of Monterey Jack)

Defrost the spinach—Mary Lou does it in her microwave, but you could be truly revolutionary and just leave it out on the counter. Make sure to squeeze out all of the liquid from the defrosted spinach.

Heat 2 tablespoons of butter in a medium-sized pan. Sauté the onion in the butter until tender. Add the drained spinach and minced garlic. Heat everything together for 5 to 10 minutes. Transfer the mixture to a casserole dish you've sprayed with nonstick cooking spray. Preheat the oven to 350°F (180°C) degrees.

In the same pan you used to sauté the onion and spinach, heat the heavy cream, cream cheese, and ½ cup (120 g) unsalted butter until all the cream cheese has melted. Add the fresh grated Parmesan cheese and stir until you have a wonderful sauce (if it gets too thick, add a little more heavy cream). Pour the Parmesan cheese mixture over the spinach; add salt and pepper to taste. Stir until the spinach and Parmesan mixture have completely blended. Sprinkle the shredded Monterey Jack cheese over the top and bake in a preheated 350°F (180°C) oven for 10 to 15 minutes until the top cheese layer is melted and bubbly. Pull out of oven and let sit for 5 minutes before serving. Delicious!

Tester's note: Julie says it's nice to sprinkle a little more grated Parmesan on top of this, and add a sprinkle of paprika. Just for presentation, don't you know?

Yield: Makes 8 servings

Each with: 413 calories; 40 g fat (84.7% calories from fat); 10 g protein; 6 g carbohydrate; 2 g dietary fiber; 4 g usable carbs.

◎ Stephanie H.'s Mushroom-Spinach Casserole

Our tester, Ray, says this is perfect if you need a hot vegetable dish to bring to a potluck or pitch-in. And Barbo, who also tested this, rated it a 10.

2–4 tablespoons (30–60 g) butter
¾–1 pound (340–455 g) fresh mushrooms, sliced
¼ cup (40 g) chopped onion
½ cup (30 g) mixed herbs of your choice (Stephanie used parsley)
1 10-ounce (280 g) package frozen chopped spinach, thawed and well-drained
1 cup (120 g) grated or finely chopped cheese (Stephanie used Swiss)
⅓ cup (80 ml) heavy cream
1 large egg
1 egg yolk
Parmesan cheese for topping (optional)

Preheat oven to 325°F (170°C).

In a skillet, melt a tablespoon (15 g) or so of butter over medium to medium-high heat, and sauté the sliced mushrooms. As you cook the mushrooms, they will begin to release their liquid. Keep cooking them until all the liquid evaporates. This is key to keeping the resulting casserole from having too much liquid. Set the cooked mushrooms aside in a mixing bowl.

In the same skillet, use another tablespoon (15 g) of butter to sauté the onion until soft. Then add the herbs and cook for a moment to release their aromas. Add this mixture to the mushrooms.

Add the spinach to the mushroom mixture and mix well. When this has cooled a bit, add the cheese (you just don't want the cheese melting from the heat of the veggies that have just been cooked). When everything has been combined, place it in a casserole dish you've sprayed with nonstick spray.

In a separate dish, whisk together the cream, egg, and egg yolk, then pour this mixture over the veggies. Top with a sprinkle of Parmesan.

Bake until the cheese is melted and bubbly, about 30 minutes, depending on your oven.

Stephanie's note: "Here are some other embellishment ideas to mix and match: garlic, ricotta cheese, sun-dried tomatoes, chopped walnuts, cooked and diced meats or seafood (chicken, ham, pepperoni, shrimp, crab, etc.). You could easily change the herbs and give it an Italian or Greek flavor."

Yield: 4 to 5 servings

Assuming 5 servings, each will have: 244 calories; 19 g fat; 12 g protein; 8 g carbohydrate; 3 g dietary fiber; 5 g usable carbs.

◉ Marilyn Olshansky's Creamed Spinach

Our tester, Julie, calls this recipe "easy and yummy!"

> 3 10-ounce (280 g) packages frozen chopped spinach
> ½ stick butter
> 2–3 cloves garlic, minced
> 1 packet Splenda or 2 teaspoons Splenda granular, or to taste
> Heavy cream

Cook the spinach, preferably in the microwave, according to package directions. Drain thoroughly, squeezing out as much water as possible.

Melt the butter in a large sauté pan and sauté the garlic until golden. Add the spinach and Splenda and stir to blend. Sauté to heat through.

Add heavy cream gradually to bring the mixture to the desired consistency.

Dana's Note: I put my spinach in a strainer, and press it hard with the back of a spoon. It's amazing how much water spinach can hold!

Marilyn's Note: " I don't really know how much heavy cream I use—I just add it until it looks right." Julie concurred—and suggested you could add more or less, depending on whether you wanted to serve this as a side dish or, her idea, a dip!

Yield: 6 servings

Analyzing for 2 cups cream, each serving will have: 377 calories; 37 g fat; 6 g protein; 8 g carbohydrate; 4 g dietary fiber; 4 g usable carbs.

◎ Grace Brown's
Spinach and Artichoke Casserole

Here's a vegetable casserole that's easy enough for the family, but elegant enough for company. Our tester, Diana, says her husband loved this!

2 10-ounce (280 g) packages frozen chopped spinach, thawed
    and squeezed dry
13 1/3-ounce (385 g) can artichoke hearts, drained and chopped
1/2 cup (120 ml) heavy cream
1/8 teaspoon salt
1/8 teaspoon pepper
2/3 cup (100 g) Parmesan cheese (reserve 1/3 cup [50 g])
1 8-ounce (225 g) package cream cheese
1 cup (240 ml) whole milk

Preheat oven to 350°F (180°C).

Combine spinach, artichokes, cream, salt, pepper, and 1/3 cup (50 g) of the Parmesan cheese. Put spinach mixture in a 1 1/2 quart (1.4 L) baking dish or 8" x 8" (20 x 20 cm) pan you've sprayed with nonstick cooking spray.

In a small bowl, beat the cream cheese till fluffy, add milk, and beat again to blend. Pour cream cheese mixture over spinach. Sprinkle remaining 1/3 cup (50 g) Parmesan cheese over the top.

Bake for 25 to 30 minutes.

Yield: Serves 8 to 10

Assuming 10 servings, each will have: 188 calories; 15 g fat; 8 g protein; 7 g carbohydrate; 2 g dietary fiber; 5 g usable carbs.

Artichokes with Curried Mock Hollandaise

4 large globe artichokes
1 batch Curried Mock Hollandaise (page 447)

Start water heating in a big darned pot over high heat. (Cover it; it'll boil faster!) While it's heating, trim the stems off of your artichokes, and trim any really ugly leaves.

When the water is hot, throw in your artichokes. I find mine want to float; I hold each one under water till it stops bubbling (i.e., all the air has escaped from between the leaves), then cover the pot to keep them in submission. Let them boil for 30 to 45 minutes.

While that's happening, you'll have plenty of time to make Curried Mock Hollandaise.

Okay, time's up. Carefully fish out your artichokes, letting the water drip back into the kettle. (Do be careful; I burnt myself a little doing this!) Put one on each of four plates. Divide the Curried Mock Hollandaise between four small dishes, and put one dish on each plate as well.

To eat, pull each leaf off the artichoke, and dip the bottom in the Curried Mock Hollandaise. Drag it between your teeth, scraping off the tender, edible bit. Discard the rest of each leaf (you'll want to give everybody a good-sized bowl to discard leaves in!).

When you get through all the leaves, you'll find a fuzzy bit—this is the choke. Scrape it out with the tip of a spoon—this is easy to do. Now use a knife and fork to cut up the yummy artichoke heart that's left, dip it in the sauce, and eat it!

Yield: 4 servings

Each with: 248 calories; 17 g fat; 9 g protein; 17 g carbohydrate; 7 g dietary fiber; 10 g usable carbs. Since much of the carbohydrate in artichokes is in the form of inulin, which has a very low glycemic index, the blood-sugar impact of this dish is less than the carb count would lead you to believe.

Artichokes with Chipotle Mayonnaise

4 large globe artichokes
1 double batch Chipotle Mayonnaise (page 446)

Start water heating in a big darned pot over high heat. (Cover it; it'll boil faster!) While it's heating, trim the stems off of your artichokes, and trim any really ugly leaves.

When the water is hot, throw in your artichokes. I find mine want to float; I hold each one under water till it stops bubbling (i.e., all the air has escaped from between the leaves), then cover the pot to keep them in submission. Let them boil for 30 to 45 minutes.

Okay, time's up. Carefully fish out your artichokes, letting the water drip back into the kettle. (Do be careful; I burnt myself a little doing this!) Put one on each of four plates. Divide the Chipotle Mayonnaise between four small dishes, and put one dish on each plate as well.

To eat, pull each leaf off the artichoke, and dip the bottom in the Chipotle Mayonnaise. Drag it between your teeth, scraping off the tender, edible bit. Discard the rest of each leaf (you'll want to give everybody a good-sized bowl to discard leaves in!).

When you get through all the leaves, you'll find a fuzzy bit—this is the choke. Scrape it out with the tip of a spoon—this is easy to do. Now use a knife and fork to cut up the yummy artichoke heart that's left, dip it in the Chipotle Mayonnaise, and eat it!

Yield: 4 servings

Each with 455 calories; 47 g fat ; 5 g protein; 14 g carbohydrate; 7 g dietary fiber; 7 g usable carbs. Since much of the carbohydrate in artichokes is in the form of inulin, which has a very low glycemic index, the blood-sugar impact of this dish is less than the carb count would lead you to believe.

◎ Susan Higgs's
Brussels Sprouts in Browned Butter

For years, I thought I didn't like brussels sprouts—and then I learned I just didn't like them boiled and plain. Thinly slicing them changes them into a whole new vegetable!

1 pound (455 g) fresh brussels sprouts, cleaned and trimmed
8 tablespoons (112 g) butter
Zest of ½ lemon
Juice of 1 lemon
Salt and pepper

First, either slice your brussels sprouts on a mandoline cutter (this is what Susan does) or run them through the slicing blade of your food processor.

Melt your butter in a big, heavy skillet and let it brown. Add thinly sliced brussels sprouts, lemon zest, and lemon juice and sauté until crisp-tender. Taste for seasonings, adding salt and pepper as desired. Serve.

Yield: Feeds 4 to 6 as a side dish

Assuming 6 servings, each will have: 167 calories; 16 g fat; 2 g protein; 7 g carbohydrate; 3 g dietary fiber; 4 g usable carbs.

Jennie's Bodacious Brussels Sprouts

Since this was sent by Karen Sonderman, I'm left wondering who Jennie is. Our tester, Diana, liked this—and she's not even a brussels sprout fan!

8 cloves garlic, chopped

2 ½ tablespoons (40 g) butter

2 ½ tablespoons (40 ml) olive oil

3 pounds (1.4 kg) brussels sprouts

1 cup (240 ml) chicken broth

Remove outer leaves and any remaining stem of brussels sprouts. Cut an X in the bottom of each sprout.

In your large skillet, sauté the chopped garlic in butter and olive oil until just turning brown. Add the brussels sprouts and stir to coat with the mixture. Now pour the chicken broth over the sprouts, and simmer 15 minutes or until sprouts are tender but not mushy. Remove the lid during the last 5 minutes of cooking time to reduce any remaining broth.

Yield: 10 servings

Each with: 115 calories; 7 g fat; 5 g protein; 12 g carbohydrate; 5 g dietary fiber; 7 g usable carbs.

Orange Mustard Glazed Sprouts

Wonderful!

> 1 pound (455 g) brussels sprouts, halved
> 3 tablespoons (45 g) butter
> 2 tablespoons (30 ml) lemon juice
> 1 1/2 teaspoons brown mustard
> 1 tablespoon (1.5 g) Splenda
> 1/2 teaspoon soy sauce
> 1/4 teaspoon orange extract

Trim the stems of your brussels sprouts, and remove any bruised leaves, then slice each one in half.

Melt the butter in your large, heavy skillet, over medium heat. Add brussels sprouts, and sauté till they're just starting to get tender and develop a few brown spots.

While the sprouts are sautéing, mix together everything else. When the sprouts are getting done, pour the mustard mixture into the skillet, and stir to coat. Cook for another 2 to 3 minutes, and serve.

Yield: 3 to 4 servings

Assuming 3 servings, each will have: 166 calories; 12 g fat; 5 g protein; 13 g carbohydrate; 5 g dietary fiber; 8 g usable carbs.

Anne Logston's Mock Fried Apples

Here's a really unique side dish. I think this would be great with pork chops or a pork roast! Our tester, Julie, said this doesn't taste exactly like apples, but it's awfully good, and her whole family liked it, so don't be nervous about that unfamiliar chayote. (She also said she found chayote at the first grocery store she tried!)

2 chayote fruits

⅓ cup (80 ml) apple cider vinegar

3–5 packets Splenda or 2–10 teaspoons granular Splenda, to taste

½ teaspoon cinnamon

1 teaspoon salt

½ stick butter

Guar or xanthan (optional)

Wash chayote thoroughly. Quarter lengthwise, removing seeds. Cut quarters crosswise into thin slices. Place slices in a bowl or zipper-lock bag. Wash your hands!

In a small bowl, combine vinegar, Splenda, cinnamon, and salt. Add to chayote slices and toss or shake to coat thoroughly. Let marinate at least 1 hour.

Melt butter in a hot skillet. When butter is sizzling, add chayote and any juice and cook until chayote is hot but still crunchy—cook until more tender if desired. (Our tester liked this cooked about 8 minutes.) If desired, thicken pan juices with your guar or xanthan shaker to create a thick, yummy glaze.

Note: When cutting up chayote, either wear plastic gloves or wash your hands with hot soapy water *immediately* afterward. The chayote juice contains a sort of starch that will form an annoying tight film on your fingertips that lasts and lasts, and once it dries it's horribly hard to scrub off.

Yield: 3 servings

Each with: 167 calories; 16 g fat; 1 g protein; 7 g carbohydrate; 3 g dietary fiber; 4 g usable carbs.

◎ Ruth Lambert's Avocado Mousse

I think this would be a great starter for any Mexican or Southwestern menu.

> 3 ripe avocados
> 6 ounces (170 g) light cream cheese (same carbs as full fat)
> 2 tablespoons (30 ml) half-and-half or cream
> Garlic salt to taste
> Medium salsa

Whip avocado pulp and cream cheese plus half-and-half with garlic salt in blender for about 2 minutes until foamy and a gorgeous light green. Serve in voluptuous scoops in little ramekins, with a bed of salsa, for a truly stunning first course that will have everyone raving.

Yield: Serves 6 generously

Each with: 280 calories; 26 g fat; 5 g protein; 11 g carbohydrate; 3 g dietary fiber; 8 g usable carbs.

Susan Higgs's Spicy Zucchini and Tomato Sauté

2 or 3 zucchinis, julienne-cut

2 tablespoons (30 g) butter

2 tomatoes, chopped

Salt and pepper to taste

1 jalapeno pepper, seeded, finely diced

⅓ cup (40 g) shredded cheese
    (cheddar or Monterey Jack is great; Parmesan is pretty good, too)

Line colander with paper towels and let julienned zucchini sit for 20 to 30 minutes to drain. Squeeze zucchini dry. Melt butter in a big darned skillet and sauté zucchini until soft but not browned. Add tomatoes, salt, pepper, and jalapeno, sautéing until heated through.

Remove from heat and add shredded cheese—scatter half over the top, stir to mix, then scatter the other half over the top, and stir again.

Tester's note: Our tester, Ray, said this overwhelmed his skillet, so consider halving this recipe unless you've got a family to feed.

Yield: Serves 4

Each with: 85 calories; 6 g fat; 2 g protein; 7 g carbohydrate; 3 g dietary fiber; 4 g usable carbs.

Leslie's Mock Kishke

When I saw this recipe, I had to look up exactly what a kishke is! Originally, kishke, a traditional Jewish dish, was made from poultry intestines, stuffed with seasoned matzoh meal. However, most of the recipes I found for kishke involved only the seasoned matzoh meal, and not the intestines—the mixture is simply formed into cylinders on its own. Leslie says this low-carb version doesn't hold together perfectly, and is more like a pilaf—great cold the next day.

> 1 onion
> 2 stalks celery
> 2 carrots
> 8 ounces (225 g) almond meal
> 4 ounces (115 g) butter, softened
> ¼ teaspoon pepper
> Salt to taste
> 1 egg

Preheat oven to 350°F (180°C).

Grind the veggies, or chop fine in your food processor, and transfer to a mixing bowl. Add everything else, and mix it all together well.

Form into two long cylinders on foil sheets. Wrap completely in the foil. Put on baking pan (jelly roll–size is good). Bake about 40 minutes.

Tester's note: Our tester, Ray, added an extra egg and found the mixture held together better. So use one egg, or two, depending on what texture you'd like.

Yield: Serves 12

Each with: 183 calories; 17 g fat; 6 g protein; 6 g carbohydrate; 2 g dietary fiber; 4 g usable carbs.

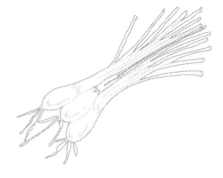

◎ Cathy Sparks's Creamed Onions

Never had creamed onions? They were a fixture at every holiday meal of my childhood. Remember that onions are a borderline vegetable, and judge your portions accordingly.

> 1 pound (455 g) bag frozen pearl onions, thawed
> 2 tablespoons (30 g) butter
> ½ cup (120 ml) chicken broth
> ½ cup (120 ml) dry white wine
> 1 cup (240 ml) heavy cream
> 1 pinch each of sea salt, white pepper, and nutmeg
> 1 teaspoon minced parsley or chives

In a large covered skillet, simmer the onions in the butter, broth, and wine about 20 minutes, until tender. Add the cream and gently simmer, uncovered, until thickened to suit. This may take 20 minutes or more for a thicker consistency. Stir in salt, pepper, and nutmeg. Place in serving dish and sprinkle with parsley or chives.

Yield: 6 servings

Each with: 209 calories; 19 g fat; 2 g protein; 6 g carbohydrate; 1 g dietary fiber; 5 g usable carbs.

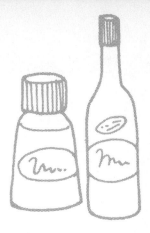

chapter six

Side Salads and Dressings

Salad, salad, beautiful salad! What a fine and glorious thing is a salad, from a simple bowl of bagged greens tossed with bottled dressing; to a gourmet offering with an exotic mix of greens, fruits, and nuts; to a bowl of down-home slaw. Especially with a simple meal of roasted, broiled, or grilled meat, fish, or poultry, an interesting salad is what will make the meal!

I've put all the dressings at the end of this chapter, just to make them easy to reference.

Vietnamese Salad

Let's start with a really exotic tossed salad from Southeast Asia!

> 1 quart (.95 L) romaine lettuce, broken up
> 1 quart (.95 L) torn butter lettuce
> 3 scallions, sliced, including the crisp part of the green shoot
> 1 ruby red grapefruit
> 1 tablespoon (1.5 g) Splenda
> 3 tablespoons (45 ml) fish sauce (nuoc mam or nam pla)
> 3 tablespoons (45 ml) lime juice
> 1 ½ teaspoons chili garlic paste
> 2 tablespoons (15 g) chopped peanuts
> ½ cup (30 g) chopped cilantro
> ½ cup (30 g) chopped fresh mint

Wash and dry your lettuce, combine it, then divide it onto 4 salad plates.

Slice your scallions, and scatter over the lettuce.

Halve your grapefruit, and using a sharp, thin-bladed knife, cut around each section to loosen. Divide the grapefruit sections between the salads.

Mix together the Splenda, fish sauce, lime juice, and chili paste. Drizzle equal amounts of the dressing over each salad; then top each portion with chopped peanuts, cilantro, and mint, and serve.

Yield: 4 servings

Each with: 101 calories; 4 g fat; 4 g protein; 14 g carbohydrate; 4 g dietary fiber; 10 g usable carbs.

Spinach-Strawberry Salad

Simply extraordinary! For my money, this is the best salad in this book. If you don't try a single other salad recipe, try this one! It's beautiful, too, and very nutritious.

> 1 pound (455 g) bagged, prewashed baby spinach
> 1 batch Sweet Poppy Seed Vinaigrette (page 214)
> 1 cup (170 g) sliced strawberries
> 3 tablespoons (25 g) slivered almonds, toasted
> ½ cup (60 g) crumbled feta cheese

Put baby spinach in your big salad bowl. Pour on the dressing, and toss well. Top with strawberries, almonds, and feta, and serve.

Yield: 4 servings

Each with: 227 calories; 19 g fat; 8 g protein; 11 g carbohydrate; 5 g dietary fiber; 6 g usable carbs.

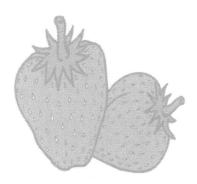

Karen Sonderman's Strawberry Romaine Salad

Dressing:
- 1 cup (240 ml) olive or canola oil
- ½ cup (12 g) Splenda
- ½ cup (100 g) polyol sweetener
- ½ cup (120 ml) red wine vinegar
- 2 cloves garlic, crushed
- ½ teaspoon salt
- ½ teaspoon paprika
- ¼ teaspoon white pepper

Mix in large shaker or lidded jar and refrigerate, shaking occasionally.

To prepare salad:

In large bowl mix:
- 2–3 packages of packaged prepared romaine, baby romaine, or romaine/radicchio greens (called Italian Blend) or wash, dry, and tear into bite-sized pieces 2–3 heads of fresh romaine

Add:
- 1 pint (340 g) strawberries, cleaned and halved
- 1 cup (120 g) shredded Monterey Jack cheese
- ½ cup (60 g) chopped walnuts, toasted

Shake dressing, pour over mixture, and toss well.

Karen's notes: "I usually start with 2 packages of lettuce and add all or part of the third package after the dressing has been added. I have used both canola oil and olive oil when preparing the dressing. Olive oil makes a lighter blend but does solidify when refrigerated and needs to be brought to room temperature to shake and before serving."

Yield: Makes 10 to 12 side salads, or 8 larger portions

With 8 servings, each will have: 398 calories; 37 g fat; 10 g protein; 12 g carbohydrate; 6 g dietary fiber; 6 g usable carbs.

Orange, Avocado, and Bacon Salad

8 cups (160 g) mixed greens
Citrus Dressing (page 209)
1/2 navel orange
1/2 California avocado
6 slices bacon, cooked and drained
1/8 red onion

Put your greens in a big mixing bowl, and pour the dressing over them. Toss well.

Peel your half-orange, and separate the sections; halve each one again. Slice the avocado, crumble the bacon, and slice the red onion paper-thin. Now strew everything artfully over the greens, and serve.

Yield: 4 servings

Each with: 189 calories; 15 g fat; 6 g protein; 9 g carbohydrate; 5 g dietary fiber; 4 g usable carbs.

Avocado-Walnut Salad

1/4 cup (30 g) chopped walnuts
2 quarts (1.9 L) romaine lettuce, broken up
Cumin Vinaigrette (page 213)
1/2 California avocado, cut in 1/2" (1.25 cm) cubes
1 stalk celery, diced
1/3 medium cucumber, diced
1/4 small red onion, sliced paper-thin

Toast your walnuts—you can simply stir them in a hot skillet, or toast them in a 300°F (150°C) oven while you're assembling the rest of the salad.

Toss the lettuce with the Cumin Vinaigrette. Top with everything else, and serve.

Yield: About 4 to 5 servings

Assuming 5 servings, each will have: 351 calories; 36 g fat; 4 g protein; 8 g carbohydrate; 3 g dietary fiber; 5 g usable carbs.

Asparagus with Chipotle Mayonnaise

This is a total rip-off of a chilled asparagus dish I was served in an extremely pricey and elegant restaurant. And it's dead simple.

> 1 pound (455 g) asparagus
> 1 batch Chipotle Mayonnaise (page 446)

Break the ends off of your asparagus where they want to break naturally. Then cook them just barely tender-crisp—I put mine in a microwaveable casserole with a lid, add a couple of tablespoons of water, and nuke 'em on high for just 3 to 4 minutes. Drain the asparagus and chill it till dinner time.

Arrange your asparagus on 4 salad plates. Now, you can add a 2-tablespoon (30 g) dollop of Chipotle Mayonnaise to each plate for dipping. Or, if you want to be truly spiffy and restaurant-like, put your mayonnaise in a squeeze bottle, and squeeze decorative random zigzag patterns over the asparagus. If you don't have a squeeze bottle, you can put the mayo in a small plastic bag and snip a tiny piece off the corner, instead.

Yield: 4 servings

Each with: 211 calories; 23 g fat; 2 g protein; 3 g carbohydrate; 1 g dietary fiber; 2 g usable carbs.

Napa Mint Slaw

Napa's distinctive texture and mild flavor are quite different from the familiar green cabbage, and mint sets this recipe apart even more! As a result, this slaw appeals even to people who aren't big fans of standard cole slaw. If you decide you like fresh mint in cooking, consider growing some. It's a snap to grow—indeed, it's so invasive, that once you plant it, you may have trouble growing anything else!

> 1 1/2 pounds (680 g) Napa cabbage
> 1/2 cup (30 g) chopped fresh mint
> 3 scallions, sliced
> Orange Bacon Dressing (page 207)
> 1/3 cup (40 g) chopped peanuts
> 5 slices bacon, cooked and drained

An average-sized head of Napa should be about 1 1/2 pounds (680 g). Remove any bruised or wilted leaves, then lay the whole head on your cutting board and cut across it at 1/4" (6.25 mm) intervals, all the way down to the bottom. Scoop your shredded Napa into a big bowl.

Add the chopped mint and sliced scallions to the cabbage.

Toss the salad with the dressing, then add your peanuts and bacon to the slaw, toss again, and serve.

Yield: 5 servings

Each with: 172 calories; 16 g fat; 5 g protein; 4 g carbohydrate; 2 g dietary fiber; 2 g usable carbs.

Cannery Row UnPotato Salad

To get 1 ½ pounds (680 g) of cauliflower, you'll need a big head or 1 ½ smaller ones. There's a scale in most produce departments.

1 ½ pounds (680 g) cauliflower
¼ cup (60 ml) olive oil
2 cloves garlic, crushed
2 tablespoons (30 g) Simple No-Sugar Pickle Relish (page 441)
¼ cup (60 g) mayonnaise
¼ cup (30 g) sliced celery
¼ cup (25 g) sliced green onions
¼ cup (25 g) sliced black olives, drained
Salt and pepper
1 ounce (30 g) pimiento
¼ cup (15 g) chopped fresh parsley

Chop your cauliflower into ½" (1.25 cm) chunks. Put it in a microwaveable casserole with a lid, add a couple of tablespoons of water, cover, and nuke it on high for 8 minutes, or until tender but not mushy. Stir together your olive oil, garlic, pickle relish, and mayonnaise. When the cauliflower is done, drain it, and put it in a big mixing bowl. Pour on the dressing, toss to coat, and let it sit until it's cooled.

When the cauliflower reaches something approaching room temperature, throw in the celery and the green onions, along with the olives. Toss, salt and pepper to taste, and toss again. You can serve this right away, or let it chill for several hours. When serving time comes, garnish with the pimento and parsley.

Yield: 5 to 6 servings

Assuming 5 servings, each will have: 224 calories; 21 g fat; 3 g protein; 9 g carbohydrate; 4 g dietary fiber; 5 g usable carbs.

Cauliflower Avocado Salad

4 cups (600 g) cauliflower
1 California avocado, peeled and diced
½ green bell pepper, diced
8 kalamata olives, pitted and chopped
4 scallions, thinly sliced, including the crisp part of the green shoot
Sun-Dried Tomato–Basil Vinaigrette (page 214)

Cut your cauliflower in roughly ½" (1.25 cm) chunks. Put it in a microwaveable bowl, add a tablespoon of water, and cover. Microwave on high for 7 minutes.

When the cauliflower is ready, drain it and dump it in a mixing bowl. Add everything else, including the Sun-Dried Tomato–Basil Vinaigrette, and toss. Serve warm, on a bed of lettuce if you like.

Yield: 6 servings

Each with: 262 calories; 25 g fat; 3 g protein; 11 g carbohydrate; 4 g dietary fiber; 7 g usable carbs.

◎ Ensalada de "Arroz"

½ head cauliflower, shredded
6 scallions, sliced, including the green
½ yellow pepper, diced
½ green pepper, diced
½ ripe tomato, diced
¼ cup (15 g) chopped fresh cilantro
¼ cup (60 ml) extra-virgin olive oil
1 tablespoon (15 ml) red wine vinegar
1 tablespoon (15 ml) balsamic vinegar
1 ½ teaspoons Dijon mustard
Salt and pepper

Put the cauliflower in a microwaveable casserole with a lid, add a couple of tablespoons of water, cover, and microwave on high for 6 minutes.

When the microwave beeps, uncover the cauliflower immediately, to stop the cooking. Drain it well, and dump it into a large mixing bowl. Let it cool for 5 to 10 minutes (stir it once or twice during this time).

Stir the chopped vegetables into your "rice." Now, mix together everything else, pour over the salad, and toss well. Chill before serving.

Yield: 5 serving

Each with: 115 calories; 11 g fat; 1 g protein; 4 g carbohydrate; 1 g dietary fiber; 3 g usable carbs.

Irene Haldeman's Czech UnPotato Salad

1 head cauliflower, boiled for 5 minutes, drained, and chopped in
$\frac{1}{2}$" (1.25 cm) pieces

$\frac{1}{2}$–$\frac{3}{4}$ cup (50–75 g) diced kosher dill pickles

1 onion, chopped (optional)

2 carrots, chopped (optional)

3 celery stalks, diced

8 hard-boiled eggs, chopped (more or less if you wish)

1–2 cups (125–250 g) hard cheese such as Jarlsberg or Swiss, cubed

1–2 teaspoons celery seed

$\frac{1}{2}$ cup (120 g) mayonnaise, or more to taste

3–4 (45–60 g) tablespoons yellow mustard, or more to taste

Salt and pepper to taste

Simply combine the vegetables, eggs, and cheese in a big mixing bowl. In a separate bowl, mix together the celery seed, mayonnaise, mustard, and salt and pepper. Pour over the vegetables, and toss.

Irene's note: "I have omitted the onion or carrots to keep the carb count to a minimum and it was great."

Yield: This makes a veritable metric boatload of unpotato salad—our testers estimate it would serve as many as 12, but say that halving the recipe works beautifully.

With 12 servings, each will have: 208 calories; 17 g fat; 10 g protein; 5 g carbohydrate; 1 g dietary fiber; 4 g usable carbs.

Pat Resler's Cauliflower and Cheese Salad

1 head cauliflower
1/4 cup (60 g) mayonnaise
8 ounces (225 g) cream cheese
16 ounces (455 g) sour cream
1/2 teaspoon salt, or to taste
1/2 teaspoon pepper, or to taste
1/2 teaspoon garlic powder, or to taste
2 cups (240 g) shredded cheddar cheese
1/2 cup (80 g) onion

Cut cauliflower into bite-sized florets. Rinse and drain.

In a medium mixing bowl, use your electric mixer to beat the mayonnaise and cream cheese until smooth. Add sour cream, salt, pepper, and garlic powder and mix.

In large bowl, combine the cauliflower, shredded cheddar, and onion. Fold dressing mixture into cauliflower. Serve.

Yield: About 6 to 8 servings

Assuming 8 servings, each will have: 391 calories; 37 g fat; 11 g protein; 5 g carbohydrate; 1 g dietary fiber; 4 g usable carbs.

◎ Susan Higgs's Cauliflower Mexican Salad

A great match with any Mexican main course.

Salad:
- 1 head cauliflower, thinly sliced
- 1 medium can of diced black olives, drained
- 1 medium can of diced mild green chilies, drained
- 1 medium jar of diced pimento, drained
- 1 small onion, finely chopped

Dressing:
- 4 tablespoons (60 ml) lemon juice
- 4 tablespoons (60 ml) red wine vinegar
- 2 teaspoons salt
- 1 teaspoon Splenda (or favorite sugar substitute)
- ½ cup (120 ml) canola oil

Place your veggies in a large bowl.

Make the dressing in your blender. Put in everything but the oil, turn on the blender, and add the oil slowly in a very thin stream, so that the dressing binds together and thickens a bit. Pour the dressing over the veggies and mix well. Taste for seasonings, modifying as you wish. Cover and chill for 3 or more hours.

Yield: 8 servings

Each with: 148 calories; 15 g fat; 1 g protein; 5 g carbohydrate; 1 g dietary fiber; 4 g usable carbs.

◎ Wendy Kaess's Cauliflower Salad

Our tester, Ray, called this "simple but good."
- 1 head cauliflower
- 2–3 scallions
- ½ cup (120 g) mayonnaise (or enough to make moist)
- Salt and pepper to taste

Chop cauliflower coarsely. Slice up scallions. Add the mayonnaise, mix well, then salt and pepper to taste. Store in a covered container—the raw cauliflower tends to brown when left out.

Yield: 5 to 6 servings

Assuming 5, each will have: 166 calories; 19 g fat; 1 g protein; 2 g carbohydrate; 1 g dietary fiber; about 1 g usable carb.

◉ Susan Higgs's Broccoli and Cauliflower Salad

Our tester, Julie, loved this salad and said that while it's a little bit of work to put together, the results are quite special.

Salad:
  1 bunch fresh broccoli
  1 head cauliflower
  1 4-ounce (115 g) can sliced mushrooms, drained
  3 stalks celery, finely chopped
  1 medium red onion, finely chopped or thinly sliced
  1 cucumber, peeled and thinly sliced
  1 lemon, juice and zest
  1/2 cup (120 ml) extra-virgin olive oil
  1/4 cup (60 ml) apple cider vinegar
  Salt and pepper to taste

Wash broccoli and trim off leaves. Remove stalks and cut florets into bite-sized pieces; place in a large bowl. Repeat process with cauliflower.

Add remaining vegetables to the bowl. Squeeze the juice of the lemon over the veggies, then add zest. Gently toss veggies. Add olive oil and vinegar, tossing while doing so. Taste the veggies and add salt and pepper to taste. Dressing should be light and should not have veggies swimming in it. Marinate 2 hours or more.

Yield: Serves 8 to 10 as a side dish

Assuming 8, each will have: 147 calories; 14 g fat; 2 g protein; 6 g carbohydrate; 2 g dietary fiber; 4 g usable carbs.

Eleanor Monfett's Cheddar Broccoli Salad

Our tester, Julie, says, "This was easy as pie, and very good! This would make a great summer salad for a picnic or something. Everyone liked this."

6 cups (1.05 kg) fresh broccoli florets
6 ounces (170 g) shredded cheddar
⅓ cup (55 g) chopped onion
1 ½ cups (360 g) mayonnaise
½–¾ cup (12–18 g) Splenda
3 tablespoons (45 ml) red wine vinegar or cider vinegar
12 bacon strips, cooked and crumbled

In a large bowl, combine the broccoli, cheese, and onion. Combine the mayonnaise, Splenda, and vinegar; pour over broccoli mixture and toss to coat. Refrigerate for at least 4 hours. Just before serving, stir in the bacon.

Eleanor's note: "Try using half cauliflower and half broccoli."

Yield: 8 servings

Each with: 455 calories; 47 g fat; 10 g protein; 4 g carbohydrate; 2 g dietary fiber; 2 g usable carbs.

Sharon Marlow's Broccoli Cashew Salad

Here's a broccoli salad with the extra crunch of cashews. I wouldn't suggest making this ahead—the cashews will get soggy.

2 tablespoons (30 ml) cider vinegar
¼ cup (6 g) Splenda
1 cup (240 g) mayo
1 large bunch (or 2 small) broccoli
2 cups (300 g) red seedless grapes
½ purple onion, chopped
1 pound (455 g) bacon, cooked (crisp) and chopped
1 cup (150 g) roasted, salted cashews

Prepare dressing by placing vinegar in a microwaveable bowl. Add the Splenda and whisk to dissolve. If needed, heat in microwave for a few seconds at a time till all Splenda is melted. Whisk in the mayo, and set aside.

Chop the broccoli into pieces about the size of a grape or smaller. Cut the grapes in half and add to broccoli. Add the onion, and crumble in the bacon. Toss the salad, add the dressing, and toss again. Finally, add the cashews, toss one last time, and serve.

Yield: 8 servings

Each with: 667 calories; 59 g fat; 23 g protein; 17 g carbohydrate; 4 g dietary fiber; 13 g usable carbs.

◉ Broccoli Sunshine Salad Low-Carb

Here's a recipe from a reader identified only as "d56alpine." Which is a shame, because our tester, Ray, says it's darned good—but then, he's inordinately fond of broccoli and bacon. If you are, too, give this a shot!

½ cup (240 g) mayonnaise
2 tablespoons (30 ml)
red wine vinegar
2 packets Splenda or 4 teaspoons Splenda granular
1 pound (455 g) broccoli florets, chopped
1 cup (120 g) shredded cheddar cheese
5 slices bacon, cooked and crumbled
3 tablespoons (30 g) red onion, or any sweet onion, chopped fine

Mix mayo, vinegar, and Splenda. Put everything else in a good-sized mixing bowl. Pour on the dressing, and toss well. Chill for about an hour before serving.

d56alpine's note: "My family will eat leftovers the next day, but I wouldn't recommend making it ahead of time as the broccoli gets kind of soft. Some people add raisins and walnuts to this recipe."

Yield: 6 servings

Each with: 264 calories; 25 g fat; 9 g protein; 5 g carbohydrate; 2 g dietary fiber; 3 g usable carbs.

Sesame-Almond Napa Slaw

I'm a big pig. I liked this so much, I ate the whole danged batch right out of the mixing bowl! I suppose there are worse things I could binge on.

> ½ big head Napa cabbage—if they've got only smallish heads
>   at the grocer, use the whole thing!
> 2 scallions
> 1 tablespoon (8 g) sesame seeds
> ¼ cup (30 g) slivered almonds
> 1 teaspoon butter
> ½ teaspoon chicken bouillon granules
> 2 tablespoons (30 ml) canola oil
> 2 tablespoons (30 ml) rice vinegar
> 1 ½ teaspoons soy sauce
> 1 ½ teaspoons sesame oil
> 1 tablespoon (1.5 g) Splenda

Shred your Napa cabbage fine, and slice your scallions; put them in a big mixing bowl.

In a medium skillet, over low heat, sauté the sesame seeds and almonds in the butter until the almonds are golden. Add to the cabbage.

Stir together everything else until the bouillon is dissolved, pour over slaw, and toss. You can eat this right away, but an hour's chilling is a fine idea. Toss again right before serving.

Yield: 5 servings, unless you're a cookbook author who waits to make dinner until 9 p.m., when she's starving.

Each with: 125 calories; 12 g fat; 2 g protein; 3 g carbohydrate; 1 g dietary fiber; 2 g usable carbs.

◉ Jill Taylor's Coleslaw

This coleslaw recipe was rated "very good, and easy to make" by our tester, Linda.

1 cup (240 ml) whipping cream
2 tablespoons (30 g) mayonnaise
6 tablespoons (90 ml) cider vinegar
Garlic and onion powder (optional)
Artificial sweetener to taste
1 pound (455 g) bag coleslaw mix

Mix the dressing ingredients together and pour over the coleslaw mix. Chill for at least an hour. Keeps well for 3 to 4 days, but bear in mind you are using fresh cream in this and it will spoil sooner than store-bought coleslaw will.

Jill's note: "In England, we always put onion in coleslaw, but my husband, Jim, doesn't like it that way. I sometimes grate an onion and press all the juice out of it. I add the juice to the coleslaw. It gives it a greater depth of taste without being overpowering."

Yield: Makes about 5 to 6 servings

Assuming 6, each has: 193 calories; 19 g fat; 2 g protein; 7 g carbohydrate; 2 g dietary fiber; 5 g usable carbs.

Marcelle Flint's Buttermilk Coleslaw

8 cups (600 g) shredded green cabbage
1/4 cup (30 g) shredded carrots

Dressing:

1/3 cup (8 g) Splenda
1/4 cup (60 ml) buttermilk
1/4 cup (60 ml) cream
1/2 cup (120 g) mayonnaise
1 teaspoon salt
1 1/2 tablespoons (25 ml) vinegar
2 1/2 tablespoons (40 ml) lemon juice

In large bowl, combine cabbage and carrots. In small bowl, combine dressing ingredients. Pour dressing over cabbage mixture and mix well. Cover and refrigerate for at least 2 hours.

Yield: Makes 8 side servings

Each with: 146 calories; 14 g fat; 2 g protein; 6 g carbohydrate; 2 g dietary fiber; 4 g usable carbs.

Snow Pea Salad Wraps

Unusual, and very good.

> 2 cups (150 g) snow pea pods
> 4 medium celery stalks, diced fine
> 1/2 cup (80 g) minced red onion
> 1/2 cup (60 g) chopped peanuts
> 1/4 cup (60 g) mayonnaise
> 1/4 cup (60 g) plain nonfat yogurt
> 1 tablespoon (15 ml) lemon juice
> 1/8 teaspoon cayenne
> 8 slices bacon, cooked and drained
> 24 lettuce leaves

Pinch the ends off your snow peas and pull off any strings, then cut them into 1/2" (1.25 cm) pieces—measure them after cutting, not before. Put the snow pea bits in a microwaveable bowl with just a teaspoon of water, cover, and microwave on high for just 1 minute. Uncover immediately!

Put your snow peas in a mixing bowl, and add the celery, onion, and chopped peanuts. Mix together the mayonnaise, yogurt, lemon juice, and cayenne; pour over the veggies; and toss. Crumble in the bacon, and toss again.

Arrange four lettuce leaves on each plate—I like Boston lettuce for this. Spoon a mound of the snow pea salad next to the lettuce. To eat, spoon the snow pea mixture onto a lettuce leaf, wrap, and eat.

Yield: 6 servings

Each with: 216 calories; 18 g fat; 8 g protein; 8 g carbohydrate; 3 g dietary fiber; 5 g usable carbs.

Michele S.'s Chunky Salad

Here's a simple salad that Julie, our tester, called "wonderful."

1 red onion
1 green pepper
1 hothouse cuke
2 tomatoes
2 tablespoons (10 g) fresh cilantro, chopped fine
2 tablespoons (10 g) fresh parsley, chopped fine
Juice of 1 lime (about 2 tablespoons[30 ml])
¼ cup (60 ml) olive oil
2 tablespoons (30 ml) red wine vinegar
Splash of Tabasco
Salt and pepper to taste

The instructions on this one are very simple: Chop veggies into big chunks (don't bother to peel cuke or tomatoes). Toss everything together.

Yield: Serves 4

Each with: 172 calories; 14 g fat; 2 g protein; 13 g carbohydrate; 3 g dietary fiber; 10 g usable carbs.

◎ Tom Budlong's Italian Olive Salad

Here's a recipe for you olive lovers. (I'm one of you!) Our tester, Ray, says that this is good alone, or you could toss a few scoops of this with mixed lettuces, for a different sort of salad. He suggests a second variation, as well: toss the Olive Salad with cauliflower.

> 1 14.5-ounce (411 g) can French-cut green beans, drained
> or 1 10-ounce (280 g) box frozen French-cut green beans, thawed.
> 1 or 2 celery stalks, thinly sliced crosswise
> 1 onion sliced
> 1 cucumber, thinly sliced
> 1 7-ounce (200 g) jar cocktail onions, drained
> 1 small lemon (slice very thinly, then quarter the slices)
> 1 4-ounce (115 g) can button mushrooms, drained
> ½ pound (225 g) black Italian or Greek olives in brine
> ½ pound (225 g) or 1 jar green cracked olives with peppers in brine
> 1 bell pepper, diced
> ½ cup (120 ml) olive oil
> 3–4 tablespoons (45–60 ml) wine vinegar

Seasonings:
Oregano
Fresh garlic, chopped
Fresh ground black pepper
Chopped parsley

Combine first 10 ingredients. Then add the oil and vinegar, and the seasonings to taste. Chill in refrigerator for a while before serving, to let flavors blend.

Tom's note: "To really taste good, you must use Mediterranean-type briny olives. Ordinary jarred black and green olives don't work as well."

Yield: 6 to 8 servings

Assuming 8 servings, each will have: 226 calories; 20 g fat; 2 g protein; 13 g carbohydrate; 5 g dietary fiber; 8 g usable carbs.

Kristy Howell's
Carrot and Cottage Cheese Salad

Here's one for all you fans of molded salads. Our tester Julie called this, "Light and fresh tasting ... a great summer salad!"

> 1 .3-ounce (8.5 g) package (4-serving size) sugar-free lime gelatin
> 1 cup (240 ml) boiling water
> 1/2 cup (60 g) chopped walnuts
> 1/2 cup (60 g) shredded carrot
> 1/2 cup (60 g) grated cucumber, juice and all
> 1/2 cup (60 g)shredded cheddar
> 1 cup (225 g) cottage cheese
> 1 cup (240 g) mayonnaise
> 1/4 teaspoon salt

Dissolve gelatin in boiling water. Chill until it starts to thicken. Add remaining ingredients. Pour into a mold or loaf pan you've sprayed with nonstick cooking spray, and chill until firm. Unmold and serve. (Alternately, you can just chill this in your mixing bowl and spoon it out.)

Yield: 6 side-dish servings

Each with: 417 calories; 41 g fat; 12 g protein; 4 g carbohydrate; 1 g dietary fiber; 3 g usable carbs.

Soy and Sesame Dressing

2 tablespoons (30 ml) soy sauce

1 ½ tablespoons (25 ml) oil

1 ½ tablespoons (25 ml) rice vinegar

1 tablespoon (1.5 g) Splenda

1 clove garlic, crushed

½ teaspoon dark sesame oil

1 ½ teaspoons lemon juice

¼ teaspoon pepper

Simply whisk everything together, or whir in your blender.

Yield: ⅓ cup (80 ml), or 3 servings of 2 tablespoons (30 ml)

Each with: 77 calories; 8 g fat; 1 g protein; 2 g carbohydrate; trace dietary fiber; 2 g usable carbs.

Orange Bacon Dressing

3 tablespoons (45 g) bacon grease

¼ cup (60 ml) white wine vinegar

1 tablespoon (15 ml) lemon juice

1 ½ tablespoons (2.25 g) Splenda

¼ teaspoon orange extract

Simply combine everything in a bowl, and whisk together.

Yield: ½ cup (120 ml), or 4 servings of 2 tablespoons (30 ml)

Each with: 92 calories; 10 g fat; trace protein; 1 g carbohydrate; trace dietary fiber; 1 g usable carb.

Big Italian Restaurant Dressing

This is my clone of the dressing from a popular Italian restaurant chain—minus the sugar, of course.

$\frac{1}{2}$ cup (120 ml) white vinegar

$\frac{1}{3}$ cup (80 ml) water

$\frac{1}{3}$ cup (80 ml) olive oil

$\frac{1}{4}$ cup (6 g) Splenda

2 $\frac{1}{2}$ tablespoons (30 g) grated Romano cheese

2 tablespoons (30 ml) beaten egg (feed the rest to the dog!)

1 $\frac{1}{4}$ teaspoons salt

1 teaspoon lemon juice

1 clove garlic, crushed

1 tablespoon (4 g) minced parsley

1 pinch dried oregano

1 pinch red pepper flakes

$\frac{1}{2}$ teaspoon guar or xanthan

This one's really easy: Just assemble everything in your blender, and run the sucker for 10 to 15 seconds. Keep in an airtight container in the fridge.

Note: If you're worried about that 2 tablespoons (30 ml) of raw egg, you can use egg substitute or pasteurized eggs instead.

Yield: 1 $\frac{1}{2}$ cups (360 ml), or 12 servings of 2 tablespoons (30 ml)

Each with: 62 calories; 6 g fat; 1 g protein; 1 g carbohydrate; trace dietary fiber, 1 g usable carb.

◎ Citrus Dressing

2 tablespoons (30 ml) lemon juice

2 tablespoons (30 ml) lime juice

1 tablespoon (15 ml) white vinegar

2 tablespoons (30 ml) canola oil

¼ teaspoon orange extract

1 tablespoon (1.5 g) Splenda

1 ½ teaspoons sugar-free imitation honey

Simply combine everything in a bowl, and whisk together. Alternately, assemble the ingredients in your blender, and run it for a few seconds.

Yield: 4 to 5 servings

Assuming 4 servings, each will have: 65 calories; 7 g fat; trace protein; 2 g carbohydrate; trace dietary fiber; 2 g usable carbs.

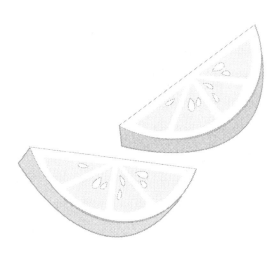

◎ Catalina Dressing

Catalina dressing and its close relative, that red stuff that calls itself "French Dressing" (I'm betting it has nothing to do with French cuisine!), are some of the more sugary dressings on the market. I kept thinking I should come up with a low-carb version, but truth is, I never liked the stuff. So when reader Emily Borman wrote me, asking me if I had a low-carb version, I jumped at the chance! I found a Catalina recipe, rewrote it with no-sugar ketchup and Splenda, and sent it to her. She promptly tried it, tweaked it with more ketchup and Splenda, and sent back the results. So here, thanks to Emily, is a Catalina dressing recipe for all you fans!

½ cup plus 2 tablespoons (150 g) Dana's No-Sugar Ketchup (page 524)
½ cup plus 2 tablespoons (16 g) Splenda
⅔ cup (160 ml) canola or peanut oil
⅔ cup (160 ml) red wine vinegar
2 cloves garlic, crushed
2 tablespoons (20 g) minced onion
Salt to taste

Simply assemble everything in a bowl or your blender, and whisk or blend it together. Store in an airtight container in the fridge.

Yield: 1 ¾ cups (420 ml), or 14 servings of 2 tablespoons (30 ml)

Each with: 107 calories; 10 g fat; 1 g protein; 4 g carbohydrate; 1 g dietary fiber; 3 g usable carbs.

Ginger Salad Dressing

¼ cup (40 g) minced onion
½ cup (120 ml) canola oil
⅓ cup (80 ml) rice vinegar
2 tablespoons (30 ml) water
2 tablespoons (20 g) grated gingerroot
2 tablespoons (20 g) diced celery
2 tablespoons (30 g) Dana's No-Sugar Ketchup (page 524)
4 teaspoons soy sauce
2 teaspoons Splenda
2 teaspoons lemon juice
½ teaspoon salt
¼ teaspoon pepper
1 clove garlic

Simply assemble everything in your blender, and run for 10 to 15 seconds. Store in a snap-top container in the fridge.

Yield: 1 ½ cups (360 ml), or 12 servings of 2 tablespoons (30 ml)

Each with: 87 calories; 9 g fat (91.7% calories from fat); trace protein; 2 g carbohydrate; trace dietary fiber; 2 g usable carbs.

Honey-Lime-Mustard Dressing

¼ cup (60 g) Dijon mustard

¼ cup (6 g) Splenda

1 tablespoon plus 1 teaspoon (20 ml) sugar-free imitation honey

1 tablespoon plus 1 teaspoon (20 ml) canola oil

1 tablespoon plus 1 teaspoon (20 ml) cider vinegar

1 tablespoon plus 1 teaspoon (20 ml) lime juice

Simply combine everything in a bowl, and whisk together.

Yield: ¾ cup (180 ml), or 6 servings of 2 tablespoons (30)

Each with: 36 calories; 3 g fat; trace protein; 1 g carbohydrate; trace dietary fiber; 1 g usable carb.

Cobb Salad Dressing

This jazzed-up vinaigrette is an obvious choice for a Cobb Salad, but it's good on any tossed salad, too.

1/4 cup (60 ml) water
1/4 cup (60 ml) red wine vinegar
1/4 teaspoon Splenda
1 teaspoon lemon juice
2 teaspoons salt
3/4 teaspoon pepper
3/4 teaspoon Worcestershire sauce
1/4 teaspoon dry mustard
1 clove garlic, crushed
1/4 cup (60 ml) olive oil
3/4 cup (180 ml) canola oil or other bland oil

Simply assemble everything in your blender and run it for a few seconds.

Yield: Makes about 1 1/2 cups (360 ml), or 12 servings of 2 tablespoons (30 ml)

Each with: 162 calories; 18 g fat; trace protein; 1 g carbohydrate; trace dietary fiber; 1 g usable carb.

Cumin Vinaigrette

Good with anything South-of-the-Border-ish, or Middle Eastern,
for that matter.

2/3 cup (160 ml) olive oil
1/3 cup (80 ml) lemon juice
2 teaspoons ground cumin
Salt and pepper to taste

Just whisk everything together, and toss with your salad.

Yield: 1 cup (240 ml), or 8 servings of 2 tablespoons (30 g)

Each with: 164 calories; 18 g fat; trace protein; 1 g carbohydrate; trace dietary fiber; 1 g usable carb.

Sweet Poppy Seed Vinaigrette

$1/2$ cup (12 g) Splenda

$1/4$ cup (60 ml) white wine vinegar

3 tablespoons (45 ml) olive oil

2 teaspoons minced red onion

1 $1/2$ teaspoons poppy seeds

1 teaspoon paprika

$1/4$ teaspoon salt

Measure everything into a bowl, whisk it together, and it's ready to go!

Yield: Makes roughly $1/2$ cup (120 ml), or 4 servings of about 2 tablespoons (30 ml)

Each with: 100 calories; 11 g fat ; trace protein; 2 g carbohydrate; trace dietary fiber; 2 g usable carbs.

Sun-Dried Tomato–Basil Vinaigrette

8 sun-dried tomato halves

2 tablespoons (30 ml) balsamic vinegar

2 tablespoons (30 ml) red wine vinegar

2 cloves garlic, crushed

$1/2$ teaspoon salt

$1/2$ cup (120 ml) extra-virgin olive oil

4 teaspoons dried basil, or 2 tablespoons fresh, minced

Chop the sun-dried tomatoes quite fine. Now simply whisk everything together, and toss with your salad.

Yield: Makes roughly $2/3$ cup (160 ml), or about 5 servings of 2 tablespoons (30 ml)

Each with: 210 calories; 22 g fat; 1 g protein; 5 g carbohydrate; 1 g dietary fiber; 4 g usable carbs.

Lemon-Mustard Dressing

¼ cup (60 ml) extra-virgin olive oil
¼ cup (60 ml) canola oil
¼ cup (60 ml) lemon juice
1 tablespoon (15 g) spicy brown mustard
Salt and pepper
½ teaspoon Splenda

Simply whisk everything together, and toss with your salad.

Yield: ¾ cup (180 ml), or 6 servings of 2 tablespoons (30 ml)

Each with: 165 calories; 18 g fat; trace protein; 1 g carbohydrate; trace dietary fiber; 1 g usable carb.

Spicy Peanut Dressing

This recipe was sent to me by no less a personage than Michael Barber, who is the executive sous chef at the Hyatt Regency DFW. This dressing is especially meant for Chef Barber's Asian Chicken Salad (page 383).

 3 tablespoons (45 g) peanut butter (natural, no sugar added)

 3 tablespoons (45 ml) vegetable oil

 1 tablespoon (15 ml) soy sauce

 2 tablespoons (30 ml) rice wine vinegar

 1/4 teaspoon cayenne

Place peanut butter in a mixing bowl and whisk in all other ingredients.

Yield: Makes 2 servings

Each with: 327 calories; 32 g fat; 5 g protein; 7 g carbohydrate; 2 g dietary fiber; 5 g usable carbs.

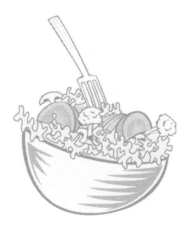

chapter seven

Chicken and Turkey

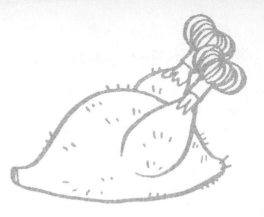

Is there a family in the country that doesn't eat chicken at least once a week? I doubt it. Chicken is reasonably priced, infinitely variable, and everyone likes it. No wonder the little jungle fowl from Southeast Asia has become a world citizen.

Turkey, our Native American bird, has gone out into the world as well. You'll find some simple things to do with ground turkey here, along with some seriously authentic Mexican turkey drumsticks, and my best recipe for using up the Thanksgiving leftovers.

Speaking of which, let me make a suggestion: Roast turkey is too good, too simple, and too cheap to save for holidays. Anytime you need to feed a crowd, consider roasting the big bird. You don't have to take the trouble to stuff it, just rub it with a little oil or mayonnaise (surprisingly good!) and roast it for 15 to 20 minutes per pound. Set it out on a buffet, and let folks carve their own, to eat plain or make sandwiches with. Sure is cheaper and spiffier than buying cold cuts at the deli!

We'll start this chapter out with a collection of chicken recipes from all around the world. These recipes tend to take some cooking time, but they're not actually terribly complex to make, and they add a satisfying variety to our low-carbohydrate cuisine.

Chicken Kampama

Greek chicken, simmered in red wine, tomatoes, and spices. If all you've had is Greek roasted chicken (wonderful, by the way!), try this!

3 pounds (1.4 kg) cut-up chicken
2 tablespoons (30 g) butter
2 tablespoons (30 ml) olive oil
1 cup (160 g) chopped onion
1 cup (240 g) canned diced tomatoes
4 tablespoons (55 g) tomato paste
1/4 cup (60 ml) dry red wine
1 clove garlic, crushed
1/4 teaspoon ground allspice
1/2 teaspoon ground cinnamon
1/4 cup (60 ml) chicken broth

In your big, heavy skillet, brown the chicken all over in the butter and olive oil. When it's golden all over, remove from the pan and pour off all but about 1 tablespoon of the fat.

In that fat, sauté the onion a bit. When it's golden, add the tomatoes, tomato paste, wine, garlic, spices, and chicken broth. Stir it all together, and bring to a simmer.

Add the chicken back to the skillet, turn the burner to lowest heat, cover, and cook for 30 minutes. Uncover and simmer for another 30 minutes, then serve.

Yield: 6 servings

Each with: 467 calories; 34 g fat; 30 g protein; 8 g carbohydrate; 1 g dietary fiber; 7 g usable carbs.

Greek Chicken with Yogurt

3 pounds (1.4 kg) chicken pieces
2 tablespoons (30 ml) lemon juice
Salt and pepper
3 tablespoons (45 g) butter
1 medium onion, sliced
2 cloves garlic, crushed
½ cup (120 ml) dry white wine
1 cup (240 ml) chicken broth
½ teaspoon ground rosemary
1 cup (230 g) plain yogurt
Guar or xanthan

Rub the chicken with the lemon juice, and sprinkle it with salt and pepper.

Melt the butter in your big, heavy skillet, over medium-high heat, and brown the chicken all over. When the chicken is brown, remove it from the skillet, pour off the fat, and put the chicken back.

Add the onion, garlic, wine, chicken broth, and rosemary to the skillet. Cover, turn the burner to low, and let the whole thing simmer for 30 minutes or so.

When time's up, pull the skillet off the heat and uncover. Let it cool for 10 minutes or so. Remove the chicken to a serving platter. Whisk the yogurt into the sauce in the skillet, stirring till it smooths out. Thicken a bit with your guar or xanthan shaker, and serve over the chicken.

Yield: 5 to 6 servings

Assuming 5, each will have: 527 calories; 37 g fat; 38 g protein; 6 g carbohydrate; trace dietary fiber, 6 g usable carbs.

Pollo en Jugo de Naranja (Mexican Chicken in Orange Juice)

The recipe I adapted this from was terribly high carb, including a cup of orange juice and a lot more raisins. The decarbed version is delicious!

3 pounds (1.4 kg) cut-up chicken, whatever you like—I like legs and thighs
Salt and pepper
2 tablespoons (30 ml) oil
1 orange
¼ cup (30 g) slivered almonds, toasted
1 tablespoon (15 ml) lemon juice
2 tablespoons (20 g) raisins
¼ cup (40 g) chopped onion
1 clove garlic, crushed
⅔ cup (160 g) canned diced tomatoes, undrained
¼ cup (60 ml) dry sherry
1 bay leaf
¼ cup snipped fresh parsley
½ teaspoon dried thyme
½ teaspoon dried oregano
Guar or xanthan gum (optional)

Sprinkle the chicken pieces with a little salt and pepper. In a large, heavy skillet, heat the oil and brown the chicken until it's lightly golden all over.

While that's happening, grate the zest of the orange and reserve. If your almonds aren't toasted, this is a good time to do that too—simply stir them in a small, heavy, dry skillet over medium heat until they start to turn golden, then set aside.

When the chicken is browned, pour off any excess fat. Squeeze in the juice of the orange, adding any pulp that may squeeze out. Add all remaining ingredients including the reserved orange zest, cover the pan, turn the burner to low, and let the whole thing simmer for 45 to 50 minutes, or until chicken is tender. Remove chicken to a serving platter

Remove bay leaf and thicken the sauce a bit with your guar or xanthan shaker, if you like; serve with the chicken.

Yield: 5 to 6 servings

Assuming 6, each will have: 448 calories; 31 g fat; 31 g protein; 9 g carbohydrate; 2 g dietary fiber; 7 g usable carbs.

Italian Chicken with White Wine, Peppers, and Anchovy

Don't be afraid of the anchovy paste in this sauce. There's no fishy taste to the recipe; it's just mellow and complex.

> 3 pounds (1.4 kg) chicken pieces
> 1/4 cup (60 ml) olive oil, divided
> 3 cloves garlic
> 1 cup (240 ml) dry white wine
> 1 tablespoon (15 g) anchovy paste
> 2 medium tomatoes, chopped
> 1 large green bell pepper, chopped
> Salt and pepper

In a Dutch oven, over medium heat, brown the chicken in 1/4 cup (60 ml) olive oil. When the chicken is golden all over, remove to a plate and set aside. Pour off the fat.

Now add the garlic, white wine, and anchovy paste to the Dutch oven, and stir until the anchovy paste is dissolved. Add the tomatoes and green pepper.

Salt and pepper your chicken, and plunk it back into the Dutch oven. Cover, set burner to lowest heat, and let simmer for 40 minutes. If you like, you can thicken the liquid in the pot a little before serving, but don't thicken too much.

Yield: 5 servings

Each with: 556 calories; 39 g fat; 36 g protein; 5 g carbohydrate; 1 g dietary fiber; 4 g usable carbs.

◎ Chicken Sancocho

This delicious, fresh-tasting Caribbean chicken stew/soup is not a quick recipe, but it's not terribly complicated, either. It's great to make over the weekend, when you're getting other things done; you'll just check in with your food every so often. And it reheats like a dream! Sadly, the fresh pumpkin needed to make it is only available for a few months in autumn, but then this makes a great chilly-evening supper anyway!

> 1 whole chicken, about 5–5 ½ pounds

Marinade:
> 4 tablespoons (60 ml) lime juice
>
> 1 ½ cups (180 g) diced celery
>
> 1 medium green pepper
>
> 1 large ripe tomato
>
> 1 medium onion
>
> ½ tablespoon (3.5 g) poultry seasoning
>
> ½ teaspoon ground nutmeg
>
> 1 tablespoon ground cumin

Stew ingredients:
> 1 quart (.95 L) chicken broth
>
> 1 large carrot, sliced
>
> 1 ½ cups (225 g) cubed rutabaga
>
> 1 ½ cups (225 g) cubed fresh pumpkin
>
> 1 small turnip, cubed
>
> 1 cup (150 g) cauliflower florets and stems, cut in small chunks
>
> 3 cups (225 g) shredded cabbage—prepared cole slaw mix works nicely
>
> 1 teaspoon to 1 tablespoon hot sauce, or to taste—use Caribbean Scotch bonnet sauce if you can get it!

Remove any giblets from the chicken's body cavity (toss them, use them in soup, or feed them to the pets, whatever you like), and place the chicken in a soup pot. Put all the marinade ingredients in a food processor with the S-blade in place (you'll want to cut everything in big chunks first, and peel your onion and core your pepper and all), and pulse until you have a coarse slurry. Pour this mixture over the chicken, and using clean hands, rub it all over, including into the body cavity. Stick the whole pot in the fridge, and let the whole thing sit overnight, turning the chicken over once or twice in that time if you think of it.

The next day, pull your pot with your chicken out of the refrigerator, put it on the stove, and pour the quart of chicken broth over the chicken. Cover it, put the whole thing over medium heat, bring it to a simmer, turn it down to low, and let it simmer for an hour. Turn it off, and let the pot sit on the stovetop and cool until you're ready to finish up the stew. (Obviously, you want this to be the same day, or no longer than the next day! If you leave the lid on, though, germs will be excluded, and it should be fine for at least 12 to 24 hours.)

When you're ready to complete your Chicken Sancocho, remove the chicken from the broth (a big tongs works well for this), put it on a platter, and set it aside. Skim the excess fat from the broth, and skim out the vegetables that were in the marinade—I used a Chinese skimmer for this, but you could just pour it through a sieve if you like. Be sure to press any broth out of the vegetables, back into the pot, before you discard them!

Put the pot of skimmed broth back on the stove, and turn the burner beneath it to medium-high. Stir in the carrot, rutabaga, pumpkin, and turnip, and let the whole thing simmer for a half an hour. While that's cooking, remove the skin from the chicken and discard it (or around here, feed it to the dog!). Then remove the meat from the bones, discard the bones, and cut the meat into bite-sized pieces. About 20 minutes before serving time, stir the meat, the cauliflower, and the cabbage into the pot, along with the hot sauce. Add water if needed, so that the broth is level with the top of the meat and vegetables. Simmer for 20 minutes, and serve.

Yield: 8 servings

Each with: 541 calories; 36 g fat; 41 g protein; 13 g carbohydrate; 3 g dietary fiber; 10 g usable carbs—but that figure is actually a tad high, since you discard some of the vegetables. I'd call it 8 g per serving. Lots of beta carotene and calcium, too.

◎ Laurence Erhili's Tagine of Chicken and Olives

Wow! I knew I wanted to have all kinds of different cuisines in this book, and it's working out even better than I planned!

> 1/2 cup (120 ml) olive oil
> 1 big onion
> 1 clove garlic
> 1 cut-up chicken (or buy 3–4 pounds [1.4–1.8 kg] skinless thighs
>   and breasts, but with the bone in)
> 1 teaspoon ground cumin
> 1 teaspoon paprika
> 1 teaspoon ginger
> 1 pinch saffron
> Salt and pepper to taste (not too much, because the olives give some salt
>   already, and if the olives are spicy, pepper is not needed)
> 1/2 bunch cilantro
> 1/2 bunch parsley
> 2 cups (480 ml) water
> 15 olives (any kind, I like the spicy ones filled with red bell peppers
>   that come in jars)

Skin the chicken. Mince your onion, and crush the garlic.

Pour your olive oil into a deep, heavy-bottomed pan (a Dutch oven would be great). Sauté the onion and garlic until they are a nice yellow color. Add the chicken pieces and spices to the pan, coat chicken with oil/spices by turning it around in the pan, and let chicken brown for a few minutes.

Wash cilantro and parsley and mince finely while the chicken is browning. Once the chicken has a nice color, add parsley, cilantro, and water. Cover and cook until boiling, and continue boiling for 20 to 30 minutes.

Reduce the heat, add the olives, and let simmer until chicken is well done, at least another 15 minutes, but I let mine cook longer (meat should almost fall off the bone). Add a little bit of water if necessary.

This is a main dish. Served on a big platter, it looks nice when you have guests. You can serve a dish of rice or potatoes on the side for people who eat more carbs. Traditionally this is eaten with bread (bread is used as a utensil and everybody helps themselves from the common dish). It is served with salads: tomatoes and cucumber salad, ratatouille, lettuce, and so forth.

Yield: About 6 servings

Each with: 721 calories; 58 g fat; 44 g protein; 4 g carbohydrate; 1 g dietary fiber; 3 g usable carbs.

◉ Orange-Five-Spice Roasted Chicken

This is my way of combining my love of Chinese food with the current trend toward citrus flavors. Good, too!

3 pounds (1.4 kg) chicken thighs
¼ cup (60 ml) soy sauce
2 tablespoons (130 ml) canola or peanut oil
1 tablespoon (30 ml) lemon juice
1 tablespoon (30 ml) white wine vinegar
1 tablespoon (3 g) Splenda
2 tablespoons (40 g) low-sugar orange marmalade
2 teaspoons five-spice powder

Place the chicken in a big zipper-lock bag. Mix together everything else, and pour into bag. Seal the bag, pressing out the air as you go. Turn the bag to coat, and throw it in the fridge. Let it sit for at least a couple of hours, and longer is fine.

Preheat your oven to 375°F (190°C). Haul the chicken out of the fridge, pour off the marinade into a small bowl, and arrange the chicken in a baking pan. Roast your chicken for 1 hour, basting 2 or 3 times with the reserved marinade.

Yield: 5–6 servings

Assuming 6, each will have: 393 calories; 27 g fat; 32 g protein; 3 g carbohydrate; trace dietary fiber; 3 g usable carbs—and that's assuming you end up consuming all of the marinade.

◉ Citrus Chicken

Don't look at this list of ingredients and turn the page! This is actually easy—
just make a marinade, marinate your chicken, and, while the
chicken's roasting, cook down the marinade for a sauce. Since you put
the chicken in to marinate long before dinnertime, the actual oh-my-God-it's-
already-six-and-the-kids-are-screaming cooking time is quite short—
just 20 to 30 minutes.

¼ cup (40 g) minced onion
2 cloves garlic, crushed
½ cup (120 g) lemon juice
½ teaspoon orange extract
1 tablespoon (15 ml) soy sauce
1 tablespoon (15 ml) rice vinegar
¼ cup (6 g) Splenda
1 tablespoon (10 g) grated gingerroot
1 tablespoon (15 g) brown mustard
3 pounds (1.4 kg) cut-up chicken
2 tablespoons (130 ml) canola or peanut oil
1 tablespoon (15 ml) sesame oil
1 cup (240 ml) chicken broth
2 teaspoons spicy brown mustard
2 teaspoons Splenda
1 teaspoon beef bouillon concentrate
Guar or xanthan

Combine the onion, garlic, lemon juice, orange extract, soy sauce, rice vinegar,
¼ cup (6 g) Splenda, gingerroot, and 1 tablespoon (15 g) mustard. Put the
chicken in a big zipper-lock bag, add this marinade, and seal the bag, pressing
out the air as you go. Turn the bag a few times to coat the chicken. Throw the
bag in the fridge for at least a few hours, and all day won't hurt a bit.

Okay, time to cook! Set your oven for 500°F (260°C). (Yes, I do mean 500°!)
Pull the chicken out of the fridge, and pour off the marinade into a saucepan.
Arrange the chicken in a roasting pan. Now mix together the canola and sesame
oils, and brush the chicken well all over with the mixture. When the oven is up to
temperature, put the chicken in, and set a timer for 20 minutes.

Put the saucepan with the marinade over a medium-high burner, and add the chicken broth, the final 2 teaspoons of mustard, the final 2 teaspoons (1 g) of Splenda, and the beef bouillon concentrate. Boil this mixture hard, till it's reduced by half. Thicken just a little—you want it about the texture of cream.

When the oven timer goes off, check the chicken. Pierce a piece to the bone—if the juices run clear, it's done. If the juices are pink, give it another five minutes, and check again. When the chicken is done, serve with the sauce.

Yield: 6 servings

Each with: 417 calories; 31 g fat; 30 g protein; 4 g carbohydrate; trace dietary fiber; 4 g usable carbs.

◉ Chinese Five-Spice Roasted Chicken

This is more traditionally Chinese than the Orange-Five-Spice Roasted Chicken, and it's equally good.

> 4 pounds (1.8 kg) cut-up chicken
> 1/4 cup (60 ml) soy sauce
> 1/4 cup (60 ml) dry sherry
> 2 teaspoons grated gingerroot
> 1 teaspoon five-spice powder
> 1/4 cup (6 g) Splenda

This is easy! Arrange the chicken in a roasting pan. Mix together everything else, and brush the chicken with it. Put the chicken in the oven at 375°F (190°C), and let it roast for 1 hour, basting every 10 to 15 minutes with the seasonings. That's it!

Yield:6 servings

Each with: 463 calories; 31 g fat; 39 g protein; 2 g carbohydrate; trace dietary fiber; 2 g usable carbs.

◎ Chunky Chicken Pie

This is a fair amount of work, but what comfort food on a cold winter night!

> 1 ½ pounds (680 g) chicken dark meat, no skin, but on the bone
> 1 quart (.95 L) water
> 1 tablespoon (10 g) chicken bouillon concentrate
> 1 pound (455 g) frozen California-blend vegetables
> 1 cup (100 g) sliced mushrooms
> 1 cup (240 ml) Carb Countdown Dairy Beverage, or half-and-half
> ½ teaspoon poultry seasoning
> Guar or xanthan
> Salt and pepper
> 1 batch Buttermilk Drop Biscuits (page 124)

Plunk chicken in a big saucepan, and add the water and chicken bouillon concentrate. Cover it, turn the burner to low, and let the whole thing simmer for 60 to 90 minutes.

Fish the chicken out with a fork or tongs, and set it on a plate until cool enough to handle (you can let it cool in the broth and do this step later, if you like— you'll just have to heat up the broth again before proceeding). In the meantime, add the California-blend vegetables and the sliced mushrooms to the broth— I actually cut mine up a little more, but you can leave everything in really big chunks if you prefer. Let this simmer for 25 to 30 minutes, or until the vegetables are tender but not mushy.

While that's happening, strip the chicken off the bones. Discard the bones, and cut the meat into bite-sized pieces. Reserve.

Okay, your veggies are cooked. Stir in the Carb Countdown Dairy Beverage and poultry seasoning. Thicken with your guar or xanthan shaker—you want a rich gravy consistency. Now, salt and pepper to taste, and stir in the chicken. Turn off the burner for the interim, while you …

Preheat the oven to 475°F (240°C), and then make a batch of Buttermilk Drop Biscuit dough, stopping right before you add the buttermilk to the dry ingredients.

Spray a 2-quart (1.9 L) casserole with nonstick cooking spray. When the oven is up to temperature, turn the burner back on under the chicken and vegetable mix-ture you want to bring it back to a boil. While that's heating, stir the buttermilk into the biscuit dough. Now, pour the boiling chicken mixture into the casserole, and spoon the dough over the top. Don't worry about covering every single millimeter of the gravy with the dough; it'll spread a bit. Just spoon it on pretty evenly, and it'll be fine. Put it in the oven immediately, and bake for 10 to 12 minutes, or until golden, then serve.

Yield: 6 servings

Each with: 481 calories; 27 g fat; 48 g protein; 13 g carbohydrate; 5 g dietary fiber; 8 g usable carbs.

◎ Black and Bleu Chicken

This is quick and easy, and very good. Why only three chicken breasts? Because that's what fits in my skillet! Once they were pounded out thin, they just barely squeezed in there together. If you want to increase this recipe, you'll need two skillets—but it will still be quick and easy and very good!

> 3 boneless, skinless chicken breasts
> Cajun seasoning, purchased or homemade
> 3 tablespoons (45 g) butter
> ¼ pound (115 g) blue cheese, crumbled

Start a large, heavy-bottomed skillet heating over medium-high heat. In the meanwhile, one at a time, place each chicken breast in a heavy zipper-lock plastic bag, and using a meat tenderizing hammer, a regular hammer, or whatever blunt object comes to hand (I use a 3-pound dumbbell!), pound each breast till it's about ¼" (6.25 mm) thick all over—this should take about 30 seconds per breast. Sprinkle both sides of each pounded breast with the Cajun seasoning. Melt the butter in the skillet, and add your chicken breasts. Sauté for 4 to 5 minutes per side, or until done through. When they're just about done, sprinkle the crumbled bleu cheese over the chicken breasts, dividing it evenly between all three. Cover the skillet for a minute more, to let the cheese melt, and serve.

Yield: 3 servings

Each with: 368 calories; 24 g fat; 36 g protein; 2 g usable carbs; a trace of fiber.

⊚ Curried Chicken "Pilau"

Back in my low-fat, high-carb day, I made a three-grain curried chicken pilau that was our very favorite supper. I hadn't had it since the day I went low carb—but this is a really convincing decarbed version, and far faster to cook, to boot. Don't omit the garnishes: chutney, chopped peanuts, and crumbled bacon. They're what make the dish!

1/2 cup (80 g) chopped onion

2 cloves garlic, crushed

2 tablespoons (20 g) curry powder

1 pound (455 g) boneless, skinless chicken breast, cut in 1/2" (1.25 cm) cubes

1 tablespoon (15 g) butter

1/2 cup (40 g) fresh snow pea pods (measure them after you cut them up!)

1/2 head cauliflower

2 teaspoons chicken bouillon concentrate

1/4 cup (60 ml) hot water

In your big, heavy skillet, over medium heat, start the onion, garlic, curry powder, and chicken sautéing in the butter. Remember to stir it once in a while during the sautéing process.

While that's happening, pinch the ends off of your snow peas, pull off any strings, and cut them into 1/2" (1.25 cm) pieces. Run the cauliflower through the shredding blade of your food processor, too—but this time, you're not going to microwave your cauli-rice. Just hang on to it. In a cup or small bowl, dissolve the bouillon in the water.

When the chicken is white all over, and the onion is translucent, stir in the cauli-rice and the dissolved bouillon, making sure everything is well combined—you want the chicken and curry flavors throughout the whole dish. Cover, turn the burner to low, and let it cook for 4 to 5 minutes. Uncover, add the snow peas, and stir again. Re-cover, and let cook for another 4 to 5 minutes. Then check to see how your cauli-rice is—you want it just barely tender, but not mushy. When it reaches that state, serve with Major Grey's Chutney (page 442), crumbled bacon, and chopped salted peanuts.

Yield: 3 to 4 servings

Assuming 3, each will have: 254 calories; 9 g fat; 36 g protein; 8 g carbohydrate; 3 g dietary fiber; 5 g usable carbs.

Easy Italian Skillet Chicken

1 pound (455 g) boneless, skinless chicken breast
1 egg
Italian Seasoned Crumbs (page 452)
1 tablespoon (15 ml) olive oil
1 tablespoon (15 g) butter
$\frac{1}{2}$ cup (60 g) shredded mozzarella cheese
$\frac{2}{3}$ cup (150 g) no-sugar-added spaghetti sauce—I use Hunt's

Put your chicken breasts, one at a time, in a heavy zipper-lock bag, and use any heavy, blunt object—I use a 3-pound dumbell—to beat them till they're $\frac{1}{2}$" thick all over. Cut into serving-sized pieces.

Crack the egg onto a plate with a rim, and beat it up with a fork. Put the crumbs on a second plate. Dip the pieces of chicken breast in the egg, then in the crumbs, pressing the crumbs in a bit, if needed, to make them stick. Set "bread-ed" chicken aside on a third plate.

Give your big skillet a squirt of nonstick cooking spray, and set it over a medium-hot burner. Add the olive oil and butter, and let them heat till the butter's melted. Tilt the skillet to swirl the two together, then add the chicken. Fry until golden and crisp on the bottom, about five minutes. Flip, and top chicken with the mozzarella. Cover with a lid you've tilted to leave a crack of about a half an inch, and let it cook until the bottom is golden and crisp, and the cheese is melted—about another 5 minutes.

While the chicken is cooking, put the spaghetti sauce in a bowl, and microwave it on 80 percent power for 60 to 90 seconds, to heat through. When chicken is done, remove to serving plates, top with spaghetti sauce, and serve.

Yield: 3 servings

Each with: 356 calories; 19 g fat; 41 g protein; 5 g carbohydrate; 1 g dietary fiber; 4 g usable carbs.

◎ Lemon Mustard Herb Chicken

⅓ cup (80 ml) lemon juice

⅓ cup (80 g) spicy brown mustard

1 tablespoon (4 g) rubbed sage

1 ½ teaspoons dried thyme

3 cloves garlic, crushed

24 ounces (680 g) boneless, skinless chicken breast

3 scallions

This is quick and easy. Just mix together the lemon juice, mustard, sage, thyme, and garlic. Put your chicken breast on a plate, and spread this mixture over both sides. Let it sit for ten minutes, and a little more won't hurt.

Heat up your electric tabletop grill, and throw the chicken breast in. Set your oven timer for 5 minutes. If there's some of the lemon-mustard mixture still on the plate, use it to baste the chicken halfway through the cooking time. Slice up the scallions, including the crisp part of the green. When the timer goes off, put the chicken on a serving plate, scatter the scallions over it, and serve.

Yield: 3-4 servings

Each with: 317 calories; 9 g fat; 53 g protein; 8 g carbohydrate; 1 g dietary fiber; 7 g usable carbs.

Chicken "Risotto" alla Milanese

This is my decarbed version of a very famous Italian dish—and it's quick and easy enough for a weeknight supper. My husband loved this—but then, any food with butter, cream, and cheese, all three, is pretty much his ideal.

1/2 head cauliflower
1 pound (455 g) boneless, skinless chicken breast
3 tablespoons (45 g) butter
3/4 cup (120 g) chopped onion
4 cup (60 ml) dry white wine
2 teaspoons chicken bouillon concentrate
1/4 teaspoon saffron threads
1 clove garlic, crushed
1/4 cup (60 ml) heavy cream
Guar or xanthan
Salt and pepper
1/2 cup (60 g) shredded Parmesan cheese

First run the cauliflower through the shredding blade of your food processor. Put it in a microwaveable casserole with a lid, add a couple of tablespoons of water, cover, and microwave on high for 5 or 6 minutes. Uncover as soon as the microwave beeps!

Cut your chicken breast in 1/2" (1.25 cm) cubes. Melt the butter in your big, heavy skillet over medium to medium-high heat, and start sautéing the chicken and onion.

When the chicken is white all over and the onion is softened, stir in the wine, bouillon concentrate, saffron threads, and garlic. Stir it around until the bouillon concentrate dissolves.

Drain your cauli-rice, and throw it in the skillet. Stir it around to blend all the flavors, and let the whole thing cook for 2 to 3 minutes. Stir in the heavy cream, and cook for another minute. If you want the whole thing a little creamier, use just a little guar or xanthan, but I didn't bother. Salt and pepper to taste.

Spoon onto plates or into bowls, and top each serving with 2 tablespoons (30 g) Parmesan, then serve.

Yield: 3 servings

Each with: 331 calories; 20 g fat; 30 g protein; 5 g carbohydrate; 1 g dietary fiber; 4 g usable carbs.

◎ Lynn Davis's
Cottage Cheese Spinach Chicken

An easy but yummy recipe for stuffed chicken.

1 10-ounce (280 g) package frozen chopped spinach, thawed
1/4 teaspoon salt
1/4 teaspoon pepper
1 teaspoon onion powder
1 cup (225 g) cottage cheese
2 pounds (1 kg) boneless, skinless chicken breast (about 4 breasts)
2 tablespoons (30 g) butter, melted
1/4 teaspoon garlic powder

Preheat oven to 350°F (180°C).

Squeeze excess water out of the thawed spinach, and put it in a large bowl. Add the salt, pepper, onion powder, and cottage cheese and mix well. Set aside.

One by one, put each chicken breast in a heavy zipper-lock bag and, using any heavy, blunt object that comes to hand, pound it to about 1/4" (6.25 mm) thick. When all the breasts are pounded thin, place 1/4 of cheese/spinach mixture in the center of each breast and fold in half. Secure with toothpicks and place in a lightly greased 9" x 13" (22.5 x 32.5 cm) baking dish.

Mix the melted butter with the garlic powder, and drizzle the resulting garlic butter over the chicken. Bake at for about 35 minutes, or until chicken is cooked through and juices run clear.

Yield: 4 servings

Each with: 402 calories; 13 g fat; 63 g protein; 6 g carbohydrate; 2 g dietary fiber; 4 g usable carbs.

Tee's Cajun Chicken and Spinach

Here's an easy and tasty slow-cooker recipe. Regarding that rice, Tee says, "This recipe would be fine without the rice, but it's an old favorite of ours that I used to make with white rice, so I didn't want to change it too much." If you call this 6 servings, the rice will add about 8 grams of usable carb to each serving.

1 cup (240 ml) water
2 teaspoons Tee's Cajun Seasoning Mix
   (page 451, or use purchased seasoning)
2 teaspoons chicken bouillon concentrate
¼ cup (60 ml) white wine (optional)
1 onion, diced
2 cloves garlic, crushed
Tabasco for added heat if desired
⅓ cup (65 g) brown rice (optional) or shredded cabbage or cauli-rice
3 pounds (1.4 kg) chicken thighs or breasts with skin removed
1 10-ounce (280 g) box frozen spinach, thawed and drained

Put 1 cup water in your slow cooker. Add seasoning, bouillon, wine, onion, garlic, Tabasco, and rice, if using it. Place chicken on top; sprinkle with a little bit of extra seasoning. Cook 6 to 8 hours on low.

When time's up, remove the lid, and turn your slow cooker up to high; if you're using the cabbage or cauli-rice, add it now. Cook for another 30 minutes to cook off some of the juices. Then add the spinach, and cook on low 10 to 15 minutes.

Yield: 8 servings

Each will have: 203 calories; 2 g fat; 33 g protein; 10 g carbohydrate; 2 g dietary fiber; 8 g usable carbs.

◎ Poppy Seed Chicken

Here's a recipe from a reader known only as H N. Too bad, too—this is really interesting and good.

4 boneless, skinless chicken breasts, cut in small cubes (about 1 1/2 lbs)
1/4 teaspoon garlic powder
1/8 cup (20 g) Parmesan cheese
2 tablespoons (30 ml) canola oil
1 1-pound (455 g) bag frozen broccoli
3/4 cup (180 g) mayonnaise
1/8 cup (30 ml) heavy cream
1 packet Splenda
1 teaspoon poppy seeds
Salt and pepper to taste (I use freshly ground black pepper)
8 ounces (225 g) shredded Colby-Jack cheese

Preheat oven to 350°F (180°C).

Dredge chicken breasts in garlic and Parmesan and stir-fry with oil in frying pan until cooked through.

While that's happening, place frozen broccoli in a 2-quart (1.9 L) casserole with lid and microwave on high for 7 minutes. Drain any excess liquid. While the chicken and broccoli are cooking, mix the mayo, heavy cream, Splenda, and poppy seeds in a small bowl using a wire whisk. Layer ingredients in casserole in this order: broccoli on bottom, then cooked chicken, then sauce mixture. Salt and pepper each layer, if you like. Top with shredded cheese and cover casserole. Bake for 30 minutes, or until bubbly.

Yield: 4 to 6 servings, assuming 6 servings

Each will have: 501 calories; 44 g fat; 28 g protein; 1 g carbohydrate; trace dietary fiber.

Terrie Shortsleeve's Lemon-Garlic Chicken

Our tester suggested taking the time to marinate the chicken breasts in the lemon juice–olive oil mixture—not a bad idea, if you think ahead!

3/4 cup (180 ml) lemon juice

6 tablespoons (90 ml) olive oil

1 teaspoon salt

1 dash ground black pepper

1 teaspoon oregano (not ground)

2 cloves garlic, crushed

4 boneless, skinless chicken breasts (about 1–1 1/2 pounds [455–680 g])

8 ounces (225 g) whole mushrooms (the smaller the better)

Preheat the oven to 400°F (200°C). Spray a 9" x 13" (22.5 x 32.5 cm) pan with nonstick spray. Whisk the lemon juice, olive oil, salt, pepper, oregano, and garlic together in a medium bowl. Dunk each of the chicken breasts into the lemon juice mixture and place in the bottom of the pan. Do the same with the mushrooms, using them to surround, but not cover, the chicken. Bake for about 35 to 45 minutes, until juices run clear, or internal temperature reaches 160°F (75°C).

Yield: Serves 4

Each having: 358 calories; 22 g fat; 33 g protein; 7 g carbohydrate; 1 g dietary fiber; 6 g usable carbs.

Donna Nisleit's
Garlic Parmesan Chicken Breasts

1/2–3/4 cup (80–120 g) grated Parmesan cheese

1 0.7-ounce (19 g) envelope dry Italian salad dressing mix
    (or 2 tablespoons [14 g] Italian seasonings)

1/4 teaspoon pepper

1/2 teaspoon garlic powder, or more to taste

6 boneless, skinless chicken breasts (about 3 pounds [1.4 kg])

1 egg, slightly mixed

Preheat oven to 400°F (200°C).

Combine cheese, salad dressing mix, pepper, and garlic powder. Dip chicken in egg, then coat with cheese mix. Place in shallow baking dish. Bake at 400°F (200°C) for 20 to 25 minutes or until juices run clear when you pierce one chicken breast.

Yield: Makes 6 servings

Each having: 175 calories; 4 g fat; 31 g protein; 1 g carbohydrate; trace dietary fiber; 1 g usable carbs.

Winnie Spicer's
Chicken in Raspberry Cream Sauce

Our tester Linda Fund called this recipe "awesome."

3 tablespoons (45 g) butter

2 tablespoons (30 ml) extra-virgin olive oil

8 boneless, skinless chicken breasts (about 4 pounds [1.8 kg])

1/2 cup (120 ml) Raspberry Vinegar (page 528, or use purchased
    raspberry vinegar)

1 cup (240 ml) chicken stock

1 cup (240 ml) heavy whipping cream

Put butter and olive oil in a large frying pan over medium heat. Once butter is melted, sauté chicken breasts on both sides. Remove and reserve chicken breasts.

Add vinegar to pan and bring to a boil, stirring well to dissolve any flavorful stuff sticking to the pan. Remove pan from the heat. Add chicken stock and stir well. Return chicken to pan, cover, and simmer 15 to 20 minutes.

Remove the chicken breasts from the pan and place in a shallow serving dish. Cover to keep warm. Boil the liquid in the pan until reduced enough to thicken a bit. Slowly add the cream and stir well over medium heat until thickened. Serve the sauce over the chicken.

Yield: 8 servings

Each with: 375 calories; 21 g fat; 43 g protein; 2 g carbohydrate; 0 g dietary fiber; 2 g usable carbs.

◉ Lauren Zizza's Mustard Chicken Dish

This dish is for those of us who like it hot and spicy!

> 2 skinless, boneless chicken breasts (about 1 lb)
> 2 teaspoons olive or canola oil
> 2 teaspoons Worcestershire sauce
> 2 tablespoons (15 g) mustard
> 1 teaspoon Adobo Seasoning (page 448), or use purchased
>   Adobo seasoning
> 2 teaspoons hot sauce
> 4 cups (300 g) chopped cabbage
> 1 tablespoon (15 g) butter

Cut chicken into ¾" (1.875 cm) cubes. Mix the oil, Worcestershire sauce, mustard, Adobo, and hot sauce in a bowl, and add chicken chunks, stirring to coat. Let the chicken marinate for at least 15 minutes.

In the meanwhile, steam the cabbage till just tender. Melt the butter in your big skillet, over medium heat. Add chicken mixture to pan.

Fry on medium heat until chicken is mostly cooked, then turn heat up a bit higher. Cook at higher temp until sauce starts to caramelize. Serve chicken mixture over steamed cabbage.

Yield: Serves 2

Each having: 288 calories; 12 g fat; 31 g protein; 14 g carbohydrate; 5 g dietary fiber; 9 g usable carbs.

◉ Gwen Meehan's Yummy Chicken Casserole

It's sometimes hard to know how to make a casserole without noodles or rice. Now you can try this family-pleasing Tex-Mex dish.

6 boneless chicken breasts (about 3 pounds)
1/4 red onion, diced
1 cup (240 ml) water
1 teaspoon salt
1 teaspoon pepper
2 teaspoons garlic powder
2 teaspoons poultry seasoning or Adobo seasoning
1 14.5-ounce (411 g) can diced tomatoes with green chilies, drained
2 cups (240 g) cheddar cheese
3 ounces (85 g) cream cheese
1 cup (230 g)sour cream

In a deep, covered skillet, simmer chicken breasts and onion in 1 cup (240 ml) water with salt, pepper, garlic salt, and poultry seasoning. Cook until chicken is no longer pink, let it cool for 10 minutes, and then cut into 1/2" (1.25 cm) cubes.

Place the chicken mixture on the bottom of a baking dish you've sprayed with nonstick cooking spray, cover with the tomatoes with chilies, a thin layer of cheddar cheese, followed by a layer of cream cheese, and finally a layer of sour cream. Top with the remaining cheddar cheese.

Bake at 350°F (180°C) for at least 15 minutes or until cheese has thoroughly melted and ingredients combine.

Yield: Approximately 6 servings

Each will have: 368 calories; 26 g fat; 26 g protein; 7 g carbohydrate; 1 g dietary fiber; 6 g usable carbs.

◎ Sophia Loren Chicken

Of all the recipes in the original *500 Low-Carb Recipes*, the one that has drawn the most favorable comment is Heroin Wings, chicken wings "breaded" with seasoned Parmesan cheese. Phillip Pickett came up with this variation. He says it's called "Sophia Loren Chicken" because it is hot, spicy, and Italian. As with the original, do not skip lining the baking pan with foil, or you'll be sorry!

6 boneless, skinless chicken breasts (about 3 lbs)
1 cup (150 g) grated Parmesan cheese
  (use the cheap stuff in the shaker for this)
2 tablespoons (8 g) dried parsley
1 tablespoon (3 g) dried oregano
2 teaspoons paprika
1 teaspoon salt
$^1/_2$ teaspoon pepper
$^1/_2$ cup (120 ml) extra-virgin olive oil
6 cloves garlic, minced
1 cup (240 ml) hot sauce
  (Phillip prefers Frank's, but any no-carb sauce would do)

Cut your chicken breasts into finger-sized pieces. Set aside.

Preheat oven to 350°F (180°C).

Combine cheese and spices in a bowl. Line a 9" x 13" (22.5 x 32.5 cm) baking pan with foil.

Combine the olive oil and garlic in a bowl. Dip each chicken finger in the olive oil, roll in the cheese/seasoning mixture, and arrange on the foil-lined pan.

Bake for 45 minutes. After removing from the oven, place the chicken fingers in shallow dish and pour hot sauce over chicken, thoroughly coating each piece. Grab a handful of napkins and enjoy.

Tester's note: Ray Stevens says you may need more cheese than this.

Yield: Makes 6 servings

Each with: 364 calories; 24 g fat; 33 g protein; 3 g carbohydrate; 1 g dietary fiber; 2 g usable carbs.

⊚ Sally Waldron's Buffalo Chicken and Slaw

Adapted from a recipe demonstrated by Sara Moulton, one of Sally's favorite chefs on the Food Network. The combination of the warm chicken and the cool, crunchy slaw is fabulous! (Our tester agrees.)

    4 boneless, skinless chicken breasts
    2 cups (480 ml) buttermilk
    2 tablespoons (30 ml) Louisiana hot sauce
        (such as Frank's or Crystal's), divided
    Salt and pepper to taste
    Spicy Blue Cheese Dressing and Dip (page 60)
    4 cups (300 g) shredded cabbage (bagged or from ¼ head of cabbage)
    2 celery ribs, sliced thinly

First, pound those chicken breasts. One by one, put them in a heavy zipper-lock bag, and using any heavy, blunt instrument that comes to hand, bash them into submission until they're ¼" (6.25 mm) thick. This is very quick and easy to do.

Now mix the buttermilk and the hot sauce in a large bowl or tall plastic container. Add chicken and marinate in the refrigerator for at least 45 minutes, or up to 2 hours.

Remove chicken from the marinade and pat dry with paper towels. (Our tester suggests you skip patting the chicken dry. If you want to keep more of the marinade flavor, that makes sense.) Season with salt and pepper to taste. Cook chicken by your preferred grilling method until juices run clear (you can fry it in a little olive oil, grill it on an electric tabletop grill, or grill it outdoors).

Just before serving, toss ¾ cup of the dressing with the cabbage and celery in a large bowl. Place one chicken breast on each serving plate, drizzle with some of the remaining dressing, and evenly divide the slaw on top of each. Serve leftover dressing on the side.

Yield: Serves 4

Each with: 510 calories; 36 g fat (64.4% calories from fat); 37 g protein; 8 g carbohydrate; 2 g dietary fiber; 6 g usable carbs.

Robin Loiselle's Teriyaki Chicken Wings

Like Japanese-style food? Here's a great recipe.

Olive oil
1 teaspoon chopped garlic
1 teaspoon grated gingerroot, or to taste
1 1/2–2 pounds (680 g–1 kg) chicken wings, cut into drummettes
   (discard the tips if you don't like them)
1/4 cup (60 ml) soy sauce
1 cup (240 ml) water
1/4 cup (6 g) Splenda
1 teaspoon liquid sweetener (Robin uses Sugar Twin)
8 drops dark sesame oil (optional, but very good)

Heat up a flat-bottomed wok and add the olive oil. Add the garlic and ginger (we use the stuff in the small jars); stir-fry for a few minutes to scent the oil.

Add the chicken wing pieces and stir-fry until there is some color happening. You don't have to spend a lot of time here! Stir-fry them just enough to get rid of that "raw" look.

Mix the rest of the ingredients, sweetening to taste, and pour into the wok. Stir the wings until everything is coated.

Cook over medium heat, covered, for about 20 minutes, stirring occasionally. The sauce will boil down and become thicker and very yummy. Serve with faux fried rice. (Try the Japanese Fried "Rice" on page 140.)

Robin's note: "If you want to make more wings, make more sauce. There are only two of us so we use one package of chicken that has about 8 whole wings in it."

Yield: Serves 3

Each will get: 422 calories; 31 g fat (66.9% calories from fat); 31 g protein; 3 g carbohydrate; trace dietary fiber.

Melissa Cathey's Jalepeno Lime Chicken

Like your food Southwestern style? Here's a really easy way to indulge your tastes. Our tester Diana Wright pronounced this "easy and delicious."

> 1 large boneless, skinless chicken breast (about 8 ounces [225 g])
> 2 teaspoons green Tabasco sauce (jalapeno flavor)
> 1 teaspoon cilantro, dried or fresh
> 1 tablespoon (15 ml) lime juice
> 1 slice jalapeno Jack cheese
> Optional: Purchased low-carb roll (not included in nutrition counts)

Spray nonstick skillet with nonstick cooking spray, and cook chicken over medium heat until golden brown, sprinkling top with Tabasco and cilantro.

After chicken is flipped, sprinkle other side with Tabasco jalapeno sauce and cilantro.

When done, sprinkle with lime juice and top with cheese; cover, reduce heat to low, and heat until cheese is melted. Serve alone or as a sandwich on a low-carb roll.

Yield: Serves 1

Not including the roll, each has: 253 calories; 12 g fat; 33 g protein; 2 g carbohydrate; trace dietary fiber; 2 g usable carbs.

◎ Amy K. Crawford's
Easy Chicken Cordon Bleu

Our tester Ray raved about these, and says he'll be making them again.

> 6 boneless, skinless chicken breasts (about 3 pounds [1.4 kg])
> 6 slices ham
> 6 slices Swiss cheese
> 3 tablespoons (25 g) low-carb bake mix (Atkins or other brand)
> 1 tablespoon paprika
> Olive oil
> 1 16-ounce (455 g) jar low-carb Alfredo Sauce

One by one, put each chicken breast in a heavy zipper-lock bag, and using any heavy, blunt object that comes to hand, beat them just to flatten slightly—don't go thinner than 1/2" (1.25 cm). Place a slice of ham and a slice of cheese on each chicken breast. Roll up, taking care to cover all of the cheese (fold the cheese a little if you need to), and secure with a toothpick.

Mix the low-carb bake mix and the paprika in a small bowl. Dredge each piece of chicken in the bake mix to lightly coat it. Brown the rolled chicken breasts in a sauté pan with the oil. When the breasts are browned, add the Alfredo sauce. Turn heat to low and simmer for 30 minutes. Remove toothpicks before serving.

Amy's Note: I serve this with asparagus and a tossed salad, and some pasta for the rest of my family.

Tester's note: Ray says to read the label on the various brands of Alfredo sauce carefully, checking not only the carb counts, but the serving sizes.

Yield: 6 very generous servings

Each will have: 611 calories; 34 g fat; 67 g protein; 6 g carbohydrate; 1 g dietary fiber; 5 g usable carbs. However, this recipe could easily serve 10.

Carol Tessman's Skillet Supper

1 pound (455 g) bulk Italian sausage

1 medium onion, cut into large chunks

½ green pepper, cut into large chunks

2–3 tablespoons (30–45 ml) olive oil

1 4-ounce (115 g) can mushrooms, drained, or 4-ounces sliced, fresh mushrooms

2 cups (110 g) diced cooked chicken

1–2 cups (225–450 g) no-sugar-added spaghetti sauce, or more to taste

In your big, heavy skillet, cook and crumble the Italian sausage. Drain, and set aside.

In the same skillet, sauté onion and green pepper in small amount of oil until onion is transparent; add mushrooms, diced chicken, and the cooked Italian sausage. Stir to combine. Add spaghetti sauce to moisten. Stir occasionally until heated through. Serve alone, or over low-carb pasta.

Tester's note: Stacey Sims suggests that if you don't have cooked chicken in the house, you can throw a couple of boneless, skinless chicken breasts in your electric tabletop grill.

Yield: 6 servings, and analyzed for using 1 cup (225 g) of spaghetti sauce total

Each serving (without the pasta) will have: 553 calories; 43 g fat; 28 g protein; 15 g carbohydrate; 5 g dietary fiber; 10 g usable carbs.

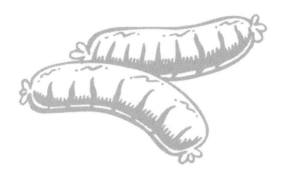

Celeste's
Chicken with Creamy Mushroom Sauce

3 tablespoons (45 g) butter, divided

4 boneless, skinless chicken breasts

1 pound (455 g) sliced mushrooms

1 cup (240 ml) heavy cream

1/4–1/2 teaspoon xanthan (or use your shaker)

Salt and pepper

Optional:

Garlic salt

2 tablespoons (30 g) sour cream

Melt 1 tablespoon (15 g) butter over medium heat, in a skillet that will fit all 4 chicken breasts. Brown the chicken until just cooked. Sprinkle both sides with garlic salt, if desired. Remove the chicken from the pan and keep warm.

Melt the remaining 2 tablespoons butter, add the sliced mushrooms, and stir until just colored. Add the cream, stir; if using sour cream, add and stir till mixed. When the cream starts to simmer, sprinkle in the xanthan gum and stir like mad. Allow to thicken to desired consistency, and salt and pepper to taste.

Return the chicken and any juices to the pan, turn to coat both sides with the sauce.

Serve with cauliflower rice, or any desired vegetables.

Celeste's note: "This sauce can also be made on its own and used with steak, but I think the chicken juices really add to the flavor."

Yield: 4 servings

Without any of the options, each of 4 servings will have: 440 calories; 33 g fat; 31 g protein; 7 g carbohydrate; 1 g dietary fiber; 6 g usable carbs.

Dorothy Markuske's Chicken Stuffed with Spinach and Goat Cheese

Our tester Diana Lee gives this gourmet recipe a 10.

2 tablespoons (30 ml) olive oil, divided

1 clove garlic, finely chopped

1 teaspoon grated gingerroot

2 1/2 cups (600 ml) white wine, divided

1 10-ounce (280 g) bag prewashed baby spinach

1 tablespoon (4 g) plus 2 1/2 teaspoons fresh tarragon, chopped, divided

1 shallot, chopped

2 scallions, chopped

8 ounces (225 g) goat cheese

1 teaspoon fresh chives, chopped

Salt and pepper

2 pounds (1 kg) boneless chicken breast

1/2 pound (225 g) sliced ham

1/2 cup (120 g) sour cream

Heat 1 tablespoon (15 ml) of the oil in your big skillet, and sauté the garlic and ginger. Add 1 cup of the white wine, the spinach, 1 tablespoon of the tarragon, the shallot, and the scallions. Cook until spinach wilts. Turn off burner.

In a bowl, mix the goat cheese with the chives, 1 1/2 teaspoons of the tarragon, and some pepper. Set aside.

One by one, put each chicken breast in a heavy zipper-lock bag, and pound it as thin as possible, without making holes. Divide goat cheese mixture between chicken breasts and spread it on them. Now cover the goat cheese with the ham. Divide the spinach mixture, and spread on top of each piece of ham. Roll up the chicken, and secure with toothpicks.

Heat the rest of the oil in a skillet, and brown the chicken rolls on all sides.

Add the salt, pepper, and the rest of the tarragon and the white wine; lower heat to simmer; cover and cook for 4 to 5 minutes until chicken is no longer pink. Remove the chicken to a platter, and keep it warm.

Raise the heat under the skillet, and boil the liquid hard to reduce, until it thickens a little. Remove the pan from the heat, and stir in the sour cream.

Remove toothpicks, and serve chicken with sauce over top.

Dorothy's note: "Enjoy with your favorite Long Island wine."

Yield: This is surely enough for 10 servings

Each with: 423 calories; 20 g fat; 36 g protein; 14 g carbohydrate; 4 g dietary fiber; 10 g usable carbs.

◎ Patti Shreiner's Chicken Continental

My sister Kim tested this one evening when she had friends coming for dinner, and everyone loved it.

> 1 pound (455 g) boneless chicken breasts, pounded thin
> 1/4 pound (115 g) ham, sliced very thin
> 1/2 pound (225 g) Asiago cheese, sliced thin

Preheat oven to 375°F (190°C). Layer chicken, ham, then cheese in casserole or stoneware pan. Be sure to cover meats with cheese as this will seal in the juices. Bake for 25 minutes or until cheese is dark golden brown. Serve immediately.

Yield: Makes 4 servings

Each with: 390 calories; 22 g fat; 44 g protein; 2 g carbohydrate; 0 g dietary fiber; 2 g usable carbs.

Brenda Theune's Cheesy Chicken

A cheesy-good, quick, and easy chicken recipe. It strikes me it would be easy to double or even triple this.

> 2 boneless, skinless frozen chicken breasts
> 4 ounces (115 g) cream cheese, softened
> 2 tablespoons (30 g) butter, softened
> 2 tablespoons (30 ml) cream
> 1 tablespoon (10 g) minced onion
> 1/4 teaspoon pepper
> 1/4 teaspoon seasoned salt
> 1/2 cup (60 g) shredded cheese

Preheat oven to 375°F (190°C).

Place the chicken breasts in a 9" x 9" (22.5 x 22.5 cm) baking pan you've sprayed with nonstick cooking spray. Mix together the cream cheese, butter, cream, onion, and spices. Spread the mixture evenly over the breasts. Put the cheese on top of the sauce. Bake for about 45 minutes or until done.

Brenda's note: "I prefer pepper Jack in this recipe, while my husband likes cheddar."

Yield: 2 servings

Each with: 607 calories; 41 g fat; 55 g protein; 3 g carbohydrate; trace dietary fiber; 3 g usable carbs.

Debbie Murawski's BBQ Chicken Breast

Ray Stevens, our tester, calls this simple recipe "quick and good."

> 1 chicken breast
> 1 tablespoon (15 g) low-carb BBQ sauce
>   (store-bought, or from the recipe on page 525)
> 2–3 slices bacon
> 1 ounce (30 g) sliced Swiss cheese

Grill or broil the chicken breast (Debbie uses an electric tabletop grill). While that's going, cook up a few slices of bacon. When the chicken breast is done, spread on the low-carb BBQ sauce, add a couple of slices of bacon, and top with a slice of Swiss cheese. Then place in microwave or under the broiler until cheese is melted.

Yield: 1 serving

With: 416 calories; 17 g fat; 59 g protein; 3 g carbohydrate; trace dietary fiber; 3 g usable carbs.

◎ Kristy Howell's Chicken Carbonara

Here's an easy Italian-style dish.

> 1 ½ pounds (680 g) boneless chicken thighs or breasts, cut into thin strips (this is easier to do with partially frozen chicken)
> 2 tablespoons (30 ml) olive oil
> 3 eggs
> ½ cup (75 g) grated Parmesan cheese
> 2 tablespoons (30 ml) milk or cream
> ¼ teaspoon salt
> ⅛ teaspoon pepper
> 8–10 slices cooked bacon, crumbled

In your big skillet, sauté chicken in oil until done. Combine eggs, cheese, milk, salt, and pepper. Pour over chicken. Cook and stir over low heat 1 to 2 minutes. Stir in bacon and serve.

Yield: About 5 servings

Each with: 372 calories; 22 g fat (53.9% calories from fat); 41 g protein; 1 g carbohydrate; trace dietary fiber; 1 g usable carb.

◉ Chicken Teriyaki Stir-Fry

Our indefatigable recipe tester Ray Todd Stevens came up with this recipe his very own self. Try it!

> 1 pound (455 g) boneless, skinless chicken breast
> 1 ½ tablespoons (25 ml) stir-fry oil
> 3 tablespoons (45 ml) soy sauce, divided
> 1 teaspoon toasted sesame oil (optional)
> 4 cloves garlic, crushed
> 2 teaspoons grated gingerroot
> 4 cups (900 g) frozen mixed stir-fry vegetables, thawed
> 1 cup (240 ml) water
> ¼ cup (6 g) Splenda

Cut up chicken breast into slices about ¼" (6.25 mm) thick. Crosscut to pieces no longer than 1 ½" (3.75 cm). Cut the biggest pieces in half.

In a big skillet or wok, over high heat, stir-fry chicken in oil till the pink is gone— about 5 minutes. Add 1 tablespoon (15 ml) soy sauce and sesame oil and stir-fry for 5 minutes.

Add the garlic and ginger, and stir fry 2 more minutes; add the vegetables.

Stir fry 5 to 10 minutes. (Depends on how tender you like the veggies.) Add the water, remaining soy sauce, and Splenda. Stir well; simmer 20 minutes. Serve.

Good as is. For those who think they need it, you can also serve these with rice.

Ray's note: "Cleaning up your wok is easy with a bamboo brush."

Yield: 2 servings

Each with: 181 calories; 6 g fat; 19 g protein; 7 g carbohydrate; 2 g dietary fiber; 5 g usable carbs.

Piernas de Guatalote en Mole de Cacahuates (Mexican Turkey Legs in Peanut Sauce)

3 turkey drumsticks, about 2¾ pounds (1.2 kg) total
1 cup (240 ml) chicken broth
1 cup (240 g) canned tomatoes with green chiles
2 tablespoons (30 g) peanut butter
¼ teaspoon ground cloves
¼ teaspoon ground cinnamon
¾ teaspoon chili powder
¼ cup (40 g) chopped onion
1 clove garlic, crushed

Place turkey legs in a Dutch oven with the chicken broth. Cover, turn burner to low, and simmer for a couple of hours. Turn off burner, and allow to cool.

Fish out the turkey legs with a tongs, and set on a platter. Ladle the broth into your blender. Add the canned tomatoes with green chiles, the peanut butter, and the spices. Blend till smooth. Pour back into the Dutch oven, add the chopped onion and crushed garlic, and stir. Put the turkey legs back in, and let the whole thing simmer together for another 20 to 30 minutes, then serve.

Yield: 3 servings

Each with: 406 calories; 16 g fat; 57 g protein; 7 g carbohydrate; 2 g dietary fiber; 5 g usable carbs.

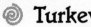 Turkey Tetrazzini

You'll thank me for this recipe the weekend after Thanksgiving!

2 tablespoons (30 g) butter

1 small onion, diced

2 4-ounce (115 g) cans mushrooms, drained

1 cup (240 ml) heavy cream

1 cup (240 ml) half-and-half

2 teaspoons chicken bouillon concentrate

2 tablespoons (30 ml) dry sherry

1 teaspoon guar or xanthan (optional, but it makes the sauce thicker)

¾ cup (120 g) grated Parmesan cheese

3 cups (675 g) cooked spaghetti squash, scraped into strings

3 cups (330 g) diced leftover turkey

Over medium heat, melt butter in a heavy skillet, and start the onions and the mushrooms sautéing in it. While that's cooking, combine the cream, half-and-half, bouillon concentrate, sherry, and guar, if you're using it, in a blender, and blend it for just ten seconds or so, to combine. Go back and stir your veggies! When the onion is limp and translucent, transfer half of the vegetables into the blender, add the Parmesan, and blend for another 20 seconds or so, to puree the vegetables. Combine this cream sauce with the spaghetti squash, the rest of the vegetables, and the turkey, and mix everything well. Put in a 10-cup (2.4 L) casserole that you've sprayed with nonstick cooking spray. Bake uncovered at 400°F (200°C) for 20 minutes, until bubbly.

This tetrazzini is wonderful; everyone who tries it loves it. However, if you have some folks in your family who are going to be unhappy about spaghetti squash, here's what you do: use half spaghetti squash, half spaghetti. Mix half of the sauce with the turkey. Divide the other half of the sauce, and the un-pureed mushrooms and onions, between 1 ½ cups (340 g) spaghetti squash and 1 ½ cups (105 g) cooked spaghetti. Put the spaghetti squash at one end of your casserole dish, and the spaghetti at the other end (it helps to use a rectangular casserole dish!). Then make a groove down the middle of the whole thing, lengthwise, and pour the turkey mixture into the groove. Bake according to the instructions above.

Assuming 6, each will have: 492 calories; 7 g carbohydrate; trace fiber; 24 g protein; 7 g usable carbs.

◉ Joan Wilson's Turkey on Spaghetti Squash

Stuck with leftover turkey? Hey, it happens to us all.

1 spaghetti squash
1/2 onion, chopped
1 pound (455 g) sliced mushrooms
Butter for sautéing
4 cups (700 g) broccoli florets
1 16-ounce (455 g) jar Alfredo sauce
Salt and pepper
2 cups (110 g) cubed or chopped leftover turkey
Grated Parmesean cheese

Cut squash in half and clean out seeds. Put it in a microwaveable dish, add 1/4 cup of water, and cover with plastic wrap. Nuke it on high for 8 to 12 minutes. When done, scrape pulp with fork to release the strings.

Spray a casserole dish with nonstick cooking spray. Spread the squash in the bottom of dish.

Sauté chopped onion and mushrooms in a little butter until onions are limp. Add the broccoli florets, then stir in the Alfredo sauce. (I add about 1/3 jar of water, just to rinse out the jar.) Bring heat up to simmer. Salt and pepper to taste.

Put diced turkey on top of squash in casserole dish. Pour sauce over turkey and sprinkle with Parmeasen cheese. Bake at 350°F (180°C) until bubbly.

Yield: Serves 6

With each serving having: 307 calories; 20 g fat; 20 g protein; 12 g carbohydrate; 2 g dietary fiber; 10 g usable carbs.

Turkey Feta Burgers

1 pound (455 g) ground turkey

2 tablespoons (20 g) minced red onion

1 teaspoon dried oregano

1 clove garlic, crushed

¾ cup (90 g) crumbled feta cheese

¼ cup (25 g) chopped kalamata olives

2 tablespoons (20 g) sun-dried tomatoes, packed in oil, chopped

Plunk everything in a mixing bowl, and with clean hands, smoosh it all together until it's very well blended. Form into four burgers—the mixture will be pretty soft, so you may want to chill them for a while before cooking.

Preheat your electric tabletop grill. When it's hot, add the burgers, and set your oven timer for 6 minutes. That's it!

Yield: 4 servings

Each with: 263 calories; 17 g fat; 24 g protein; 4 g carbohydrate; 1 g dietary fiber; 3 g usable carbs.

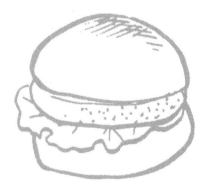

Turkey Chorizo with Eggs

Here's how to turn a pound of ground turkey into a quick-and-easy Mexican dinner!

 1 pound (455 g) ground turkey
 2 tablespoons (30 ml) olive oil
 4 cloves garlic, crushed
 2 teaspoons dried oregano
 ½ teaspoon ground cinnamon
 ½ teaspoon ground cloves
 1 teaspoon pepper
 2 tablespoons (30 ml) dry sherry
 1 teaspoon Splenda
 1 teaspoon salt or Vege-Sal
 8 eggs
 1 cup (240 g) canned diced tomatoes, drained
 ¼ cup (40 g) minced onion

Start the turkey browning in the olive oil, crumbling it as you go. When it's mostly browned, add the garlic, oregano, cinnamon, cloves, and pepper. Cook it for 2 or 3 more minutes, then stir in the sherry, Splenda, and salt or Vege-Sal. Remove from the heat.

Now scramble the eggs, and stir in the tomatoes and onion. Put the skillet back on the heat, pour the eggs over the turkey, and scramble till the eggs are set.

Yield: 4 servings

Each with: 399 calories; 25 g fat; 32 g protein; 8 g carbohydrate; 1 g dietary fiber; 7 g usable carbs.

Thai Turkey Burgers

1 pound (455 g) ground turkey
1 tablespoon (15 ml) lemon juice
1 tablespoon (15 ml) lime juice
1/2 cup (60 g) grated carrot
2 teaspoons chili paste
4 scallions, minced
2 tablespoons chopped cilantro
1 teaspoon fish sauce
1 batch Chili Lime Mayo (page 447)

This is very straightforward. Start your electric tabletop grill heating. Then dump everything except the Chili Lime Mayo in a bowl, smoosh it all together really well with clean hands, and make three burgers—the mixture will be pretty soft. When the grill is hot, slap the burgers in it, and set your oven timer for 5 minutes.

Top with Chili Lime Mayo, and serve.

Yield: 3 servings

Each with: 382 calories; 29 g fat; 27 g protein; 6 g carbohydrate; 1 g dietary fiber; 5 g usable carbs.

Cat's Chili

Cat says this turkey chili is very popular with her friends and family. Our tester Barbo liked this a lot and says it's good made with ground sirloin, too.

1/2 bell pepper, diced
1/2 Vidalia or other sweet onion, cut into chunks
1 teaspoon minced garlic
2–3 tablespoons (30–45 ml) olive oil
1 pound (455 g) ground turkey (or use ground beef or ground chicken)
1 15-ounce (420 g) can diced tomatoes with green chilies

Season with:
Red pepper flakes
Ground ginger

In your big, heavy skillet, sauté the pepper, onion, and garlic in the olive oil. Add the ground turkey. Brown and crumble it. Then add the canned tomatoes, and one can of water. Simmer for 20 to 30 minutes, until it starts to thicken up. Add red pepper flakes and ground ginger to taste, and allow it to simmer for 10 more minutes.

Note: Optional additions are shredded cabbage, sliced zucchini, or green beans. Barbo added the green beans and said it was a good choice!

Yield: Without the options, this will serve 3

With each having: 272 calories; 13 g fat; 28 g protein; 11 g carbohydrate; 2 g dietary fiber; 9 g usable carb.

◎ Sloppy Toms

This is an easy way to add interest to a pound of plain old ground turkey. You can serve this on low-carb rolls, if you can get them locally. I prefer to serve it over cauli-rice or, better yet, in omelets!

 1 pound (455 g) ground turkey
 1 tablespoon (15 ml) olive oil
 ⅓ cup (55 g) chopped onion
 1 clove garlic, crushed
 1 Anaheim chili pepper, diced
 ½ cup (120 g) Dana's No-Sugar Ketchup (page 528)
 1 tablespoon (15 g) yellow mustard
 2 tablespoons (30 ml) cider vinegar
 1 tablespoon (1.5 g) Splenda
 1 tablespoon (15 ml) Worcestershire sauce

In your big, heavy skillet, start browning and breaking up the ground turkey in the olive oil. Throw in your onion, garlic, and diced pepper, too.

When all the pink is gone from the turkey, stir in the ketchup, mustard, vinegar, Splenda, and Worcestershire sauce. Simmer the whole thing for 5 minutes before serving.

Yield: 4 to 5 servings

Assuming 5, each will have: 202 calories; 11 g fat; 17 g protein; 10 g carbohydrate; 2 g dietary fiber; 8 g usable carbs.

⊚ Jody Leimbek's Low-Carb Wraps

Julie our tester suggests a variation: slices of jalapeno or pepperoncini in place of the olives. Julie also says, "This is quick, easy, made with things commonly found in the fridge, and is very filling. It doesn't feel like a 'diet' food or even a 'low carb' food. It's just plain good food." What more could you want?

- 1 slice deli-sliced turkey or chicken
- 1 tablespoon sliced black olives
- 1 or 2 strips of bacon, cooked and drained
- 1 slice Swiss cheese (Parmesan is great, too!)
- 1 tablespoon ranch dressing
- 1 low-carb tortilla (La Tortilla, or other brand)

Roll up all ingredients in tortilla and enjoy!

Yield: 1 serving

Each one will give you: 804 calories; 59 g fat; 60 g protein; 14 g carbohydrate; 8 g dietary fiber; 6 g usable carb.

chapter eight

Fish and Seafood

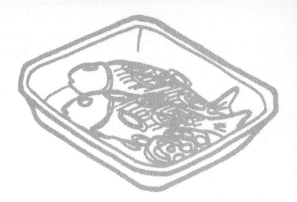

Detractors of our low-carb lifestyle like to point out that this is "that diet where you can eat all the steak and bacon cheeseburgers you want." That is, theoretically speaking, true, though it sounds terribly monotonous to me. But it is equally true that this is a diet on which you can eat all the shrimp, lobster, scallops, salmon, sole, catfish—and any other fish or seafood—that you want. With a big salad on the side. But nobody ever says that, do they? Because everybody accepts that fish is healthy, so pointing out that we can have all we like doesn't yank any chains.

Here are two big advantages of fish: First of all, if you're one of the many folks who have discovered that you need to keep an eye on calories along with carbs, fish is a bargain. And second, most fish dishes are very quick-cooking.

Feel free, by the way, to play mix and match with fish recipes. If a recipe calls for swordfish, you can use sea bass, grouper, or any firm-fleshed fish. If a recipe calls for sole, tilapia, or flounder, any mild white fish should be fine. Tell the fish guy at your market what sort of a recipe you're making, and ask what's good that day. Your recipe should come out fine.

◎ Ceviche

Most countries in Latin America have a version of this classic dish, in which the fish is "cooked" in lime juice, instead of by heat. This makes a posh appetizer or, if you want to increase the serving sizes, a light main course. This is not only low carb, it's also very low calorie—and except for squeezing all those limes, very simple.

> 1 ½ pounds (680 g) fish fillets
>
> 8 limes
>
> 2 tomatoes
>
> 1 fresh jalapeno (optional)
>
> 1 California avocado
>
> ¼ red onion, diced
>
> ¼ cup (15 g) chopped fresh oregano
>
> ¼ cup (15 g) chopped fresh cilantro
>
> Salt and pepper to taste

This dish lends itself to endless variation, but one thing remains constant: Everything must be perfectly fresh, especially the fish. Talk to the fish guy at your grocery store, and tell him you'll be using the fish for ceviche (that's "seh-vee-chay"). Tell him you need fish that has never been frozen, and choose from what he has, rather than going into the store with the idea of buying a particular kind of fish and ending up buying something that's been thawed. You can use seafood as well as fish fillets—shelled shrimp, scallops, baby squid, and chunks of lobster tail all lend themselves to this treatment. Or you can use fin fish like mackerel, red snapper, grouper, halibut, cod, or flounder. It is customary to use two to four kinds, rather than just one, but suit yourself.

Cut any fish fillets into serving-sized pieces. Put your fish or seafood in a glass or crockery dish. Squeeze 7 of your limes—you should have about 1 ¼–1 ½ cups (300–360 ml) lime juice—and pour the lime juice over the fish. Turn the fish to make sure it's completely coated. Cover the dish with piece of plastic wrap, and refrigerate for 8 to 12 hours or overnight. If at all possible, it's best to turn the fish at least a few times during the marination time, to make sure it "cooks" evenly.

Drain the fish or seafood, and put it in a fresh bowl.

Cut the tomatoes in half across the equator, and squeeze them gently to get rid of the seeds. Dice them fairly fine. Seed the jalapeno, if you're using it, and dice it fine, too. Cut your avocado in half, remove the seed, peel it, and cut it into dice as well. Put all of these vegetables and the diced red onion in the bowl with the fish. Throw in the fresh herbs, too. Squeeze the last lime over the whole thing, season with salt and pepper, toss gently, and serve.

Yield: 8 appetizer servings

Each with: 123 calories; 4 g fat; 16 g protein; 5 g carbohydrate; 2 g dietary fiber; 3 g usable carbs. This analysis assumes you discard all but about ¼ cup (60 ml) of the lime juice used to marinate the fish.

◎ Orange-Sesame Salmon

> 1 ½ pounds (680 g) salmon fillet
> ¼ cup (60 ml) sesame oil
> 1 teaspoon orange extract
> ⅓ cup (80 ml) lemon juice
> 4 teaspoons Splenda
> 2 teaspoons Dijon mustard
> 2 teaspoons dried tarragon, crumbled

Cut your salmon into serving-sized pieces, and lay it in a glass pie plate or any big plate with a rim.

Mix together everything else, and pour it over the salmon fillets, turning them to coat. Stick the plate in the fridge, and let the fish marinate for at least 30 minutes, and an hour's fine.

Spray your big, heavy skillet with nonstick cooking spray, and put it over medium heat. When it's hot, add the fish, reserving the marinade. Give the salmon about 4 minutes on each side—you want it opaque almost clear through. Then add the marinade, and let the two cook together for another couple of minutes. Serve with the liquid from the pan scraped over the fish.

Yield: 4 servings

Each with: 329 calories; 20 g fat; 34 g protein; 2 g carbohydrate; trace dietary fiber; 2 g usable carbs.

◉ Flo Conklin's Salmon with Heavenly Topping

Our tester, my sister Kim, tried this with catfish, too, and said it was great!

> 2 pounds (1 kg) boneless, skinless salmon fillet
> 4 tablespoons (60 ml) lemon juice, divided
> ½ cup (75 g) grated Parmesan cheese
> 4 tablespoons (60 g) butter, melted
> 3 tablespoons (45 g) mayonnaise
> 3 tablespoons (20 g) green onion, chopped
> 1 teaspoon prepared mustard
> ¼ teaspoon salt
> Dash Tabasco sauce

Rinse and pat fish dry. Place in a shallow baking pan you've greased well or sprayed with nonstick cooking spray. (Flo lines the pan with foil for a quick cleanup.) Brush the fish with 2 tablespoons (30 ml) of the lemon juice. Bake for 30 to 40 minutes at 350°F (180°C).

While the fish is baking, combine your remaining ingredients, including the final 2 tablespoons (30 ml) of lemon juice. Remove the fish from the oven when the time's up. Spread it with the cheese mixture, and put under the broiler for 2 to 3 minutes or until cheese mixture is golden brown and fish flakes easily.

Yield: 6 servings

Each with: 327 calories; 21 g fat; 33 g protein; 1 g carbohydrate; trace dietary fiber; 1 g usable carb.

Nancy Zarr's Pan-Seared Salmon

Here's a simple but flavorful salmon recipe.

> Olive oil
> 2 pounds (1 kg) salmon, in one large piece or in individual servings,
>   as desired (our tester suggests salmon steaks)
> 2 teaspoons black pepper
> 2 teaspoons chili pepper
> 1/4 teaspoon cayenne pepper
> 1 teaspoon cumin
> 1 1/2 teaspoons kosher salt
> 4 cloves garlic, minced
> Lime wedges

Preheat oven to 350°F (180°C).

Rub olive oil on both sides of fish. Combine all the peppers, cumin, and salt. Divide garlic and divide pepper mixture so that half will be put on each side of fish. Sprinkle 1/2 of garlic on one side of fish, then sprinkle half of pepper mixture over fish. Repeat on the other side. Fish may be refrigerated at this point, if you'd like to do this part in advance and cook it later.

Heat small amount of olive oil in pan. Sear fish for 2 minutes per side. Transfer to a baking dish and bake up to 12 minutes for thick fish. Serve with fresh lime wedges to squeeze on fish as desired.

Nancy's note: I have gone to the trouble of grilling the fish after searing instead of baking in the oven and I really like it in the oven better. This is such an easy recipe and good enough for company.

Yield: With 4 servings

Each will have: 277 calories; 8 g fat; 46 g protein; 3 g carbohydrate; 1 g dietary fiber; 2 g usable carbs.

◎ Leslie's Pickled Salmon

1 pound (455 g) salmon steaks or skinned fillets
1 teaspoon salt
1 1/2 cups (360 ml) water
1/2 cup (120 ml) white vinegar
1/4 cup (6 g) Splenda
1/2 bay leaf
2-inch piece cinnamon stick
1 slice fresh ginger, crushed
1/2 lemon, sliced
1 medium onion, thinly sliced

Rub fish with salt, cover, and refrigerate for 1 hour.
Rinse fish with cold water and set aside.

In a 2-quart (1.9 L) saucepan, combine water, vinegar, Splenda, bay leaf, cinnamon stick, ginger, and lemon. Bring to a boil, reduce heat, and simmer for 5 minutes. Add fish and simmer, uncovered, for another 7 minutes.Place your onion slices in a large jar or glass casserole with lid. Place fish on top and cover with the hot vinegar mixture. Cool, cover, and refrigerate at least 4 hours and preferably overnight.

Yield: 4 servings

Each with: 170 calories; 4 g fat; 23 g protein; 11 g carbohydrate; 4 g dietary fiber; 7 g usable carbs. This analysis assumes that you are eating all the pickling lquid, which you probably won't. So assume you probably get fewer carbs than this.

◎ Salmon Stuffed with Lime, Cilantro, Anaheim Peppers, and Scallions

This is impressive for how simple it is, and it will feed a crowd.

1 whole salmon, cleaned and gutted, about 6 pounds (2.7 kg)
1 lime, sliced paper-thin
1 bunch cilantro, chopped
1 Anaheim chili pepper, cut in matchstick strips
3 scallions, sliced thin lengthwise
2 tablespoons (30 g) olive oil

This is simple. Preheat your oven to 350°F (180°C). Lay your salmon in a great big roasting pan you've sprayed with nonstick cooking spray. Now stuff everything else except the oil into the salmon, distributing everything evenly along the length of the body cavity.

I like to sew Mr. Fishy up, using a heavy needle and thread. Now rub him with olive oil on both sides, and thow him in the oven for 30 to 40 minutes. It's a good idea to stick a thermometer in the thick part of the flesh to see if he's done; it should read between 135°F and 140°F (about 60°C).

Cut into slices, with some of the stuffing in each serving.

Yield: 12 servings

289 calories; 10 g fat; 45 g protein; 1 g carbohydrate; trace dietary fiber; 1 g usable carbs.

◎ Baked Sole in Creamy Curry Sauce

This is simple, and the curry makes it a pretty yellow color.

> 1 cup (230 g) plain yogurt
> 1/2 cup (120 g) mayonnaise
> 1 tablespoon (15) lemon juice
> 1 teaspoon curry powder
> 2 pounds (1 kg) sole fillets

Mix together everything but the sole fillets, to make a sauce. Pat your fish fillets dry. Spray an 8" x 8" (20 x 20 cm) baking dish with nonstick cooking spray.

Now, spread each fillet with some of the sauce—you want to use up about half the sauce, total, in this process. As each fillet is spread with sauce, roll it up and place the roll, seam-side down, in the baking pan.

Spoon the rest of the sauce over and around the fish. Bake at 350°F (180°C) for 30 minutes, and serve.

Yield: 6 servings

Each with 296 calories; 19 g fat; 30 g protein; 2 g carbohydrate; trace dietary fiber; 2 g usable carbs.

◎ Sautéed Sole in White Wine

This simple but elegant dish is very Italian.

  1 pound (455 g) sole fillets
  Salt and pepper
  2 tablespoons (30 g) butter
  1 tablespoon (15 ml) olive oil
  ¼ cup (60 ml) dry white wine
  1 teaspoon dried oregano
  3 tablespoons (30 g) shredded Parmesan cheese
  3 lemon wedges

Pat the sole fillets dry with a paper towel, and sprinkle them on both sides with a little salt and pepper. Lay them on a plate while you spray your big skillet with nonstick cooking spray and set it over medium heat. Add the butter and the olive oil, and swirl them together as the butter melts. When the fat is hot, lay the fillets in the pan, and sauté them just a few minutes on each side, turning carefully.

Pour the wine into the skillet—pour it in around the edge, rather than pouring it right over the fish. Sprinkle the oregano over the fish, and set your timer for 5 minutes. Let the fish simmer in the wine till the timer goes off—if it browns slightly on the bottom, all the better. Remove to serving plates, sprinkle each serving with a tablespoon of Parmesan cheese, and serve with a lemon wedge to squeeze over it.

Yield: 3 servings

Each with: 284 calories; 16 g fat; 31 g protein; 1 g carbohydrate; trace dietary fiber; 1 g usable carb.

◎ Kim's Tilapia Provençal

  1 tablespoon (15 ml) olive oil
  16 ounces (455 g) tilapia fillets
  1 cup (240 g) canned diced tomatoes
  12 kalamata olives, pitted and chopped
  ¼ cup (60 ml) lemon juice
  ¼ cup (15 g) chopped parsley

Heat the olive oil in your big, heavy skillet, over medium heat. Add the tilapia fillets, and sauté for about 3 to 4 minutes per side. Now stir together the tomatoes, chopped olives, and lemon juice, and pour over tilapia. Let the whole thing simmer for five minutes or so, then top with parsley and serve.

Note: The easiest way to pit an olive, assuming you don't care about keeping it whole, is to just press down on it with your thumb.

Note: This one's for my sister, who's a huge fan of the cooking of Provence. I made this with tilapia only because it's consistently inexpensive at my market. Feel free to try this with another fish, if you prefer—I suspect cod would work well.

Yield: 3 servings

Each with: 233 calories; 10 g fat; 28 g protein; 9 g carbohydrate; trace dietary fiber; 9 g usable carbs.

◎ Susan Higgs's Tilapia in Browned Butter

Be aware that the baking time may vary some with the thickness of your fillets, so check early for doneness.

> 1 stick butter
> 2 pounds (1 kg) tilapia fillets (or other favorite fish)
> Juice and zest of 1 lemon
> Fresh thyme to taste, optional
> Salt and pepper to taste
> Paprika to taste

Preheat oven to 450°F (230°C). Put butter in a 9" x 13" (22.5 x 32.5 cm) baking dish and place in hot oven until butter is melted and browned. (The browned butter is the flavor maker in this dish.) Reduce heat to 400°F (200°C). Place fish in hot butter and bake for 10 to 15 minutes. Turn fillets quite carefully and baste with pan juices. Sprinkle fillet with lemon juice, lemon zest, thyme (if using), salt, pepper, and paprika. Bake for another 5 minutes. Serve with pan juices.

Yield: Makes 4 servings

Each with: 392 calories; 25 g fat; 41 g protein; 1 g carbohydrate; trace dietary fiber; 1 g usable carb.

◎ Pan-Barbecued Sea Bass

This has a lot of flavor for something so quick and easy! Feel free to cook any firm-fleshed fish this way.

   1 pound (455 g) sea bass fillets
   1 tablespoon (7 g) Classic Barbecue Rub
      (page 538, or use purchased barbecue rub)
   4 slices bacon
   2 tablespoons (30 ml) lemon juice

Cut your sea bass fillets into serving portions. Sprinkle both sides liberally with the barbecue rub.

Spray your big, heavy skillet with nonstick cooking spray, and place over medium-low heat. Using a sharp kitchen shears, snip your bacon into small pieces, straight into the skillet. Stir it about for a moment. As soon as a little grease starts to cook out of the bacon, clear a couple of spaces for the fish, and put the fish in the pan. Cover, and set your oven timer for 4 minutes.

When time is up, flip the fish, and stir the bacon around a bit, so it will cook evenly. Re-cover the pan, and set the timer for another 3 to 4 minutes. Peek at your fish at least once; you don't want to overcook it!

When the fish is flaky, remove to serving plates, and top with the browned bacon bits. Pour the lemon juice in the skillet, stir it around, and pour over the fish. Serve.

Yield: 3 servings

Each with: 202 calories; 7 g fat; 31 g protein; 2 g carbohydrate; trace dietary fiber; 2 g usable carbs.

◎ Zijuatenejo Sea Bass

   1 1/2 pounds (680 g) sea bass fillets
   Salt and pepper
   1 teaspoon ground cumin
   2 tablespoons (30 ml) olive oil
   Easy Orange Salsa (page 440)
   1/4 cup (15 g) chopped fresh cilantro

Cut your fish into individual portions, if needed. Sprinkle it on both sides with salt and pepper and the cumin. Heat the olive oil in your big heavy skillet, over medium-low heat, and throw in the fish. Give it 4 to 5 minutes per side, or until opaque clear through. Remove each portion to a serving plate; top each with 2 tablespoons (30 g) Easy Orange Salsa and 1 tablespoon chopped cilantro.

Yield: 4 servings

Each with: 236 calories; 10 g fat; 32 g protein; 2 g carbohydrate; 1 g dietary fiber; 1 g usable carb.

◉ Orange Swordfish Steaks with Almonds

16 ounces (455 g) swordfish steak
¼ cup (60 ml) lemon juice
2 tablespoons (30 ml) olive oil
½ teaspoon orange extract
2 teaspoons Splenda
2 tablespoons (30 g) butter
2 tablespoons (15 g) slivered almonds

Put the swordfish in a zipper-lock bag. Combine the lemon juice, olive oil, orange extract, and Splenda, and pour into the bag. Seal the bag, pressing out the air as you go, and turn the bag once or twice to coat the fish. Throw it in the fridge. Let your fish marinate for an hour, turning it when you think of it.

Now, spray your skillet with nonstick spray, and add half the butter. Melt over low heat, then add the swordfish steak. Reserve the marinade. Let the fish cook for 5 minutes, then turn it over and let it cook for another 5.

While the fish is cooking, melt the other half of the butter in a small skillet. Add the almonds, and sauté, stirring frequently, until golden. If they're done before the fish is, remove from the heat.

When the 10 minutes of cooking time for the fish is up, add the marinade to the pan. Let the fish cook another 2 to 3 minutes in the marinade, turning once. Remove to a serving plate, pour the marinade over it, and top with the almonds. Serve.

Yield: 3 servings

Each with: 372 calories; 26 g fat; 31 g protein; 3 g carbohydrate; trace dietary fiber; 3 g usable carbs.

◎ Curried Swordfish and Cabbage

I'll curry anything that stands still long enough! This is a fast and simple yet elegant meal, all made in one big skillet. But if you want to make more than 1 or 2 servings, you'll need to do it twice, or get a really, really huge skillet!

2 tablespoons (30 g) butter

1 ½ teaspoons curry powder

2 cups (150 g) shredded cabbage (you can used bagged cole slaw mix, if you like)

¼ medium onion, sliced thin

1 clove garlic, crushed

8 ounces (225 g) swordfish steak, 1 ½" (3.75 cm) thick

Spray your big skillet with nonstick cooking spray. Melt the butter in it, over low heat, and add the curry powder. Let it cook for just a minute, then add the cabbage, onion, and garlic. Sauté the vegetables, stirring frequently, for 3 or 4 minutes.

Make a hole in the middle of the cabbage big enough to lay your swordfish steak on the pan. Cover the pan, and set the oven timer for 5 minutes.

When the timer beeps, turn the fish over, and stir the cabbage. Re-cover the pan, and set the timer for another 5 minutes. When time's up, serve swordfish with the cabbage heaped around it.

Yield: 1 to 2 servings

Assuming 1, it will have: 538 calories; 33 g fat; 48 g protein; 13 g carbohydrate; 5 g dietary fiber; 8 g usable carbs.

⦿ Broiled Orange Chili Lobster

If you ever manage to get tired of lobster with lemon butter, or lobster with curried mayonnaise, try this.

4 lobster tails, split down the back of the shell

2 tablespoons (30 g) butter

1 1/2 teaspoons chili garlic paste

1/4 teaspoon orange extract

1/2 teaspoon Splenda

1 teaspoon lemon juice

Your lobster tails should have their shells split along the back. Put them on a broiler rack.

Melt the butter, and stir in everything else. Baste the lobster tails with this mixture, being sure to get some down into the shell. Place tails 5" (13 cm) to 6" (15 cm) under broiler, set on high.

Broil for 7 to 8 minutes, basting every couple of minutes with the butter mixture, ending the basting about 2 minutes before the end of cooking time. Serve.

Yield: 4 servings

Each with: 308 calories; 8 g fat; 53 g protein; 2 g carbohydrate; trace dietary fiber; 2 g usable carbs.

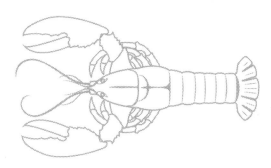

◎ Coquilles St. Jacques

This is a seafood classic!

1 tablespoon (15 g) butter
1 ½ teaspoons minced onion
½ clove garlic, crushed
½ cup (50 g) chopped mushrooms
Salt and pepper
8 ounces (225 g) bay scallops
¼ cup (60 ml) dry white wine
½ cup (120 ml) heavy cream
Guar or xanthan
⅓ cup (40 g) shredded Gruyere

In a medium-sized saucepan, melt the butter over medium-low heat. Add the onion and garlic, and sauté for just a minute or so. Now add your mushrooms and sauté, stirring frequently, until mushrooms have changed color and are limp. Salt and pepper a little, and add scallops and wine. Heat to just a bare simmer, and let simmer just until scallops are opaque; do not overcook.

Using a slotted spoon, scoop out the scallops and mushrooms, and divide between two large scallop shells, or two ovenproof ramekins.

Turn up the heat under the liquid remaining in the saucepan, and let it boil hard for just a minute or so, to reduce. Turn heat back down, and stir in cream. Now, using a whisk and your guar or xanthan shaker, thicken the sauce up a bit. Add half the cheese, and whisk until it's melted.

Divide the sauce between the two shells or ramekins, and divide the remaining cheese between the two servings. Run the shells or ramekins under a low broiler, about 4" (10 cm) from the heat, until the tops have gotten golden—just 4 or 5 minutes. Serve.

Yield: 2 servings

Each with: 453 calories; 34 g fat; 26 g protein; 6 g carbohydrate; trace dietary fiber; 6 g usable carbs.

⊚ Scallops Vinaigrette

Fast and simple.

>   2 tablespoons (20 g) minced onion
>   ½ red bell pepper, cut in matchstick strips
>   4 teaspoons olive oil
>   2 cups (350 g) bay scallops
>   4 tablespoons (60 ml) Italian salad dressing—I used Paul Newman's
>   Guar or xanthan

In your big skillet, sauté the onion and pepper in the olive oil for a couple of minutes. Add the scallops, and sauté until they're white clear through. Stir in the salad dressing, and simmer for a couple of minutes. Thicken a little if you like, and serve. Cauli-rice is nice with this, though not essential.

Yield: 2 servings

Each with: 437 calories; 25 g fat; 40 g protein; 11 g carbohydrate; 1 g dietary fiber; 10 g usable carbs.

Stir-Fried Scallops and Asparagus

This stir-fry has a light, springlike flavor.

>10 asparagus spears
>10 scallions
>¼ cup (60 ml) canola oil
>2 cups (350 g) bay scallops
>½ cup (60 g) shredded carrot
>2 teaspoons soy sauce

Snap the bottoms off of your asparagus where the stalks break naturally. Slice on the diagonal into ½" (1.25 cm) pieces. Slice your scallions, too.

Heat the oil in your big skillet, or in a wok if you have one, over high heat. Add the scallops, asparagus, scallions, and carrot. Stir-fry until the asparagus is tender-crisp and the scallops are done through. Stir in the soy sauce, and serve.

Yield: 2 to 3 servings

Assuming 2, each will have: 508 calories; 29 g fat; 43 g protein; 18 g carbohydrate; 5 g dietary fiber; 13 g usable carbs.

Now we come to the shrimp recipes. It's a funny thing about writing a cookbook; you go along for months, cooking this, cooking that, and entering it into your recipe management program. Then you get around to copying and pasting it all into book form, and suddenly you realize you've got a lot of some kinds of recipes. I have a lot of shrimp recipes. And for a few very simple reasons: Shrimp are quick and easy to cook, just as easy to vary, and my husband really likes them. So here you are—a whole big pile of shrimp recipes. Hope you like shrimp as much as my husband does!

Curried Shrimp in Coconut Milk

Exotic!

14 ounces (400 g) coconut milk

1 1/2 tablespoons (11 g) curry powder

1 clove garlic, crushed

1 teaspoon chili garlic paste

1 pound (455 g) large shrimp, shelled

1 tablespoon (14 ml) fish sauce

2 teaspoons Splenda

3 scallions, sliced thin

1/4 cup (15 g) chopped cilantro

In a large, shallow pan combine the coconut milk, curry powder, garlic, and chili garlic paste. Heat over medium-low flame, and let simmer 7 to 10 minutes.

Add shrimp, fish sauce, and Splenda. Stir, and let simmer for 5 to 7 more minutes, or until shrimp are pink clear through.

Stir in scallions, let simmer for another minute, and serve—spoon over cauli-rice if desired, or eat as is. Top each serving with chopped cilantro.

Yield: 3 servings

Each with: 450 calories; 34 g fat; 29 g protein; 12 g carbohydrate; 4 g dietary fiber; 8 g usable carbs.

Easy Shrimp in Garlic Herb Cream Sauce

Too easy! You may use full-fat garlic and herb cheese—Boursin or Allouette—if you prefer. Your calorie count will go up, but not your carb count.

        1 pound (455 g) large shrimp, shelled
        2 tablespoons (30 g) butter
        ½ cup (115 g) light garlic and herb spreadable cheese
        ¼ cup (60 ml) heavy cream
        4 tablespoons (15 g) chopped fresh parsley

Make sure your shrimp are shelled and ready to go. Melt the butter in your big skillet, over medium heat, and throw in the shrimp. Sauté for 2 to 3 minutes per side, or until pink. Add the cheese, and stir until it melts. Your sauce will look like a gloppy mess. Do not panic. Stir in the cream, and the whole thing will smooth out beautifully as you stir. Transfer to serving plates, top with parsley, and serve.

Yield: 3 servings

Each with: 340 calories; 23 g fat; 29 g protein; 3 g carbohydrate; 1 g dietary fiber; 2 g usable carbs.

Hot Paprika Shrimp

        1 pound (455 g) large shrimp, shelled
        ¼ cup (60 ml) oil
        4 teaspoons paprika
        4 teaspoons chili garlic paste
        4 cloves garlic, crushed

Just sauté your shrimp in the oil for about 5 minutes, until it's pink. Sprinkle the paprika over it, and stir in the chili garlic paste and garlic. Cook for another minute or so, and serve.

Yield: 2 to 3 servings

Assuming 3, each will have: 297 calories; 20 g fat; 26 g protein; 4 g carbohydrate; 1 g dietary fiber; 3 g usable carbs.

◎ Shrimp and Artichoke "Risotto"

Not only is it lower carb and lower calorie to use cauli-rice to make "risotto," but it's tremendously quicker and easier, too. I adapted this recipe from one of Emeril's, and it's fabulous. You can use precooked or raw shrimp in this—since you're using the tiniest shrimp you can find, the cooking time is next to nothing anyway. Just make sure your shrimp are pink before you serve this—which should take approximately a minute and a half.

½ head cauliflower, shredded
½ cup (80 g) chopped onion
4 cloves garlic
1 tablespoon (15 ml) olive oil
1 tablespoon (2.5 g) dried basil, or ¼ cup (15 g) chopped fresh basil
1 tablespoon (15 ml) lemon juice
1 teaspoon salt or Vege-Sal
½ teaspoon pepper
1 14-ounce (400 g) can artichoke hearts, drained and chopped
1 teaspoon Creole seasoning, purchased or homemade
½ pound (225 g) teeny-weeny shrimp
½ cup (120 ml) heavy cream
¾ cup (120 g) grated Parmesan cheese
4 scallions, sliced, including the crisp part of the green shoot
Guar or xanthan

Put the cauliflower in a microwaveable casserole with a lid. Add a couple of tablespoons of water, cover, and microwave on high for 6 minutes.

While that's happening, throw the onion and garlic in your big, heavy skillet along with the olive oil. Sauté over medium-low heat until the microwave beeps—you want the onion to be turning translucent.

Okay, cauliflower's done. Pull it out, drain it, and add it to the onions and garlic. Stir in the basil, lemon juice, salt or Vege-Sal, pepper, chopped artichoke hearts, Creole seasoning, shrimp, and cream. Let the whole thing simmer for a minute or two, to blend the flavors. Stir in the Parmesan and scallions, thicken just until good and creamy with your guar or xanthan shaker, and serve.

Yield: 4 servings

Each with: 321 calories; 20 g fat; 22 g protein; 14 g carbohydrate; 2 g dietary fiber; 12 g usable carbs.

Shrimp in Sherry

This calls for 18 ounces (500 g) of shrimp because the big shrimp I get at my grocery run just about 1 ounce (30 g) apiece, and 6 big shrimp seemed a good serving size. But if you only have a pound of shrimp, don't sweat it.

18 ounces big darned shrimp—about an ounce apiece—shelled
3 tablespoons (45 ml) olive oil
3 tablespoons (45 ml) dry sherry
1/4 teaspoon hot sauce
Guar or xanthan

Have your shrimp shelled and ready to go. In your big skillet, sauté the shrimp in the olive oil over medium-high heat until it's pink almost all over. Add the sherry and hot sauce, and stir. Let cook another minute or two. Thicken the pan juices just a tiny bit with your guar or xanthan shaker, and serve.

Yield: 3 servings

Each with: 267 calories; 15 g fat; 28 g protein; trace carbohydrate; trace dietary fiber; trace usable carb.

Spicy Shrimp in Beer and Butter

6 tablespoons (90 g) butter
3/4 teaspoon salt
1 1/2 teaspoons cayenne
3/4 teaspoon dried thyme
1/2 teaspoon dried rosemary, ground
1/2 teaspoon dried oregano
6 cloves garlic, crushed
1 tablespoon (15 ml) Worcestershire sauce
24 ounces (680 g) great big shrimp, shelled
3/4 cup (180 ml) light beer—I used Miller Lite or Milwaukee's Best Light

In your big, heavy skillet, over very low heat, start the butter melting. As it melts, stir in the seasonings. When the butter is all melted, add the shrimp—I like to use good, big ones, about an ounce apiece. Let the shrimp sauté 2 to 3 minutes per side, letting them get acquainted with the seasoned butter.

Now pour the light beer into the skillet. Cover the skillet, and let the shrimp cook for 2 to 3 minutes. Uncover, and let them cook for another 2 minutes or so.

Remove the shrimp to serving plates, and turn up the heat under the skillet. Let the sauce boil hard until it's reduced by about half, and pour over the shrimp. Serve.

Yield: 3 to 4 servings

Assuming 3, each will have: 412 calories; 25 g fat (56.6% calories from fat); 38 g protein; 5 g carbohydrate; 1 g dietary fiber; 4 g usable carbs.

◎ Scallops with Morroccan Spices

Fast, easy, tasty, and different enough to be interesting! You can use bay scallops if you prefer, I just think the big sea scallops make for a more impressive presentation.

> 1 pound (455 g) sea scallops
> 2 tablespoons (30 ml) olive oil
> 2 tablespoons (30 ml) butter
> 2 cloves garlic, crushed
> 1 teaspoon ground cumin
> 1/2 teaspoon ground ginger
> 2 teaspoons paprika
> 1/2 teaspoon hot sauce
> 1/2 lemon
> 1/4 cup (12 g) chopped fresh cilantro

In your big, heavy skillet, heat the olive oil and butter over medium heat, and swirl them together. Add the garlic, and let it cook for just a minute, then add the cumin, ginger, paprika, and hot sauce. Now add the scallops, and saute, stirring frequently for about 5–7 minutes, or until they're opaque.

Squeeze the lemon over the scallops, and transfer to 4 serving plates. Scatter a tablespoon of cilantro over each plate, and serve.

Yield: 4 servings, each with: 220 Calories; 14g Fat; 19g Protein; 5g Carbohydrate; trace Dietary Fiber; 5 g usable carbs.

Sweet and Spicy Shrimp

2 tablespoons (30 ml) oil

½ teaspoon cayenne pepper

1 ½ teaspoons five-spice powder

2 cloves garlic, crushed

1 tablespoon (6 g) grated gingerroot

2 tablespoons (20 g) minced onion

2 tablespoons (30 ml) rice vinegar

2 tablespoons (3 g) Splenda

⅛ teaspoon blackstrap molasses

1 pound (455 g) large shrimp, shelled

Salt and pepper

2–3 lime wedges

In a large, heavy skillet over medium-low flame, heat the oil, and add the cayenne, five-spice, garlic, ginger, and onion. Stir for about 2 minutes, or until fragrant, taking care not to let garlic turn brown.

Stir in the rice vinegar, Splenda, and blackstrap. Now add the shrimp, and stir to coat with the seasonings. Sauté shrimp, turning frequently, until they're pink clear through. Salt and pepper lightly, transfer to serving plates, and serve with a lime wedge.

Yield: 2 to 3 servings

Assuming 2, each will have: 315 calories; 15 g fat; 38 g protein; 6 g carbohydrate; trace dietary fiber; 5 g usable carbs.

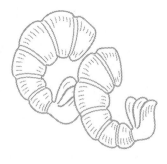

Marlene D. Wurdeman's Easy Tuna Casserole

Here's a casserole for all of us tuna fans.

2 6-ounce (170 g) cans chunk-style tuna
½ cup (60 g) chopped celery
⅓ cup (35 g) sliced scallions, including the crisp part of the green shoot
1 large head cauliflower
½–⅔ cup (115–160 g) sour cream
½ cup (120 g) mayonnaise
2 teaspoons yellow mustard
½ teaspoon Dried thyme
Salt and pepper to taste
1–2 small zucchini, scrubbed, sliced
1–2 cups (180 g) shredded Monterey Jack or chedder cheese
1 small tomato, chopped (optional)

Preheat oven to 350°F (180°C).

Drain and flake the tuna. In a large bowl, combine tuna, celery, and green onion.

Using only the white tops of the cauliflower, slice the cauliflower completely from stems and stalks. Steam until fork tender (don't allow to get too soft) and add to tuna.

In a small bowl, combine sour cream, mayonnaise, mustard, thyme, and salt and pepper. Blend into the tuna mixture.

Spoon half the mixture into a buttered 2-quart (1.9 L) casserole. Top with half the zucchini. Repeat layers. Top with cheese. Bake for 30 to 40 minutes or until hot and bubbly.

Sprinkle with the chopped tomato, and serve.

Yield: 4 to 6 servings

Assuming 4, each will have: 539 calories; 44 g fat; 32 g protein; 9 g carbohydrate; 3 g dietary fiber; 6 g usable carbs.

◎ Susan Higgs's Tuna Roll-Ups

> 1 7-ounce (200 g) package vacuum-packed tuna (Susan loves this stuff because you don't have to drain it!)
>
> 1 tablespoon (15 g) mayonnaise
>
> 1/2 teaspoon lemon juice
>
> 1/2 teaspoon dried parsley flakes
>
> Salt and pepper to taste
>
> 1 8-ounce (225 g) package hard salami (the smaller round ones)
>
> 1 6-ounce (170 g) package sliced Swiss cheese

Mix tuna, mayo, lemon juice, parsley, and salt and pepper together in a bowl, tasting for seasoning and adjusting as desired. Lay down a slice of salami and put a piece of Swiss cheese on it, trimming so that it fits the round salami. Place a teaspoonful or two of tuna on the cheese and roll it up jellyroll–style, securing with one or two toothpicks. (One if you are going to use these for lunch or a snack. Two if you are going to make appetizers.) Repeat until you're out of tuna, salami, and cheese. Refrigerate at least 2 hours. If serving as appetizers, cut jellyrolls in half, ensuring that there is a toothpick in each piece. Serve.

Yield: About 4 servings

Each with: 384 calories; 26 g fat; 33 g protein; 3 g carbohydrate; trace dietary fiber; 3 g usable carbs.

◎ Leslie's Crab-Stuffed Poblano Peppers

Here's an easy but impressive recipe. Our tester, Ray, says to tell you they're pretty hot, but then, some of us like that! He also says this would impress a dinner date, should you have someone you'd like to cook for, fellas.

> 6 large poblano peppers
>
> 1 pound (455 g) crab, picked over for shells
>
> 8 ounces (225 g) cream cheese, softened
>
> 2 cloves garlic, pressed
>
> 1 cup (120 g) shredded sharp cheddar cheese
>
> 1 teaspoon Splenda

Broil peppers on all sides until charred. Place in paper bag to steam. Peel off skins. Make a slit in the side of each pepper and remove seeds. For filling, combine all other ingredients. Carefully stuff into peppers. Place seam-side up in a baking dish that has been sprayed with butter-flavored or olive oil nonstick cooking spray. Spray tops of peppers with spray. Bake for 30 minutes at 350°F (180°C) or until filling is bubbly.

Yield: Serves 3

Each getting: 599 calories; 41 g fat; 45 g protein; 15 g carbohydrate; 2 g dietary fiber; 13 g usable carbs.

◎ Winnie Spicer's Favorite Imperial Crab Casserole

    1 egg, well beaten
    1 cup (240 g) mayonnaise
    1–2 teaspoon Old Bay Seasoning
       (look for this in the spice aisle, it's widely distributed)
    3 dashes Worcestershire sauce
    1 pound (455 g) lump backfin crabmeat
       (our tester just used what crabmeat she could find, and said it was great)
    1/3 cup (40 g) grated white cheddar cheese
       (optional, or use yellow cheese)
    1 tablespoon (15 g) butter for topping

To beaten egg, add mayonnaise and seasonings. Mix well and carefully fold in the crabmeat so as not to break up the lumps. Put in a buttered casserole dish. If using the cheese, sprinkle on top. Dot with 1 tablespoon butter. Bake in preheated 350°F (180°C) oven for 25–30 minutes. Ovens vary so be sure to check early!

Yield: 4 servings

Each with: 587 calories; 55 g fat; 28 g protein; trace carbohydrate; 0 g dietary fiber; a trace usable carbs.

Susan Higgs's Deviled Crab

Our tester, Ray, said this was easy, if a bit pricey. He also says that if you can afford to spring for a full pound of crab, you should!

1/2 pound (225 g) claw or backfin crabmeat
4 tablespoons (60 g) mayonnaise
1/2 teaspoon paprika
1 hard-boiled egg, diced
2 tablespoons (30 g) butter, melted
2 tablespoons (30 g) Worcestershire sauce
2 tablespoons (30 ml) very dry sherry
1/4 teaspoon Tabasco
1/4 teaspoon salt
1 tablespoon (15 g) Dijon mustard
3 tablespoons (45 g) grated Parmesan cheese
1/4 teaspoon nutmeg, fresh grated if possible

Preheat oven to 350°F (180°C).

Clean crabmeat and ensure there aren't any shell fragments in it. Reserve 1 tablespoon of mayonnaise and the paprika. Combine all other ingredients, mixing well, and placing in a small casserole or 4 seafood baking dishes or 4 clean crab shells. Frost the top of the crab mixture with mayo and then sprinkle with paprika. Bake 20 minutes. Place dish(es) under the broiler for 1 minute or until the mayo topping puffs up and browns slightly.

Yield: 4 servings

Each with: 261 calories; 21 g fat; 15 g protein; 2 g carbohydrate; trace dietary fiber; 2 g usable carbs.

Grilled Fish with Caper Sauce

This is more of a method for grilling a wide variety of fish fillets, and adding a simple but elegantly piquant sauce. The main element of this recipe is the sauce. Ingredient amounts are not important, you can vary to taste. The resulting mixture should be something you spoon over the fish, not a pourable sauce. (Our tester said he used 2 tablespoons of each of the following for 1 pound of fish fillets, and it worked very well.) This is a very piquant sauce, not for the timid of palate, but most delicious!

As for grilling the fish, some people prefer to do it in the Spanish style of first salting the fillets, letting them sit for 15 minutes or so, then rinsing and drying them, brushing them with olive oil, and grilling them on a cast-iron griddle. Swordfish and sea bass are wonderful this way; so are tilapia fillets (which are much cheaper).

Garlic, finely chopped
Parsley, flat-leaf preferable, finely chopped (or half parsley, half cilantro)
Anchovies, finely chopped (if omitting, salt to taste)
Capers, drained
Fresh lemon juice
Olive oil

Mix the above ingredients, spoon over grilled fish, and serve.

Yield: 4 servings

If sauce is made with the suggested 2 tablespoons of each ingredient, each serving will have: 177 calories; 8 g fat; 23 g protein; 2 g carbohydrate; trace dietary fiber; 2 g usable carbs.

◎ Susan Higgs's Shrimp-Stuffed Fish

This can be done ahead and then baked later.

> ½ cup (120 g) butter, divided
> 2 cloves garlic, crushed
> 1 small onion, very finely chopped
> ¼ green pepper, very finely chopped
> 12 cooked, peeled medium shrimp, divided
> 4 ounces (115 g) cream cheese, cut into 1-ounce (30 g) cubes
>   so that it will melt more quickly
> 1 tablespoon (4 g) fresh parsley, chopped
> ½ teaspoon salt
> ¼ teaspoon pepper
> ½ teaspoon lemon zest (save the lemon for the sauce recipe;
>   you'll need the juice)
> 4 large fillets of flounder or sole (or favorite thin fish)
>   —about 1 ½ pounds (680 g)

Heat skillet and add ¼ cup (60 g) butter. Once butter is melted, add garlic, onion, and green pepper, sautéing until golden. Dice 8 shrimp and add to skillet. Add cream cheese, parsley, salt, pepper, and lemon zest. Mix well and remove from heat once cream cheese has melted.

Put 2 to 3 tablespoons (30 g) of stuffing mixture on a fillet and roll it up, securing with toothpick if necessary. Place in pan for baking or zipper-lock bag for chilling. If chilling, remove from refrigerator 30 minutes before baking.

When ready to bake, preheat oven to 350°F (180°C). Butter a 9" x 13" (22.5 x 32.5 cm) pan, or spray it with nonstick spray, and arrange fish rolls in it. Melt the other ¼ cup (60 g) of butter and pour evenly over fish rolls. Bake 25 to 30 minutes.

While fillets are baking, sauté or boil your remaining 4 shrimp for a garnish, cooking just until pink. Then make the following sauce to pour over fillets before serving.

Sauce:

- 1/2 cup (60 g) butter, softened
- 3 egg yolks
- 2 tablespoons (30 ml) lemon juice—from the lemon whose zest you grated
- 1/4 teaspoon cayenne pepper (or to your desired heat level)
- 1/4 teaspoon salt
- 1/8 teaspoon white pepper (optional)

Combine sauce ingredients in pan and heat over low heat. Remove the toothpicks from the fish rolls, pour on the sauce, garnish each with a whole shrimp, and serve.

Yield: Makes 4 servings

Each with: 721 calories; 61 g fat; 39 g protein; 5 g carbohydrate; 1 g dietary fiber; 4 g usable carbs.

◎ Naked Shrimp Stir-Fry

Here's another stir-fry from our recipe tester, Ray Stevens. He says, "This is basically stir-boiling the veggies. Have everything ready and measured out—it happens fast and requires attention the whole time. This has no sauce to it. It is basically just the veggies and meat. That is what is good about it."

- 12 ounces (340 g) medium-sized shrimp, shelled
- 1/2 tablespoon (7 g) peanut or canola oil
- 2 tablespoons (30 ml) soy sauce
- 1 teaspoon dark sesame oil
- 1 teaspoon garlic
- 4 cups (600 g) frozen stir-fry mix vegetables, thawed
- 1 cup (240 ml) water in a ceramic cup by the stove

In a wok or big skillet, over high heat, stir-fry the shrimp in the oil for about 2 minutes. Add the soy sauce, sesame oil, and garlic. Stir-fry 2 minutes.

Add veggies. Stir-fry, adding about 1 tablespoon of water. Keep "stir-frying," adding water a couple of tablespoons at a time as needed to keep a noticeable pool in the center till cooked. Remove from heat and continue to stir and add water till steam stops appearing. Take care not to burn. Serve.

Yield: 2 servings

With: 215 calories; 6 g fat (24.2% calories from fat); 27 g protein; 13 g carbohydrate; 4 g dietary fiber; 9 g usable carbs.

Susan Higgs's Broiled Fish with Creamy Topping

Our tester, Ray, says this recipe is easy and really good!

> 3 tablespoons (45 g) sour cream
> 2 tablespoons (30 g) mayonnaise
> ½ teaspoon lemon zest
> ½ teaspoon dill (or curry powder), optional
> 4 swordfish or halibut steaks, ½ pound each (or other fish you prefer)
> Seasoned salt
> Lemon wedges

Mix together sour cream, mayo, lemon zest, and dill (or curry powder) if using. Broil your fish until it's almost done—about 4 to 5 minutes per side. Remove pan, and frost pieces of fish evenly with the sour cream/mayo mixture. Sprinkle the top with seasoned salt. Return to broiler and cook until fish is done. Serve immediately with lemon wedges.

Yield: Makes 4 servings

Each having: 349 calories; 17 g fat; 45 g protein; 1 g carbohydrate; trace dietary fiber; 1 g usable carb.

chapter nine

Beef

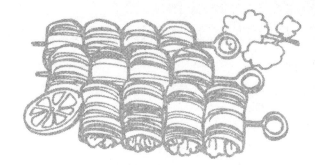

One of the most persistent images people have of a low-carb diet is that it consists of wall-to-wall steaks and bunless burgers. We know that's not true; we eat a fantastic variety of foods. But the idea persists, largely because we've had it drilled into our heads that beef is evil and unhealthy and bad for us, so the idea of eating it without fear is exotic.

I don't believe in a steady diet of any one food, but my fear and guilt about eating beef are gone, and a beautiful thing it is. Still, who wants to eat plain bunless burgers and naked broiled steaks day after day? Here is a whole stampede of ideas of what to do with beef!

Portobello Fillets

Here's a very simple way to make those wonderful but pricey little fillets mignon seem bigger, while impressing the heck out of your company.
Add a big tossed salad and a loaf of crusty bread for the carb eaters, and you've got an elegant meal that takes practically no work.

> 4 large portobello mushrooms
> 1 cup (240 ml) balsamic vinaigrette dressing
> 4 fillets mignon, about 5 ounces (140 g) each
> Olive oil for brushing

Lay your portobellos in a shallow baking dish, gill-side up, and pour the balsamic vinaigrette over them. Turn them over once or twice, to make sure they're thoroughly coated in the dressing, then let them sit for 10 to 15 minutes.

Okay, now you're going to multitask: Heat up the broiler to high, and brush your steaks with a little olive oil. Also heat up your electric tabletop grill.

Start your fillets broiling close to the heat, and set your oven timer—I'd probably give them about 5 to 5 ½ minutes per side, but cook them to your own preference. When you turn them over, put the marinated mushrooms in your electric grill. Let them cook for about 5 minutes. Your steak and your mushrooms should be done right about the same moment!

Put each mushroom on a plate, and put a fillet on top of each, then serve piping hot.

Dana's note: Feel free to cut a larger steak into individual portions to serve on your mushrooms, if you prefer. Those fillets just come exactly the right size. Do, however, use a good thick steak for this—at least 1 ¼" (3.125 cm).

Yield: 4 servings

Each with: 717 calories; 64 g fat; 28 g protein; 9 g carbohydrate; 2 g dietary fiber; 7 g usable carbs. However, this analysis assumes you consume all of the balsamic vinaigrette, while in actuality some will be left in the dish you marinated the mushrooms in. So you'll actually get fewer carbs and calories than this.

Marco Polo Steak

Far tastier than the simplicity of this recipe would imply—and it comes with its very own easy vegetable dish! (See page 158 for Marco Polo Stir-Fried Vegetables.)

> 1 batch Marco Polo Marinade (page 445)
> 1 ¹/₂–2 pounds (680 g–1 kg) steak—rib eye, sirloin,
>   or whatever you have that's tender and fit for broiling

First make your marinade. Using a fork, pierce the steak all over. Then put it in either a big zipper-lock plastic bag or a shallow, nonreactive pan. Either way, pour the marinade over it. If you're using the bag, press the air out as you seal the bag. Turn your steak over a few times to make sure it's coated, then let it marinate for at least an hour, and more won't hurt.

When dinnertime rolls around, pull out your steak, and pour off the marinade into a bowl. Broil your steak as close as you can to your broiler, set on "high," basting it once or twice with the reserved marinade. Your timing will depend on the thickness of your steak, and how well done you like it. I have my steaks cut 1 ¹/₄" (3.125 cm) thick, and give them about 6 to 6 ¹/₂ minutes per side.

Yield: Assuming 2 pounds (1 kg) of steak, you'll have 5 servings

Each with: 596 calories; 6 g of carbohydrate per serving, but that's assuming you eat all the marinade, which you don't, by any means. I'd guess no more than 3 g per serving; 34 g protein; 4 g fat; trace fiber. Carb and calorie count will be lower because you will not eat all of the marinade.

◎ Orange Tequila Steak

Here's a Southwestern twist for your steak. I'd probably serve this with Chipotle Cheese Fauxtatoes (page 137) and a salad with avocados in it.

> 1 pound (455 g) beef steak—rib eye is my choice, but sirloin or T-bone should do fine
>
> 3 cloves garlic
>
> 1/4 cup (60 ml) lemon juice
>
> 1/4 cup (60 ml) lime juice
>
> 1 shot tequila
>
> 1 1/2 teaspoons chili powder
>
> 1 tablespoon (3 g) Splenda
>
> 1 1/2 teaspoons dried oregano
>
> 3 tablespoons (45 ml) olive oil
>
> 1/4 teaspoon orange extract

Throw your steak in a big darned zipper-lock bag. Mix together everything else, and pour it into the bag. Seal the bag, pressing out the air as you go. Turn the bag to coat the steak, then throw it in the fridge and let the steak marinate for at least a few hours, and a whole day is fine.

Pull the steak out of the fridge, and pour off the marinade into a bowl. Now you get to decide—outside on the grill or inside in the broiler? Either way, grill or broil your steak fast, close to high heat (but if you're using a charcoal grill, keep down flare-ups; they char, not cook). If your steak is 1 1/4" (3.125 cm) thick (that's how I have the meat guys cut mine), about 6 to 6 1/2 minutes per side will be right for medium to medium-rare. Baste at least 2 or 3 times with the marinade during cooking—but quit with at least 2 or 3 minutes of cooking time to go; you want the heat to kill any raw beef germs!

Yield: 2 to 3 servings

Assuming 3, each will have: 560 calories; 46 g fat; 26 g protein; 6 g carbohydrate; 1 g dietary fiber—but this assumes you consume all of the marinade, which you won't. I'd guess no more than 3 g per serving.

Pepper Steak with Whiskey Sauce

1 tablespoon (15 g) butter

2 tablespoons (20 g) minced onion

1 cup (240 ml) beef broth

1/2 teaspoon beef bouillon granules

1/4 teaspoon pepper

1 clove garlic

1 1/2 ounces (45 ml) bourbon

Guar or xanthan

1 1/2 teaspoons coarsely ground pepper

1 pound (455 g) steak, 1 1/4" (3.125 cm) thick
  —rib eye, sirloin, or T-bone would all be fine

1 tablespoon (15 g) butter

1 tablespoon (15 ml) oil

Melt 1 tablespoon (15 g) butter in a medium saucepan, and add the onion. Sauté 4 or 5 minutes, till it's just turning golden. Add beef broth, bouillon granules, pepper, garlic, and bourbon, and let the whole thing boil until it's reduced by about half. Thicken just a little with your guar or xanthan shaker— you want it about the texture of heavy cream—right before you serve the steak.

While the sauce is cooking down, sprinkle the pepper evenly over both sides of the steak, and press it into the surface. Put your big, heavy skillet over medium-high heat, and add 1 tablespoon (15 g) butter and oil. As soon as the butter and oil are hot, throw in the steak. Assuming your steak is 1 1/4" (3.125 cm) thick, I think 6 1/2 minutes per side is about right—that gives me a steak that's medium-rare—but cook it to your liking. Serve with the whiskey sauce.

Yield: 3 servings

Each with: 503 calories; 39 g fat; 26 g protein; 3 g carbohydrate; trace dietary fiber; 3 g usable carbs.

◎ Lori Herbel's Country Fried Steak

I'm glad Lori came up with this! I tried, but being from New Jersey originally, I lack the requisite experience with "the real thing," and the results were dismal. But our tester, Julie, a Texan, liked this a lot!

> 1 ¼ pounds (680 g) round steaks (or other similar steak cuts)
> 1–2 eggs
> Pork rind crumbs
> Oil for frying

Tenderize the round steak by pounding it with a tenderizer hammer or other blunt object. Whisk egg in a shallow bowl. Dip steaks into beaten egg and then into the pork rind crumbs. Fry on both sides in a small amount of oil in a nonstick frying pan until done.

Tester's note: Julie says that if you want to, you can simply pound a small, unopened bag of pork rinds with a hammer until they're finely crushed, and avoid dirtying your food processor.

Yield: Serves 4

Each with: 286 calories; 19 g fat; 26 g protein; trace carbohydrate; 0 g dietary fiber.

Gwen Meehan's Delicious Peppers and Onions with Cheesy Steak

Our tester, Ray Stevens, didn't have leftover steak, so he used chuck steak he cooked for the occasion, and said, "I have eaten a lot worse than this at fancy restaurants!"

1 red pepper, cut into strips
1 orange pepper, cut into strips
½ red onion, sliced
3 tablespoons (45 g) butter
½ cup (120 ml) water
Leftover steak, sliced (about 6 ounces [170 g])
1 cup (120 g) shredded pepper Jack cheese

Sauté the peppers and onion in the butter in a large skillet over medium-high heat. Once the veggies are a little brown (almost a grilled look) and the onion is translucent, add the water and cover. Cook for about 10 minutes, until the peppers get soft and their skins are almost peeling off.

Take the lid off to let water evaporate. Push the pepper mix to the side and add your sliced leftover steak to the skillet, just to warm it. Put the mixture in bowls and top it with pepper Jack cheese.

Yield: 2 servings

Each with: 597 calories; 49 g fat; 29 g protein; 13 g carbohydrate; 2 g dietary fiber; 11 g usable carbs.

◎ Smoky Marinated Steak

This has a subtle but great smoky flavor that really enhances the meat.

    1 pound (455 g) T-bone steak at least 1″ (2.5 cm) thick
        (sirloin or rib eye would do, too)
    1 tablespoon (15 ml) liquid smoke flavoring
        (most big grocery stores carry this)
    1 teaspoon salt or Vege-Sal
    1 clove garlic, crushed
    1 dash pepper
    1 teaspoon olive oil
    1/8 teaspoon onion powder
    1/4 cup (60 ml) water

Put your steak in a zipper-lock plastic bag. Mix together everything else, pour into the bag, and seal, pressing out the air as you go. Turn the bag once or twice to coat, and throw your steak in the fridge for a few hours at least, and a day won't hurt a bit.

When dinnertime rolls around, pull out the steak, and drain off the marinade into a bowl, for basting. Broil very close to a high broiler—for a steak about 1 1/4″ (3.125 cm), I like about 6 minutes per side, but do it to your liking. Baste halfway through cooking each side, using the reserved marinade.

Note: If you like, sautéed mushrooms would be great on top of this, but they're hardly necessary; it's great as is.

Yield: 3 servings

Each with: 276 calories; 20 g fat; 23 g protein; 1 g carbohydrate; trace dietary fiber; 1 g usable carb.

◎ Steak with Brandy-Stilton Cream Sauce

This is decadent beyond belief, and absolutely magnificent. Stilton, if you haven't tried it, is a very strong blue cheese from England. If you can't find it, use whatever blue cheese you've got kicking around, and I'm sure it will be fine.

> 1 pound (455 g) beef rib eye steak, 1 1/4" (3.125 cm) thick (or use any tender, broilable cut)
> 1 tablespoon (15 ml) olive oil
> 2 tablespoons (30 ml) brandy
> 1/2 cup (120 ml) heavy cream
> 2 ounces (55 g) Stilton cheese, crumbled

In your big, heavy skillet, over medium-high heat, start pan-broiling the steak in the olive oil. About 6 minutes per side is right for my tastes, but do it to your preferred degree of doneness.

When the steak is done, remove to a platter and keep it warm!

Pour the brandy into the skillet, and stir it around, dissolving all the brown bits stuck to the skillet. Now pour in the cream, and stir it around. Add the Stilton, and stir till it's melted and the sauce smooths out. Pour over the steak, and serve.

Yield: 3 servings

Each with: 597 calories; 51 g fat; 26 g protein; 1 g carbohydrate; 0 g dietary fiber; 1 g usable carb.

◎ Bacon Chili Burgers

Something interesting to do with your ground beef when you're weary of plain burgers!

    1 pound (455 g) ground chuck
    2 tablespoons (30 g) chili garlic paste
    ¼ cup (40 g) minced onion
    6 slices bacon, cooked and drained

Put your ground chuck and chili garlic paste in a mixing bowl. Add your onion, too. Crumble the bacon into the bowl as well. Now, using clean hands, smoosh everything together until it's well mixed. Form into 3 burgers. Put them on a plate, and chill for half an hour or so—this isn't strictly necessary, but it makes them easier to handle.

Now you can cook your burgers—I like to give mine 6 minutes in my electric tabletop grill, but you can broil them for 4 to 5 minutes per side, or even cook them on your grill outdoors.

Yield: 3 servings

Each with: 485 calories; 38 g fat; 31 g protein; 2 g carbohydrate; trace dietary fiber; 2 g usable carbs.

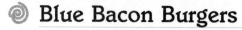 # Blue Bacon Burgers

Here's a bacon cheeseburger with the bacon and cheese cooked in!

> 1 ⅓ pounds (590 g) ground chuck
> 4 tablespoons (30 g) blue cheese, crumbled
> 4 tablespoons (60 g) blue cheese salad dressing
> 4 tablespoons (40 g) minced red onion
> 6 slices cooked bacon, crumbled

Assemble everything in a mixing bowl. Using clean hands, smoosh everything together well. Form into 4 to 6 burgers. It's good to chill these for 30 minutes before cooking, but it's not essential.

I like to cook my burgers in my electric tabletop grill for about 5 to 6 minutes, but you could cook these about 5 minutes per side under the broiler or in a hot skillet, or even cook them on your grill outside.

Yield: 4 to 6 servings

Assuming 4, each will have: 565 calories; 46 g fat; 32 g protein; 2 g carbohydrate; trace dietary fiber, 2 g usable carbs.

◎ Linda Magsaysay's Chili Burgers

A truly original, hot and spicy way of varying your ground beef. Our tester, Julie, called this "good stuff," and said she'd order it at a restaurant.

2 teaspoons Worcestershire sauce

2 teaspoons raspberry vinegar

2 tablespoons (30 ml) olive oil

8 ounces (225 g) crimini mushrooms, sliced

1 1/2 pounds (680 g) hamburger

1 small onion, chopped

2 cloves garlic, chopped

1 pickled jalapeno, chopped

3 tablespoons (45 g) tomato paste

2 1/2 tablespoons (25 g) chili powder

Good pinch salt and pepper

1 egg, beaten

1 cup (120 g) shredded mozzarella cheese

In a bowl, mix the Worcestershire sauce and raspberry vinegar, and whisk in the olive oil. Pour this mixture into a big skillet, sauté the mushrooms in it till soft. Set aside.

Mix meat with onion, garlic, jalapeno, tomato paste, chili powder, salt and pepper, and beaten egg; shape into 4 large patties, and grill for 8 minutes (Linda uses her trusty electric grill).

When burgers are done, top with cooked mushrooms, then add cheese and allow to melt.

Serve with tossed salad or coleslaw.

Linda says: "Really easy and fast to make, and absolutely delicious, and everybody has hamburger in their freezer."

Yield: 6 servings

Each will have: 508 calories; 41 g fat; 26 g protein; 10 g carbohydrate; 3 g dietary fiber; 7 g usable carbs.

Salisbury Steak

Talk about your old-time comfort food! Our tester said she'd happily pay for this in a restaurant.

2 pounds (1 kg) ground round
¼ cup (25 g) oat bran
¼ cup (12 g) crushed pork rinds
4 tablespoons (60 ml) heavy cream, divided
½ cup (65 g) minced onion, divided
1 ½ tablespoons (22 ml) Worcestershire sauce, divided
½ teaspoon salt or Vege-sal
¼ teaspoon pepper
8 ounces (225 g) sliced mushrooms
1 cup (240 ml) beef broth
½ teaspoon beef bouillon granules
1 clove garlic
1 teaspoon tomato paste
½ cup (120 ml) Carb Countdown Dairy Beverage
guar or xanthan
salt and pepper to taste

In a big mixing bowl, combine your ground round, oat bran, pork rind crumbs, 2 tablespoons of the heavy cream, ¼ cup of the minced onion, 1 tablespoon Worcestershire, and the first salt and pepper. Using clean hands, smoosh these together until they're well-blended. Form into 6 oval patties. Brown them on either side in a hot skillet, then remove to a baking dish.

Pour off all but about 1 tablespoon grease from the skillet. Add your mushrooms and onion to the skillet, and sauté till the mushrooms soften.

Add the beef broth, beef bouillon granules, garlic, and tomato paste, and stir until the bouillon and tomato paste blend in. Now stir in the Carb Countdown and the remaining 2 tablespoons cream. Thicken to a gravy consistency with your guar or xanthan shaker, stir in the remaining ½ tablespoon Worcestershire, and salt and pepper to taste.

Pour the gravy over the patties, distributing the mushrooms evenly. Bake at 300 for 1 hour. Serve with fauxtatoes for that gravy!

Yield: 6 servings, each with: 427 calories; 28 g fat; 35g protein; 7 g carb; 1 g dietary fiber; 6 grams usable carbs.

Southwestern Stuffed Peppers

This was one of those recipes you just come up with out of what's in the house at the time—and it turned out so well, I'd be willing to go buy the ingredients to make it!

> 1 pound (455 g) ground beef
> 1/2 cup (80 g) chopped onion
> 1 clove garlic, crushed
> 1 14.5-ounce (411 g) can tomatoes with green chilies, divided
>   1 egg
> 1/2 cup (120 ml) half-and-half
> 1/2 cup (25 g) pork rind crumbs
> 1 teaspoon ground cumin
> 1 teaspoon salt or Vege-Sal
> 1/2 teaspoon pepper
> 3 big, nicely shaped green peppers

In a large bowl combine the ground beef, onion, garlic, 1/2 cup of the tomatoes with chilies, the egg, half-and-half, pork rind crumbs, and seasonings. Using clean hands, combine very well. Cut your peppers in half from top to bottom, and scoop out the seeds and core. Form the meat mixture into 6 equal balls, and press each into a pepper half, mashing it down a little to fill the peppers. Arrange peppers in a baking pan as you stuff them. Spoon the remaining tomatoes over the top, and bake at 350°F (180°C) for 75 to 90 minutes.

Yield: This makes 6 servings from 1 pound (455 g) of ground beef, which is pretty impressive! Filling, too.

Each serving has: 413 calories; 30 g fat; 9 g carbohydrate; 2 g fiber; for a usable carb total of 7 g; 27 g protein.

◉ Sheryl McKenney's Stuffed Tomatoes

This is a tasty and attractively presented recipe. Our tester liked that it didn't call for anything out of the way or hard to find—and that her son liked it, too!

6–8 large tomatoes
1 pound (455 g) lean ground beef
1 cup (175 g) frozen "seasoning blend" vegetables (frozen chopped onion, celery, green and red peppers)
1 8-ounce (225 g) can tomato sauce or 1 cup (240 ml) tomato juice
1 tablespoon (15 ml) apple cider vinegar
1 tablespoon (1.5 g) Splenda
1 teaspoon Italian seasoning
1/8 teaspoon cinnamon
1/4 teaspoon curry powder
Salt and pepper to taste
Shredded cheese of your choice (I used Colby/mozzarella)

Preheat oven to 375°F (190°C).

Cut off the tops of the tomatoes and scoop out the insides of the tomatoes, leaving a 1/2" (6.25 mm) shell.

In a large skillet, start cooking and crumbling ground beef with the seasoning blend vegetables. Cook until ground beef is browned. Add tomato sauce or juice, apple cider vinegar, Splenda, Italian seasoning, cinnamon, curry powder, and salt and pepper. Simmer until all ingredients are well blended.

Salt the insides of the tomato shells and place in baking pan you've sprayed with nonstick cooking spray. Sprinkle a layer of shredded cheese in the bottoms of the tomatoes. Fill the tomatoes with the meat mixture. Sprinkle more cheese on the top.

Bake for 30 minutes.

Sheryl's note: "For a variation, add 1 cup (150 g) of cauli-rice to the meat filling."

Yield: 8 servings

Each will have: 273 calories; 20 g fat; 15 g protein; 9 g carbohydrate; 2 g dietary fiber; 7 g usable carbs.

Kathryn Luzardo's
Stuffed Poblano Peppers

Here's a Mexican favorite. Our tester, Julie, raves, "I live on Mexican food, and this was heavenly. My son loved this as well. The recipe is right, the smell is wonderful, and it tastes like something you could get in a nice Mexican restaurant. It doesn't taste low carb in the slightest. Wonderful!" Olé!

4 poblano peppers (medium-sized Mexican peppers)
1 pound (455 g) ground beef
1 tablespoon (10 g) chopped garlic
¼ cup (40 g) chopped onion or ¼ cup (25 g) chopped scallions
2 tablespoons chile powder
1 teaspoon paprika
1 tablespoon (1 g) cilantro
1 teaspoon salt or Vege-Sal
1 cup (120 g) shredded cheddar or Mexican cheese blend

Put your peppers directly on a stove burner and turn them until they are mostly black all over. Set aside to cool, then slip the skins and take off the stem and cut down the side and remove the seeds and seed membranes. Rinse and set in a heavy baking pan or ovenproof skillet (Catherine uses a cast-iron skillet) that has been lightly oiled to keep things from sticking.

Brown the hamburger with the garlic and onions or scallions. When browned, drain and then add the chile powder, paprika, cilantro, and salt or Vege-Sal. You can add a little water to moisten the mixture and mix the spices through the beef if it is necessary. Simmer for 5 minutes.

Put ¼ of the hamburger mixture in each pepper and lay the peppers on their side, open side up. Top with ¼ of the cheese, and place in oven at 350°F (180°C) for approx 20 minutes, or until cheese is melted and bubbly.

Catherine's Note: Serve topped with sour cream and chopped scallions, maybe a black olive for luck. A little lettuce, tomato, and guacamole on the side make a wonderful addition. For my kids I also serve with a small amount of Spanish rice. The peppers are not usually too hot and the smell is wonderful.

Yield: Makes 4 servings

Each with: 512 calories; 40 g fat; 28 g protein; 10 g carbohydrate; 3 g dietary fiber; 7 g usable carbs.

Kristy Howell's Zucchini Moussaka

This version of moussaka is perfect for you eggplant-haters! Our tester, Julie, really liked this, and adds that it would be great for a buffet dinner.

1 pound (455 g) ground beef or lamb
1 small onion, chopped
3 cloves garlic, minced
1 6-ounce (170 g) can tomato paste
1/2 teaspoon cinnamon
1/2 teaspoon oregano
1/2 teaspoon salt
1/4 teaspoon pepper
1/4 teaspoon nutmeg
3 medium zucchini, halved lengthwise and sliced

Sauce:
3 tablespoons (45 g) butter
3 tablespoons (25 g) flour
1/4 teaspoon cinnamon
3/4 cup (180 ml) heavy cream
3/4 cup (180 ml) water
1 beaten egg
1/4 cup (40 g) grated Parmesan cheese

In your big, heavy skillet, brown meat, onion, and garlic over medium heat. Drain the fat. Add tomato paste, cinnamon, oregano, salt, pepper, and nutmeg, and simmer 10 minutes.

Stir in the sliced zucchini. Place in greased 9" x 9" (22.5 x 22.5 cm) or 11" x 7" (27.5 x17.5 cm) pan.

Now, make your sauce. In a saucepan, melt the butter, and stir in flour and cinnamon until smooth. Cook and stir 1 minute. Combine cream and water, whisk into flour mixture. Heat to simmering, cook and stir 2 minutes or until thickened. Let cool slightly. Stir a little of the sauce into the beaten egg; return all to pan and whisk together. Cook and stir 2 minutes, remove from heat, and stir in cheese. Pour over meat/zucchini mixture.

Bake at 350°F (180°C) for about 30 minutes or until sauce is lightly browned. Let sit 10 minutes before serving.

Kristy's note: "The meat sauce will appear very thick, but don't be tempted to add water or other liquid. The zucchini releases lots of water as it cooks."

Dana's note: That flour adds about 4 g of carb per serving. If you'd like to cut 4 g off each serving, heat the cream and water with the cinnamon, then thicken with your guar or xanthan shaker. Per Kristy's admonition that the zucchini releases a lot of water, you'll want to make it fairly thick.

Yield: Makes 4 servings

Each with: 714 calories; 58 g fat; 28 g protein; 22 g carbohydrate; 5 g dietary fiber; 17 g usable carbs.

⊚ Melisa McCurley's Good Stuff Casserole

Our tester, Barbo Gold, rated this a 10. She suggests using different varieties of canned tomatoes and cheeses to make this Mexican, Italian, or Greek, as you like.

> 1 ½ pounds (680 g) lean ground beef
> ½ onion, chopped
> 1 1-pound (455 g) bag frozen cut spinach, thawed and water squeezed out
> Salt to taste
> 1 8-ounce (225 g) block cream cheese or Neufchatel cheese, softened
> 1 14.5-ounce (411 g) can Mexican-style diced tomatoes,
>   medium or hot, your choice, drained
> Shredded cheddar or Colby cheese

Preheat oven to 350°F (180°C).

Brown and crumble the beef in a large skillet. When almost done, add the onions and continue cooking until translucent. Drain the grease.

Add the thawed, drained spinach to the meat mixture in the skillet, and cook for a few minutes more. Salt to taste. Stir in the cream cheese and drained tomatoes.

Spray a 2-quart (1.9 L) casserole dish with nonstick cooking spray and top with shredded cheese. Bake for 20 minutes.

Melisa's note: "Use hot tomatoes, and this becomes Hot Stuff Casserole."

Yield: 4 servings

Each with: 826 calories; 70 g fat (76.1% calories from fat); 39 g protein; 10 g carbohydrate; 4 g dietary fiber; 6 g usable carbs.

Hamburger Curry

I adapted this recipe from Peg Bracken's Appendix to *The I Hate to Cook Book*. Peg's cookbooks stand as the funniest ever written, and they're full of simple but tasty recipes, many of which have been easy to adapt. They're out of print, so if you see a Peg Bracken cookbook at a used-book store, grab it!

1 1/2 pounds (680 g) ground beef
1/2 cup (80 g) chopped onion
2 teaspoons curry powder
1 clove garlic
16 ounces (455 g) tomato sauce
1 cup (240 ml) water
1 tablespoon (15 ml) lemon juice
1/2 head cauliflower

In your big, heavy skillet, start browning and crumbling your ground beef. When it's mostly browned, pour off the fat, and stir in the onion, curry, garlic, tomato sauce, and water. Cover, turn the burner to low, and let the whole thing simmer for 30 minutes.

In the meanwhile, shred the cauliflower in your food processor. Put it in a microwaveable casserole with a lid, add a couple of tablespoons of water, cover, and nuke on high for 6 minutes. Uncover your cauliflower as soon as the microwave beeps, or you'll get overcooked mush!

When the half hour is up, stir the lemon juice into the curry, let it simmer another five minutes, and serve over the cauli-rice, with chopped peanuts, crumbled bacon, sugar-free chutney, or whatever other garnishes you wish.

Yield: 4 servings

Each with: 578 calories; 46 g fat; 30 g protein; 12 g carbohydrate; 3 g dietary fiber; 9 g usable carbs. Carb count does not include garnishes.

Chili-Glazed Meat Loaf

Meatloaf:

1/4 cup (30 g) minced green bell pepper

1/4 cup (30 g) shredded carrot

1/3 cup (55 g) minced onion

1 pound (455 g) ground chuck

1 egg

2 tablespoons (30 g) Dana's No-Sugar Ketchup (page 528)

1 teaspoon chili garlic paste

2 tablespoons (15 g) oat bran

1/4 teaspoon dried oregano

1/4 teaspoon dried basil

1/2 teaspoon salt or Vege-Sal

1/4 teaspoon pepper

Glaze:

1/4 cup (60 g) Dana's No-Sugar Ketchup

1 tablespoon (1.5 g) Splenda

1/4 teaspoon blackstrap molasses

1 teaspoon apple cider vinegar

1 tablespoon (15 ml) olive oil

1/2 teaspoon chili garlic paste

First, put all your vegetables in a big mixing bowl. Add the ground chuck, egg, 2 tablespoons (30 g) ketchup, 1 teaspoon of the chili garlic paste, oat bran, oregano, basil, salt or Vege-Sal, and pepper. Using clean hands, smoosh everything together until it's all very well mixed. Pack it into a loaf pan to mold it, then turn your meat loaf out onto your broiler rack. Bake at 350°F (180°C) for 50 to 60 minutes. For glaze, combine the 1/4 cup (60 g) ketchup, Splenda, molasses, vinegar, 1/2 teaspoon chili garlic paste, and olive oil. About 20 to 30 minutes before baking time is up, take your meat loaf out of the oven and spread the glaze over it. Return it to the oven till done.

Yield: 4 to 5 servings

Assuming 5, each will have: 310 calories; 23 g fat; 19 g protein; 8 g carbohydrate; 2 g dietary fiber; 6 g usable carbs.

◎ Philippa's Meat Loaf

Philippa was my grandmother, and this is the meat loaf she made, and the meat loaf my mom made (and still makes). Or rather, it's my sister Kim's decarbed version, because the original had cereal in it. Kim says to tell you that this recipe doubles or even triples well.

> 1 pound (455 g) ground beef
> 1/2 cup (25 g) crushed pork rinds
> 1/2 cup (120 ml) Carb Countdown Dairy Beverage
> 1 egg
> 1 medium onion, diced
> 1 tablespoon (7 g) poultry seasoning
> 1 teaspoon salt or Vege-Sal

Just plunk everything into a big mixing bowl, and use clean hands to smoosh it all together very well. Pack it into a loaf pan, then turn it out onto your broiler rack. Bake at 400°F (200°C) for 40 minutes.

Yield: 4 to 5 servings

Assuming 5, each will have: 318 calories; 26 g fat; 18 g protein; 3 g carbohydrate; trace dietary fiber; 3 g usable carbs.

Homestyle Meat Loaf

1 pound (455 g) ground chuck

2 tablespoons (15 g) oat bran

1 egg

1/4 cup (60 ml) V8 vegetable juice

1/4 cup (40 g) minced onion

1/2 cup plus 1 tablespoon (135 g) Dana's No-Sugar Ketchup (page 524)

1 teaspoon spicy mustard

1/2 teaspoon salt or Vege-Sal

1/4 teaspoon pepper

3 tablespoons (4.5 g) Splenda

1/2 teaspoon blackstrap molasses

2 teaspoons spicy mustard

Plop your ground chuck, oat bran, egg, V8, onion, 1 tablespoon of ketchup, mustard, salt, and pepper into a big mixing bowl, and using clean hands, just smoosh it all together really well. Pack it into a loaf pan to mold it, then turn it out onto your broiler rack. Bake at 350°F (180°C) for 1 hour.

Twenty minutes before it's done, combine the remaining 1/2 cup (120 g) of ketchup, the Splenda, blackstrap, and the other 2 teaspoons of mustard, and brush over the meat loaf to glaze.

Yield: 4 to 5 servings

Assuming 5, each will have: 284 calories; 20 g fat; 19 g protein; 8 g carbohydrate; 1 g dietary fiber; 7 g usable carbs.

Famous Meat Loaf

Here's Sharyn Taylor's easy and delicious meat loaf—our tester says it will impress people!

2 pounds (1 kg) ground beef

2 eggs

3/4 cup (170 g) picante sauce

1 1 1/4-ounce (35 g) envelope dry onion soup mix

1 cup (50 g) pork rind crumbs (see page 452)

Preheat oven to 350°F (180°C).

Put everything in a big mixing bowl, and use clean hands to mix it all thoroughly. Form into a loaf freehand in a 9" x 13" (22.5 x 32.5 cm) pan or pack into a loaf pan. Bake 1 hour, or 1 hour 15 minutes if cooking in a loaf pan. Let stand 10 minutes before serving.

Dana's note: I like to form my meat loaf by molding it in a loaf pan, then turning it out on a broiler pan. I get a nicely shaped loaf, and the fat drips away as it cooks, so the meat loaf isn't greasy.

Yield: Makes 8 servings

Each having: 551 calories; 41 g fat; 39 g protein; 4 g carbohydrate; 1 g dietary fiber; 3 g usable carbs.

◎ Jen Holling's Cream Cheese Meat Loaf Surprise

This meat loaf looks pretty, with those yellow-and-white slices of egg in the middle of every serving! Our tester, Doris, really liked this, and said her husband did, too, despite disliking cream cheese.

> 1 pound (455 g) ground beef
> 1 pound (455 g) ground pork
> 1 8-ounce (225 g) package cream cheese, softened
> 2 raw eggs
> 1 medium onion, chopped
> 2 teaspoons salt
> 1 teaspoon pepper
> 5 hard-boiled eggs
> ½ cup (120 g) Dana's No-Sugar Ketchup (page 528)

Dump everything but the boiled eggs and ketchup in a big bowl, and using clean hands, mix it all very well. Place half the mixture in a greased loaf pan. Now peel your hard-boiled eggs, and lay them lengthwise along the pan, touching end to end. Cover with other half of meat loaf and form over it so eggs are hidden and totally enclosed. Cover with ketchup. Bake at 350°F (180°C) for 1 hour and 15 minutes

Yield: 8 servings

Each will have: 512 calories; 42 g fat; 27 g protein; 7 g carbohydrate; 1 g dietary fiber; 6 g usable carbs.

Barb Thompson's Meatballs Arrabiata

Arrabiata means "angry" in Italian and refers to the intense flavor combinations. Our tester, Ray, says these definitely did not make him angry!

½ pound (225 g) Italian sausage

½ pound (225 g) lean ground beef

2 tablespoons (18 g) garlic powder

1 tablespoon (18 g) salt

½ cup (60 g) green pepper, seeded, cut in thin strips

½ cup (80 g) coarsely chopped onion

1 14-ounce (400 g) can diced tomatoes, with juice

½ cup (120 ml) chicken stock or water

2 tablespoons (12 g) crushed red pepper, or to taste

Combine the Italian sausage and ground beef in a bowl. Add the garlic powder and salt. Mix well and roll into meatballs.

In a large skillet, brown the meatballs over medium heat.

After meatballs are browned all over (about 5 to 7 minutes), add remaining ingredients, stirring well. Cover and simmer 15 minutes.

Barbara's note: "This is great as a meat dish or can be served on top of spaghetti squash. I have even made larger patties and grilled them."

Yield: 4 servings

Each with: 397 calories; 30 g fat; 20 g protein; 11 g carbohydrate; 2 g dietary fiber; 9 g usable carbs.

Spicy Orange Meatballs

1 pound (455 g) ground round

1 teaspoon Worcestershire sauce

½ teaspoon salt or Vege-Sal

¼ teaspoon pepper

¼ medium onion, minced fine

¼ teaspoon chili powder

1 clove garlic, crushed

1 egg

½ cup (120 g) Dana's No-Sugar Ketchup (page 528)

2 tablespoons (30 ml) Worcestershire sauce

2 tablespoons (40 g) low-sugar orange marmalade

1 pinch cayenne

½ teaspoon chili powder

¼ teaspoon orange extract

2 tablespoons (30 ml) lemon juice

2 tablespoons (30 ml) white vinegar

1 ½ tablespoons (2.25 g) Splenda

½ cup (120 ml) beef broth

Guar or xanthan

Plunk your ground round into a mixing bowl, and add the next 7 ingredients—everything through the egg. Using clean hands, smoosh everything together until it's well blended, then form 1" (2.5 cm) meatballs. You should have about 40 of 'em.

Spray your big skillet with nonstick cooking spray, and put it over medium heat. Add the meatballs, and let them brown all over. Remove them to a plate, and pour off the grease.

Measure everything from the ketchup through the beef broth into your skillet, and whisk it all together over medium heat until it's smooth. Thicken just a little with your guar or xanthan shaker. Put the meatballs back in the skillet, turning to coat with the sauce, and simmer for 10 minutes.

You can serve this as is, or over cauli-rice. Also very good as a party nibble; keep them in a chafing dish, and have a supply of toothpicks on hand for spearing.

Yield: 3 servings

Each with: 407 calories; 27 g fat; 32 g protein; 6 g carbohydrate; trace dietary fiber; 6 g usable carbs.

Cranberry Meatballs

1 1/2 pounds (680 g) ground beef
1 egg
1/2 cup (80 g) minced onion
3/4 teaspoon salt or Vege-Sal
1/4 teaspoon pepper
1 teaspoon dry mustard
8 ounces (225 g) tomato sauce
1/2 cup (50 g) cranberries
3 tablespoons (4.5 g) Splenda
1 tablespoon (15 ml) lime juice
1/4 cup (60 ml) water

In a big bowl, combine the ground beef, egg, minced onion, salt or Vege-Sal, pepper, and mustard. Using clean hands, smoosh everything until well combined. Form into meatballs about 1 1/2" (3.75 cm) in diameter.

Put everything else in your food processor, with the S-blade in place, and pulse until the cranberries are chopped fairly fine.

Now spray your big, heavy skillet with nonstick cooking spray, and put it over medium-high heat. Brown the meatballs all over. Pour off the fat, and add the sauce. Turn the burner to low, cover, and simmer for 30 minutes. Serve over cauli-rice if you want something to sop up the sauce, but they're fine alone.

Yield: 4 to 5 servings

Assuming 4, each will have: 577 calories; 47 g fat; 31 g protein; 8 g carbohydrate; 2 g dietary fiber; 6 g usable carbs.

Swedish Meatballs

This traditional Swedish favorite usually has mashed potatoes in it, but the Ketatoes mix works very well. Serve this with Jansson's Temptation (page 145) for a Swedish feast! Or keep these warm in a chafing dish, with a supply of toothpicks, for a great hot hors d'oeurve.

1 pound (455 g) ground chuck
1/4 large onion, minced
6 tablespoons (20 g) Ketatoes mix
1/3 cup (80 ml) heavy cream
1 tablespoon (ml) water
1 egg
1/2 teaspoon salt or Vege-Sal
1/4 teaspoon pepper
2 tablespoons (8 g) minced parsley
2 tablespoons (30 g) butter

Assemble everything but the butter in a mixing bowl. Using clean hands, smoosh it all together until it's very well blended. Form into meatballs about 1" (2.5 cm) in diameter.

Put your heavy skillet over medium heat. Melt the butter, and brown the meatballs all over—you'll have to do this in a couple of batches, unless your skillet is a lot bigger than mine!

You can serve these as is, and they're very nice. Or, if you like, you can pour another cup of heavy cream over them, let them simmer for 10 minutes or so, and serve them over Ultimate Fauxtatoes (page 136), or even keep them hot in a chafing dish and serve them as a hot hors d'oeurve.

Yield: Assuming this is dinner, not an hors d'oeurve, it's 4 servings

Each with: 523 calories; 40 g fat; 30 g protein; 12 g carbohydrate; 6 g dietary fiber; 6 g usable carbs. (Analysis does not include adding the extra cup of cream. Add about 1.5 g carbs per serving and 200 calories if you use the cream.)

◎ Sesame Orange Beef

An unusual sort of stir-fry!

    1 pound (455 g) beef chuck
    2 teaspoons dark sesame oil
    ¾ cup (180 ml) white wine vinegar
    2 tablespoons (3 g) Splenda
    1 teaspoon orange extract, divided
    1 tablespoon (15 ml) soy sauce
    3 tablespoons (45 ml) peanut or canola oil
    ½ medium onion, sliced
    ½ cup (60 g) shredded carrots
    2 cups (300 g) frozen cross-cut green beans, thawed
    Guar or xanthan shaker

Slice the beef thin, across the grain, and put it in a large zipper-lock bag. Combine the sesame oil, white wine vinegar, Splenda, and ½ teaspoon of the orange extract, and pour over the beef. Press the air out of the bag, seal, and turn it over a few times to coat the beef. Throw the bag in the fridge for a few hours, and all day won't hurt. This would be a good time to pull your green beans out of the freezer to thaw, too!

Okay, it's dinnertime. Pull your beef out of the fridge and pour off the marinade into a little bowl. Stir the soy sauce and the rest of the orange extract into the marinade, and have this waiting by the stove.

Put your big, heavy skillet, or a wok if you have one, over highest heat, and add the oil. When it's hot, throw in the beef, and stir-fry it until all the pink is gone. Remove from the skillet to a bowl or plate. Add a little more oil, if needed, and let it heat. Throw in the veggies, and stir-fry until they're just tender-crisp. Add the beef back to the skillet or wok, stir in the marinade, thicken a tiny bit with your guar or xanthan shaker if you think it needs it, and serve alone or over cauli-rice.

Yield: 4 servings

Each with: 388 calories; 30 g fat; 20 g protein; 10 g carbohydrate; 2 g dietary fiber; 8 g usable carbs.

Ropa Vieja

This is a basic recipe for Mexican shredded beef, which can be used in many ways. The name means "old clothes," and refers to the shredded texture of the meat.

> 2 pounds (1 kg) boneless beef roast (chuck or round is good)
> 1 carrot, cut in chunks
> 1 onion, sliced ¼" (6.25 mm) thick
> 1 stalk celery, whacked into 3 or 4 pieces
> Water

Place the beef, carrot, onion, and celery in a Dutch oven, or in your slow cooker. Add just enough water to cover. If using a slow cooker, set to "low"; if using a Dutch oven, cover and set on a very low burner. Either way, let your beef and vegetables simmer until the beef wants to fall apart when you stick a fork in it—about 3 to 4 hours on the stove, and at least 7 or 8 in a slow cooker. When the beef is very tender, turn off the heat, and let it cool in the broth.

Now, fish your beef out of the broth, and put it on a big plate. Using clean hands or two forks, shred it until it's a big pile of little beef threads. Now you're ready to use this very tasty beef in a number of ways. Be sure and save the broth, too.

Yield: 5 servings

Each with: 394 calories; 28 g fat; 29 g protein; 4 g carbohydrates; 1 g fiber; 3 usable carbs (if you eat all of the vegetables).

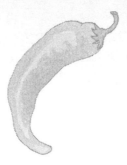

Now, here are a couple of ways to use your Ropa Vieja (see also Inauthentic Machaca Eggs, page 83).

◎ Ropa Vieja Chili

¹⁄₂ medium onion, diced fine

1 green pepper, diced fine

1 clove garlic, crushed

3 cups (600 g) Ropa Vieja (page 319)

1 cup (240 g) canned tomatoes with green chilies

2 cups (480 ml) Ropa Vieja broth

2 tablespoons (30 g) tomato paste

1 tablespoon oil

In your big, heavy skillet, over medium heat, sauté the onion and green pepper in the oil until onion is translucent. Stir in everything else, and let it simmer for 20 minutes or so, then serve.

Yield: 3 servings

Each with: 474 calories; 33 g fat; 31 g protein; 13 g carbohydrate; 3 g dietary fiber; 10 g usable carbs.

◎ Ropa Vieja Hash

This is a great Mexican take on hash, bound to be popular with the family!

> 1 cup (150 g) turnip, diced small
> 1 cup (150 g) cauliflower, diced small
> 1 medium onion, diced
> 1 pasilla chili, diced, or 1 green bell pepper, diced,
>   plus red pepper flakes to taste
> 1 clove garlic, crushed
> 2 tablespoons (30 ml) oil
> 4 cups (800 g) Ropa Vieja (page 319)
> 1 cup (240 ml) Ropa Vieja broth (page 319)
> 1 cup (60 g) chopped cilantro

First, put your turnip and cauliflower in a microwaveable container with a lid, add a tablespoon or so of water, cover, and nuke it on high for 7 minutes.

While that's happening, start sautéing the onion, pepper, and garlic in the oil over a medium flame. After a couple of minutes, add the Ropa Vieja, and stir everything together. Continue sautéing for about 10 minutes, stirring often, at which time your turnip and cauliflower will be ready to add to the skillet.

So add them! Stir them in, and keep sautéing! Give it another 5 minutes or so, then add 1 cup (240 ml) of the broth from the Ropa Vieja, along with some of the vegetables in it. Stir this into the hash, chopping up the boiled vegetables with the edge of your spatula or spoon.

Let the whole thing cook, stirring from time to time, until the broth has evaporated, and the whole thing is fairly dry. Serve topped with cilantro.

Yield: 5 servings

Each with: 392 calories; 28 g fat; 24 g protein; 9 g carbohydrate; 3 g dietary fiber; 6 g usable carbs.

◎ Thai Beef Lettuce Wraps

This is fast to make, yet interestingly exotic. And it's fun to eat wrapped-up stuff, whether you use tortillas or lettuce leaves!

1 pound (455 g) ground round

1 teaspoon red pepper flakes

1/2 cup (80 ml) chopped onion

1 clove garlic

1 medium yellow pepper, diced
   (if you don't have a yellow one, a green or red one will do!)

1/4 cup (60 ml) lemon juice

2 teaspoons chopped fresh mint

1 teaspoon beef bouillon granules

1/2 head cauliflower, shredded

1 tablespoon (15 ml) fish sauce (nuoc mam or nam pla)

2 teaspoons soy sauce

1/2 cup (60 g) chopped peanuts

1/2 cucumber, diced small

16 lettuce leaves

In your big, heavy skillet, start browning and crumbling the ground round along with the pepper flakes.

When the beef is browned, tilt the pan and spoon off any fat that's accumulated. Stir in the onion, garlic, pepper, lemon juice, mint, and beef bouillon granules. Stir until the bouillon dissolves. Turn the burner to low, and let the whole thing simmer.

While that's happening, put the cauliflower in a microwaveable casserole with a lid, add a couple of tablespoons of water, cover, and microwave on high for 6 minutes.

By the time the cauliflower's done, your pepper and onion should be tender. Drain the cauli-rice, and stir it into the beef mixture. Stir in the fish sauce and soy sauce, too.

Put your peanuts and the cucumber in small dishes. Arrange 4 good-sized lettuce leaves on each of 4 plates, and spoon a mound of the meat mixture next to them. To eat, spoon some of the meat mixture into a lettuce leaf, and sprinkle with cucumber and peanuts. Wrap in the lettuce, and eat as you would a burrito.

Yield: 4 servings

Each with: 413 calories; 29 g fat; 28 g protein; 12 g carbohydrate; 3 g dietary fiber; 9 g usable carbs.

◉ Kim's Boeuf Bourguignonne

My sister Kim is a huge fan of French cooking—classical French, rustic French, you name it, she digs it. This is her version of Boeuf Bourguignonne.

    2 pounds (1 kg) beef stew meat
    2 cups (480 ml) dry red wine
    4 tablespoons (60 g) butter
    ³⁄₄ cup (180 ml) water
    2 medium onions, sliced
    1 clove garlic, crushed
    1 teaspoon salt
    ¹⁄₄ teaspoon pepper
    1 ¹⁄₂ teaspoons dried parsley
    ¹⁄₂ teaspoon dried sage
    ¹⁄₂ teaspoon dried thyme
    ¹⁄₂ teaspoon dried marjoram
    2 medium turnips, peeled and sliced thin
    ³⁄₄ teaspoon guar or xanthan
    ¹⁄₂ pound (225 g) sliced mushrooms

Cut your beef stew meat into 1" (2.5 cm) cubes. If time allows, marinate the beef overnight in the red wine, but this is not essential.

Melt the butter in your large, heavy skillet over medium heat. If you've marinated the beef, drain it, retaining the wine. Either way, start the meat browning in the butter.

While the meat is browning, combine the wine and the water in a saucepan. Put it over a burner set to medium-high. You're going to bring this to a boil, then turn it off.

When the beef is looking brown, add the onions, and sauté until they're starting to soften. Add the garlic, and sauté a few more minutes. Transfer the meat, onions, and garlic to a large casserole you've sprayed with nonstick cooking spray (or, if you prefer, you can use your Dutch oven). Sprinkle the salt and pepper and all the dried herbs over this mixture. Now layer the sliced turnips over the meat.

Put ¹⁄₂ cup (120 ml) of the wine in your blender, and add the guar or xanthan. Blend briefly to get rid of any lumps. Pour this over the beef, then pour in the rest of the wine.

Cover and bake at 300°F (150°C) for 1 hour and 45 minutes.

Open the lid, and stir in the mushrooms. Re-cover. Return to the oven for another 15 minutes, then serve.

Yield: 6 servings

Each with: 416 calories; 21 g fat; 34 g protein; 9 g carbohydrate; 2 g dietary fiber; 7 g usable carbs.

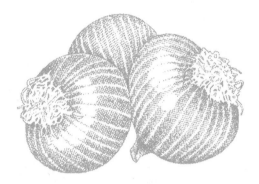

Nancy O'Connor's Greek Shepherd's Pie

Here's a family-pleasing supper.

1 pound (455 g) ground beef

1 medium onion, chopped

1–2 tablespoons (10–20 g) minced garlic

1 14.5-ounce (411 g) can diced tomatoes, drained

1 14.5-ounce (411 g) can crushed tomatoes
    or an 8-ounce can of tomato sauce

2–3 packets of Splenda, or 4-6 teaspoons granulated Splenda

1 teaspoon cinnamon or allspice

1 teaspoon oregano

1 tablespoon (15 ml) Worcestershire sauce

Salt, pepper and Tabasco to taste

2 cups (300 g) frozen cross-cut green beans, thawed (or 1 cup frozen
    peas, thawed, but this is higher carb!)

1/2 cup (75 g) grated Parmesan or 1 cup (120 g) shredded cheddar
    or a mixture of the two

1 batch Nancy O'Connor's Creamy Garlic-Chive Fauxtatoes (page 137)

In a big, heavy skillet or Dutch oven, brown the ground beef, then drain it. Add the chopped onion, and cook till the onion softens.

Add the garlic, tomatoes, Splenda, seasonings, and green beans. Mix together in skillet and let simmer for about 20 minutes. Add some water if it seems too dry and let it cook down.

Spread thickened mixture in the bottom of a large casserole—about 12" x 16" (30 x 40 cm) or so. Sprinkle the top with the cheese, and top with the Garlic-Chive Fauxtatoes.

Bake at 375°F (190°C) for about 20 minutes or until bubbly and starting to brown. Sprinkle top with a little more grated or shredded cheese.

Yield: Serves 4 to 6

Assuming 4 servings, each will have: 580 calories; 42 g fat; 31 g protein; 21 g carbohydrate; 6 g dietary fiber; 15 g usable carbs.

◎ Nancy O'Connor's Low-Carb Moussaka

Eggplant is very low carb!

    1 large eggplant
    Olive oil for brushing
    1 pound (455 g) ground beef
    1 medium onion, chopped
    1–2 (10–20 g) tablespoons minced garlic
    1 8-ounce can diced tomatoes, drained
    1 8-ounce can crushed tomatoes or tomato sauce
    2 or 3 packets of Splenda, or 4–6 teaspoons Splenda
    1 teaspoon cinnamon or allspice
    1 teaspoon oregano
    1 tablespoon Worcestershire sauce
    salt, pepper and Tabasco to taste
    1 batch Nancy O'Connor's Creamy Garlic-Chive Fauxtatoes
       (see page 137)
    ½ cup (75 g) Parmesan cheese

Slice your eggplant about ¼" (6.25 mm) to ½" (1.25 cm) thick. Brush it with a little olive oil, and grill or broil it till tender.

In a big, heavy skillet or Dutch oven, brown the ground beef, then drain it. Add the chopped onion, and cook till the onion softens.

Add the garlic, tomatoes, Splenda, and seasonings. Mix together in skillet and let simmer for about 20 minutes. Add some water if it seems too dry, and let it cook down.

Now, layer the meat and the eggplant in a big casserole. Top with the Garlic-Chive Fauxtatoes, with ½ teaspoon nutmeg added.

Bake the moussaka about 40 minutes at 375°F (190°C). Then sprinkle with grated Parmesan and return to the oven for about 5 minutes or until the cheese browns a little.

Yield: Assuming 4 servings

Each will have: 589 calories; 42 g fat; 31 g protein; 23 g carbohydrate; 7 g dietary fiber; 16 g usable carbs.

Susan Higgs's Piquant Ground Beef

3 tablespoons (45 g) butter

1 large onion, thinly sliced

1 pound (455 g) ground beef

3 tablespoons (45 ml) Worcestershire sauce

2 tablespoons (30 ml) apple cider vinegar

3 tablespoons (4.5 g) Splenda (or your favorite sugar substitute)

16 ounces (455 g) tomato sauce

Melt butter in a skillet, add onion. Once the onion starts to soften, add the ground beef and cook until done, breaking up any large chunks. Once beef is cooked, add all other ingredients and bring to a boil. Reduce heat and simmer for 20 minutes. Serve over cauliflower rice, fauxtatoes, French-cut green beans, finely sliced zucchini, or your favorite cooked veggie.

Yield: Makes 4 main-dish servings

Each with: 483 calories; 39 g fat; 21 g protein; 13 g carbohydrate; 2 g dietary fiber; 11 g usable carbs.

George Hollenbeck's Hamburger Stroganoff

You could try this over cooked spaghetti squash or fauxtatoes. And our recipe tester, Ray, says to tell you this might impress a girl!

1 pound (455 g) lean ground beef
1 small onion, chopped (½ cup [80 g])
1 clove garlic, minced
½ cup (120 ml) beef broth
1 cup (240 ml) dry red wine
1 cup (230 g) sour cream
Guar or xanthan (optional)

In your big, heavy skillet, brown beef with onion and garlic till meat is brown and veggies are soft. Add beef broth and wine and simmer about 15 minutes. Add sour cream and heat through, but don't let it boil again or your sour cream will "crack." Thicken a little more with your guar or xanthan shaker if you think it needs it, then serve.

Yield: Makes about 6 generous servings

Each having: 323 calories; 24 g fat; 16 g protein; 4 g carbohydrate; trace dietary fiber. And George says it works out to about 12 g usable carbs per serving when he serves it with spaghetti squash. Without spaghetti squash, it would be 4 g usable carbs.

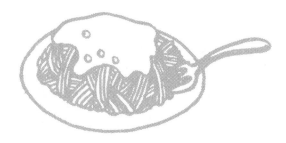

◉ Pat Best's Chili Con Carne

Here's your family's favorite chili with beans, decarbed.

> 1 pound (455 g) lean ground beef
> 1 14.5-ounce (420 g) can stewed tomatoes
> 1 15-ounce (420 g) can black soy beans
> 1 medium yellow onion, diced
> 2 tablespoons (14 g) chili powder
> 1 teaspoon salt
> ¼ teaspoon cumin
> ¼ teaspoon red pepper (optional—if you like your chili hot)
> 1 bay leaf
> 3 whole cloves

Toppings:
> Diced onion
> Sour cream
> Shredded cheddar cheese

Brown the ground beef in a heavy saucepan or Dutch oven. Drain off the excess fat. Return to heat and add the remaining ingredients. Cover and simmer on low for at least 1 hour—check halfway through, and add a little water if it needs it. Remove bay leaf and discard. Serve warm with diced onion, sour cream, and shredded cheddar cheese as toppings.

Pat says her family's never noticed the switch to soybeans! She also notes that you may as well make a double or triple batch and freeze the extra for a busy night.

Yield: Serves 4

Each having: 457 calories; 30 g fat; 31 g protein; 19 g carbohydrate; 10 g dietary fiber; 9 g usable carbs. (Counts do not include optional toppings.)

Kathy Monahon's Baked Penne

A low-carb version of a family favorite.

> 2 cups (300 g) dry low-carb penne pasta
>
> 1 1/2 pounds (680 g) ground beef
>
> Salt and pepper
>
> 15 ounces (420 g) ricotta cheese
>
> 1 quart (.95 L) jar spaghetti sauce, lowest carb you can find, divided
>   (Dana's note: I like Hunt's No Sugar Added.)
>
> 1/2 cup (75 g) grated Parmesan cheese
>
> 1 egg
>
> 1 tablespoon (4 g) dried parsley
>
> 1/2 cup (60 g) mozzarella cheese, shredded

Cook pasta in a Dutch oven according to the package directions. Drain pasta and set aside. In the same Dutch oven, brown and crumble the ground beef. Drain. Season with salt and pepper to taste. To browned beef add ricotta, half of the spaghetti sauce, Parmesan, egg, and parsley. Mix thoroughly. Add pasta and mix.

Coat a 13" x 9" x 2" (32.5 x 22.5 x 5 cm) baking dish with nonstick cooking spray. Put meat, cheese, and pasta mixture into dish. Pour remaining spaghetti sauce evenly over mixture. Sprinkle mozzarella cheese on the top.

Bake at 350°F (180°C) for 30 minutes or until hot and bubbly and cheese just begins to brown.

Yield: Makes 6 generous servings

Each with: 657 calories; 46 g fat; 46 g protein; 16 g carbohydrate; 4 g dietary fiber; 12 g usable carbs. This will vary some depending on which brand of low-carb pasta you use.

Nanci Messersmith's Low-Carb Lasagna Recipe Using Zucchini for Noodles

Missing lasagna? Try this recipe.

Ingredients:

  5–6 medium zucchini
  Italian seasoning
  1 ¾ pounds (795 g) ground chuck
  Salt and pepper
  1 26-ounce (780 g) can Hunt's Garlic and Herb spaghetti sauce
  1 ½ pounds (680 g) ricotta cheese
  1 ½ pounds (680 g) grated mozzarella cheese
  1 cup (150 g) grated Parmesan cheese

Prepare zucchini by cutting off ends. Slice lengthwise into ¼" (6.25 mm) thick slices. Place on ungreased cookie sheet. Sprinkle with Italian seasoning. Bake at 425°F (220°C) degrees for about 20 minutes until tender. Set aside.

In a skillet, brown ground chuck until crumbly. Drain excess fat and season with salt and pepper.

Stir in spaghetti sauce.

In a 9" x 13" (22.5 x 32.5 cm) baking pan (pan must be at least 2" [5 cm] deep) spread a thin layer of the meat sauce.

Top with a layer of zucchini slices (approximately 8 to 10 slices per layer). Top with ⅓ of the ricotta cheese. Top that with ⅓ of the mozzarella cheese. Top with ⅓ of the meat sauce.

Top with ⅓ of the Parmesan cheese.

Repeat layering 2 more times ending with Parmesan cheese.

Bake in a preheated oven at 350°F (180°C) for about 45 minutes or until brown and bubbly.

Cool about 10 minutes before cutting into squares to serve.

Yield: Assuming 12 servings

Each will have: 520 calories; 38 g fat; 35 g protein; 11 g carbohydrate; 3 g dietary fiber; 8 g usable carbs.

Marcelle Flint's Zucchini Lasagna

Our tester, Ray, says this is as good as restaurant lasagna!

  1 pound (455 g) ground beef

  1 garlic clove, minced

  1 15-ounce (420 g) can tomato sauce

  1 teaspoon salt

  1 teaspoon dried basil

  1 teaspoon dried oregano

  1/2 teaspoon dried thyme

  1/2 teaspoon dried marjoram

  1 14-ounce (400 g) container whole milk ricotta cheese

  1/2 cup (75 g) grated Parmesan cheese

  1 egg

  4 medium zucchini

  2 tablespoons (16 g) low-carb bake mix

  1 cup (120 g) shredded mozzarella cheese

In a large skillet, brown beef with garlic, breaking the beef up well. Drain off any fat. Stir in tomato sauce, salt, basil, oregano, thyme, and marjoram; simmer uncovered, 10 minutes.

In bowl, combine ricotta cheese, 1/2 of Parmesan cheese, and egg.

Scrub zucchini; slice lengthwise into approximately 1/8" (3.125 mm)-thick slices. (Ray noted that this was not simple with a knife. If you have a mandoline cutter—the sort of thing with a stationary blade that you just slide the food over—use it!)

Preheat oven to 350°F (180°C). Lightly oil a 13" x 9" (32.5 x 22.5 cm) baking dish.

Layer 1/2 of zucchini in oiled baking dish; sprinkle with 1/2 of bake mix. Top with 1/2 of ricotta cheese mixture and 1/2 of meat mixture, then with 1/2 of mozzarella cheese. Top with remaining zucchini; sprinkle with remaining bake mix. Top with remaining ricotta cheese mixture, meat mixture, and mozzarella cheese. Sprinkle remaining Parmesan cheese over top. Bake, uncovered, 1 hour. Let stand about 15 minutes before serving.

Yield: Makes 8 big servings at Marcelle's house

Each having: 377 calories; 27 g fat; 24 g protein; 10 g carbohydrate; 2 g dietary fiber; 8 g usable carbs.

☉ Susan Higgs's Imperial Beef

This is the sort of thing you'd pay big money for at a restaurant if it were made with fillets—and even with chopped meat patties, it rises above the ordinary!

Salt and pepper
4 7-ounce (200 g) beef fillets or chopped sirloin patties
   or ground round patties
1/2–3/4 stick butter (Susan's family likes the extra butter)
1 medium onion, chopped
1/4 cup mushrooms, chopped
1 teaspoon garlic powder (optional)
1/4 cup chicken livers, chopped
3/4 cup dry red wine
Toasted almonds

Salt and pepper the beef on both sides. Melt the butter in your big, heavy skillet over medium-high heat, then add the onion. Once onion is softened, add mushrooms, garlic powder, and chicken livers. Stir in wine while the skillet is hot so it deglazes the pan. Cook until volume is reduced by half.

Broil, grill, or fry the beef until your desired doneness. (My family likes the fillets medium-rare, but the patties cooked through.) Put about 2 tablespoons of sauce on 4 plates and top with the meat. Divide the remaining sauce over the 4 pieces of beef. Garnish with toasted almonds; serve.

Yield: Makes 4 servings

Each with: 550 calories; 45 g fat; 23 g protein; 6 g carbohydrate; 2 g dietary fiber; 4 g usable carbs.

◎ Rita Eichman's Shepherd's Pie

    1 1/2 pounds (680 g) ground chuck or round

    Salt and pepper to taste

    2 14-ounce (400 g) cans green beans, drained

    1–2 jars Ragu Light Parmesan Alfredo cheese sauce

    1 batch Fauxtatoes Deluxe (page 533)

    1/2 cup (60 g) shredded cheddar or other cheese

Brown the ground beef, with onions if desired. Add salt and pepper to taste.

Mix the drained green beans with the cooked meat, and add the Ragu cheese sauce. Pour into a buttered 2-quart (1.9 L) casserole or baking dish. Top with the fauxtatoes. Sprinkle with shredded cheese. Bake at 350°F (180°C) for 20 to 30 minutes.

Yield: 6 servings

Assuming 6 servings, and 1 jar of Alfredo sauce, each serving will have: 578 calories; 48 g fat; 26 g protein; 11 g carbohydrate; 3 g dietary fiber; 8 g usable carbs.

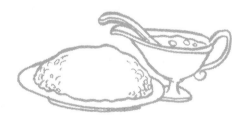

Patty Southard's Festiva Beef Italiano

A simple slow-cooker recipe. It makes plenty!

   2 pieces tri-tip beef roast, totaling about 4 1/2 pounds (2 kg)
   3 10 1/2-ounce (315 ml) cans beef broth 1–2 cups (240–480 ml)
      water—enough so the beef is covered
   2 cloves garlic, minced
   2 teaspoons Italian seasoning
   1 teaspoon basil
   1 0.7-ounce (19 g) envelope Italian dressing (dry mix)
   1 1.25-ounce (35 g) envelope onion soup mix

Put roast in a 5-quart (4.75 L) slow cooker. Mix remaining ingredients together, pour over beef. Cook for 8 to 10 hours on low. Remove roast, shred with two forks; put back in the slow cooker, and mix well. Enjoy!

Yield: 10 servings

Each will have: 459 calories; 32 g fat; 36 g protein; 4 g carbohydrate; 1 g dietary fiber; 3 g usable carbs.

Nancy Machinton's Pot Roast

½ teaspoon garlic powder

1 teaspoon salt or Vege-Sal

3–4 pound (1.4–1.9 kg) rump roast

1 8-ounce (225 g) can tomato sauce

½ onion, chopped

1 garlic clove, pressed

2 teaspoons Italian seasoning

1 cinnamon stick

¼ teaspoon ginger

½ cup (120 ml) of sweet red wine such as Mogen David (optional)

Rub the garlic powder and salt or Vege-Sal into the roast and let it sit for about ½ hour, coming to room temperature.

Put your meat in a Dutch oven, and cover with tomato sauce and all the other ingredients. Cover the pot and simmer for 90 minutes. Then turn your meat and simmer another 60 to 90 minutes, or until fork tender.

Remove meat and allow it to cool before slicing. Skim the fat from pan. Once meat is sliced, return it to the pan and reheat with sauce. This is better the next day!

Nancy's note: "This would be especially good for Jewish holidays like Passover when sweet wine is often used. (If you're wary of that sweet wine, keep in mind that it won't add more than about 1 gram of carbohydrate per serving.)"

Yield: Serves about 6 and is great with fauxtatoes

Not including the fauxtatoes, each serving will have: 401 calories; 13 g fat; 59 g protein; 6 g carbohydrate; 1 g dietary fiber; 5 g usable carbs.

Pamela Merritt's Marinated Pot Roast

Use an oven bag for easy cleanup!

> 5 small turnips
> 3 stalks celery
> 1/2 small onion
> 2 cups (300 g) carrots/zucchini/cauliflower/peppers
>   (depending on tastes and carbs), cut into bite-sized pieces
> 2 pounds (1 kg) London broil
> 1 cup (240 ml) Italian dressing (Pamela uses Paul Newman's)

Cut the turnips, celery, and onion into bite-sized pieces. Put all vegetables and the meat into an oven bag. Mix it all up with the Italian dressing. Throw it in the fridge, and let it marinate for 6 to 24 hours—it's great to make this one night and roast it the next.

Bake at 350°F (180°C) for 1 hour and 15 minutes.

Note: For a south-of-the-border flavor, vary the marinade by using salsa, and for an Asian twist, try low-sugar Teriyaki Sauce instead (page 531).

Yield: 6 servings

Each with: 668 calories; 55 g fat; 29 g protein; 14 g carbohydrate; 3 g dietary fiber; 11 g usable carbs.

Dorothy Keefe's Marinated Chuck Roast

½ cup (120 ml) strong coffee (prepared)
½ cup (120 ml) soy sauce
1 tablespoon (15 ml) Worcestershire sauce
1 tablespoon (15 ml) vinegar (I use wine vinegar)
5 pounds (2.3 kg) chuck roast
Guar or xanthan

Mix coffee, soy sauce, Worcestershire, and vinegar, and pour over roast in a non-reactive bowl. Let stand in refrigerator several hours or overnight, basting several times—turning the roast over is a good idea!

The next day put meat in a Dutch oven or other covered roaster. Pour marinade over, cover. Place in preheated oven and bake at 325°F (170°C) for about 2 ½ hours. Baste a few times while cooking.

When it's done, you can remove the roast from the Dutch oven, put it on a platter, and keep it hot while you thicken up the liquid in the pot with your guar or xanthan shaker, for gravy.

You can also cook this in your slow cooker—cook on low for 7 to 8 hours.

Dorothy's note: "This can be portioned into meal-sized servings, covered with a little marinade, and frozen. It is so handy to get out when you need a quick meal."

Yield: About 10 servings

Each with: 482 calories; 35 g fat; 37 g protein; 2 g carbohydrate; trace dietary fiber; 2 g usable carbs.

Rho's Slow-Cooker Chuck Roast

This roast drew raves from our tester, Patty Mishler. She said she "freaked out" that there was no salt or pepper listed, but rated the sauce not just a 10, but an 11!

2 8-ounce (225 g) packages sliced mushrooms

1 medium onion, cut into large dice

1 tablespoon (10 g) chopped garlic

½ cup (120 ml) red wine

1 14.5-ounce (411 g) can diced tomatoes with green chilies

4 pounds (1.8 kg) chuck roast

½ cup (115 g) sour cream

Thickener—guar, xanthan, or Rho's choice, ThickenThin from Expert Foods.

Spray your slow cooker with nonstick cooking spray. Put your mushrooms in the bottom of the pot, then your onion on top of that, and your garlic spread over it all. Pour the wine and canned tomatoes over everything, and give it a stir.

Place your chuck roast on top. Cover the slow cooker and set to high. Cook for about 8 hours. Remove the roast, stir the sour cream into the stuff in the pot, and thicken to taste.

Rho's note: "I used Del Monte Zesty Tomatoes with Mild Green Chili."

Tester's note: Patty was serving non–low carbers, so she served Garlic Mashed Potatoes with this, and said it was a good match. Consider serving Nancy O'Connor's Creamy Garlic-Chive Fauxtatoes (page 137).

Yield: About 8 servings

Each with: 423 calories; 30 g fat; 29 g protein; 6 g carbohydrate; 1 g dietary fiber; 5 g usable carbs.

⊚ Sharon Palmer-Brownstein's Fantastic Brisket of Beef

This recipe is a simple way to cook a darned big piece of meat—and have left-overs for quick meals for several days.

> 3–4 pounds (1.4–1.9 kg) brisket
> 1 large onion, diced fine
> Salt (to taste)
> Pepper (to taste)
> Garlic powder (to taste)
> 1 cup (240 ml) water

Horseradish sauce:
> 1 cup (230 g) sour cream
> White prepared horseradish, to taste

Place brisket in a large Dutch oven. Sprinkle onion, spices, and water over brisket. Cover and cook for approximately 2 1/2 hours on medium heat, turning the brisket every half hour. Once cooked, remove from pot and slice thin. Mix sour cream and horseradish together. You will need to taste as to how hot or mild you want your horseradish sauce to be.

Serve brisket with horseradish sauce.

Yield: Easily serves 10

Each getting: 622 calories; 53 g fat; 32 g protein; 2 g carbohydrate; trace dietary fiber; 2 g usable carbs.

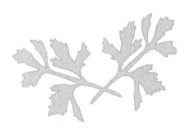

◎ Janette Kling's
Bourbon Glazed Cajun Tenderloin

This recipe strikes me as something I'd order at a fancy restaurant!
Our tester, Diana Lee, says this is definitely worth the work.

　　　1 2 ½–3-pound (1–1.4 kg) center-cut beef tenderloin
　　　Extra-virgin olive oil

Marinade:
　　　¼ cup (60 ml) Worcestershire sauce
　　　2 tablespoons (30 ml) blackstrap molasses
　　　2 tablespoons (30 g) Dijon mustard

Meat Rub:
　　　1 tablespoon (6 g) cracked black pepper
　　　1 tablespoon (9 g) garlic powder
　　　1 tablespoon (7 g) paprika
　　　2 teaspoons salt
　　　½ teaspoon cayenne red pepper

Glaze:
　　　¼ cup (60 ml) bourbon
　　　¼ cup (60 g) Dijon mustard
　　　2 tablespoons blackstrap molasses

Whisk marinade ingredients together.

Trim meat of excess fat and silver skin. Place meat and marinade in a zipper-lock plastic bag and refrigerate for 8 to 24 hours.

When time comes to cook, remove meat from plastic bag and discard marinade. Preheat oven to 425°F (220°C) degrees.

Combine all meat rub ingredients together in a small bowl. In another bowl, whisk all meat glaze ingredients together thoroughly.

Lightly blot meat with paper towels. Press meat rub into meat and let stand for 20 to 30 minutes.

Lightly brush meat with olive oil. Sear meat in a hot skillet on all sides, approximately 3 to 5 minutes per side. Insert a meat thermometer in thickest part of meat. Place meat on rack in a roasting pan and cook for approximately

1 to 1 ¼ hours or until internal meat thermometer reaches 135°F (60°C) degrees for 10 to 20 minutes. During last 10 minutes, turn and baste meat with glaze.

Remove meat from oven and allow to rest for 10 minutes. The internal meat thermometer will rise 5 to 10 degrees during this rest time. Remember, approximately 140°F (60°C) equals medium-rare.

Cut into slices and serve.

Yield: 8 servings

Each will have: 551 calories; 40 g fat; 31 g protein; 10 g carbohydrate; 1 g dietary fiber; 9 g usable carbs.

chapter ten

Pork and Lamb

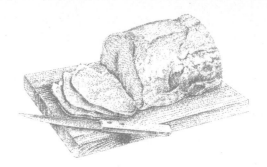

I live in Indiana, home of the breaded pork tenderloin. If most of your recipes for pork have to do with breaded chops and tenderloins, or ribs with sugary sauce, you may be wondering what to do now that bread crumbs and sugar are no longer a part of your life. Wonder no more! You're bound to find at least four or five new favorites here, from all around the world.

I adore lamb, and for the life of me I can't figure out why so many Americans have never even tried it—it's perhaps the most popular meat in the rest of the world. If you haven't tried lamb, do. And if you're already a lamb lover, like me, try some of these great new ideas for your old favorite.

Ginger Sesame Pork

You can serve this simple stir-fry over cauli-rice, if you like, but it's nice just as it is.

12 ounces (340 g) boneless pork top loin
2 tablespoons (20 g) grated ginger root
4 teaspoons soy sauce
1 teaspoon Splenda
2 teaspoons toasted sesame oil
4 scallions, sliced, including the crisp part of the green
2 tablespoons (30 ml) dry sherry
2 cloves garlic, crushed
2 tablespoons (30 ml) peanut oil

Slice your boneless pork loin as thinly as you can—it helps to have it half-frozen.

Mix together everything else in a medium-sized bowl. Add the pork, stir to coat, and let it marinate for at least a half an hour.

Over high flame, heat the oil in a heavy skillet or wok. Add the pork with all of the marinade, and stir-fry until meat is done through, about 4 to 5 minutes. Serve.

Yield: 2 servings

Each with: 393 calories; 25 g fat; 31 g protein; 5 g carbohydrate; 1 g dietary fiber; 4 g usable carbs.

Carnitas

These brown and tender cubes of pork are a Mexican classic. Serve them over a salad, or make a simple soft taco by piling your carnitas on a low-carb tortilla.

3 pounds (1.4 kg) pork shoulder, skin and bone removed
Water
1 tablespoon (15 ml) lime juice
2 teaspoons salt

Cut your pork into 1" (2.5 cm) cubes, and put them in your big, heavy skillet. Add just enough water to barely cover the cubes, add the lime juice, sprinkle with salt, and bring to a boil. Do not cover the pan.

Turn the heat down to medium-low, and let the meat continue to boil until all the water has evaporated.

Turn the burner down even lower, and let the meat continue to cook, stirring often, until the meat cubes are browned all over, which may take as long as an hour.

Yield: 6 servings

Each with: 402 calories; 31 g fat; 29 g protein; 0 g carbohydrate; 0 g dietary fiber; 0 g usable carb.

◎ Island Pork Steaks

Caribbean-style seasonings!

> 1 ½ (680 g) pounds pork shoulder steaks
> 1 teaspoon ground allspice
> ¼ teaspoon ground nutmeg
> ½ teaspoon dried thyme
> ⅛ teaspoon cayenne
> 2 tablespoons (30 ml) olive oil
> ¼ cup (40 g) chopped onion
> ¼ cup (60 ml) lime juice
> ¼ cup (60 ml) chicken broth
> 1 teaspoon Splenda
> 3 cloves garlic, minced

Put your pork steaks on a big plate. Mix together the allspice, nutmeg, thyme, and cayenne, and sprinkle the mixture over both sides of the pork. Let the steak sit for 30 to 45 minutes.

Heat the olive oil in your big, heavy skillet, over medium flame, and throw in the pork steaks. Give 'em 6 or 7 minutes per side—you want them golden on the outside and just done through on the inside. Remove to a plate, and cover with a spare pot lid to keep warm.

Throw your onion in the skillet, and sauté it until it's just translucent. Add the lime juice, chicken broth, Splenda, and garlic. Turn up the heat, and boil the sauce hard until it's reduced by about half. Pour over pork and serve.

Yield: 2 to 3 servings

Assuming 3, each will have: 503 calories; 40 g fat; 30 g protein; 5 g carbohydrate; 1 g dietary fiber; 4 g usable carbs.

◉ Pork Chili

The pumpkin seed meal used to thicken this chili is an authentically Mexican touch.

3/4 cup (120 g) chopped onion

4 cloves garlic, crushed

2 tablespoons (30 ml) olive oil

1 1/2 pounds (680 g) boneless pork loin, cut in 1/2" (1.25 cm) cubes

2 1/2 teaspoons chili powder

1 teaspoon ground cumin

1 green pepper, chopped

1 cup (240 ml) chicken broth

1/4 cup (60 g) picante sauce

3 chipotle chiles canned in adobo, minced

2 teaspoons adobo sauce from the chili can

1/4 cup (60 g) pumpkin seed meal (page 24)

Salt to taste

In your big heavy skillet, or better yet, in a Dutch oven, sauté the onion and garlic in the olive oil until the onions are translucent.

Add everything else except the ground pumpkin seeds and the salt, turn the burner to low, cover the pan, and let the whole thing simmer for 45 minutes to an hour.

Now stir in the pumpkin seed meal, and let it simmer another 10 to 15 minutes. Salt to taste, and serve.

Yield: 3 to 4 servings

Assuming 4, each will have: 335 calories; 17 g fat; 34 g protein; 11 g carbohydrate; 3 g dietary fiber; 8 g usable carbs.

Pork Stew

This winter-night supper is not only low carb, it's quite low calorie, too. Pork loin is a very lean meat.

1 tablespoon (15 ml) olive oil

1 tablespoon (15 g) butter

1 medium onion, sliced ¼" (6.25 mm) thick

4 cloves garlic, crushed

1 cup (130 g) sliced carrot

2 pounds (1 kg) boneless pork loin, cut in 1" (2.5 cm) cubes

8 ounces (225 g) sliced mushrooms

2 14-ounce (400 ml) cans chicken broth

1 pinch ground cloves

1 teaspoon salt

¼ teaspoon pepper

Guar or xanthan

In a Dutch oven, over a medium burner, heat the olive oil and the butter. Add the onion and garlic, and sauté for a few minutes. Add everything else, and stir to combine. Cover, turn the burner to low, and let the whole thing simmer for 90 minutes to 2 hours.

Thicken the gravy with your guar or xanthan shaker, and serve.

Yield: 6 servings

Each with 257 calories; 12 g fat; 30 g protein; 7 g carbohydrate; 1 g dietary fiber; 6 g usable carbs.

◉ Seriously Simple Roasted Ribs

We've come to think of pork ribs solely in terms of barbecue—sweet and spicy sauces, outdoor cooking, or Chinese restaurants. So it surprised me to discover how great they are simply roasted, plain. Give this a try—it takes a couple of hours of cooking time, but almost no work. Feel free to do a whole slab, by the way—I just figured most of you don't have eight people to feed!

> 3 pounds (1.4 kg) pork spareribs (about half a slab)
> Salt or Vege-Sal and pepper

This is ridiculously simple. Turn your oven on to 325°F (170°C). While it's heating, put your ribs on your broiler rack, and sprinkle both sides with salt and pepper. Put 'em in the oven, and roast 'em for 2 to 2 1/2 hours. That's it.

Note: I find a good sharp kitchen shears is better than a knife for cutting ribs apart, either before or after cooking.

Yield: 3 to 4 servings

Assuming 4, each will have: 604 calories; 50 g fat; 36 g protein; 0 g carbohydrate; 0 g dietary fiber; 0 g usable carb.

Oven Barbecued Ribs

1 tablespoon paprika

1 teaspoon salt or Vege-Sal

2 teaspoons spicy brown mustard

1 bay leaf

$1/2$ teaspoon chili powder

$1/4$ teaspoon cayenne

2 tablespoons (30 ml) Worcestershire sauce

$1/4$ cup (60 ml) cider vinegar

$1/3$ cup (75 g) tomato sauce

2 tablespoons (30 g) Dana's No-Sugar Ketchup (page 528)

$1/2$ cup (120 ml) water

1 teaspoon lemon juice

2 tablespoons (20 g) minced onion

1 clove garlic, crushed

$1/2$ teaspoon molasses

3 pounds (1.4 kg) pork spareribs (about a half a slab)

In a large, nonreactive saucepan combine everything but the ribs. Stir together, bring to a boil, turn down to a simmer, and let it cook for 10 to 15 minutes.

Preheat your oven to 450°F (230°C). While the sauce is cooking, I like to cut in between the ribs, about halfway up, but that's optional—it just gives more surface for the sauce to coat! Place the ribs on your broiler pan.

Paint the ribs thoroughly with the sauce, and let them roast at 450°F (230°C) for 30 minutes. Now turn the oven down to 350°F (180°C), baste the ribs with the sauce, turn them over, and baste the other side. Continue roasting your ribs for 90 minutes, basting every 20 to 30 minutes, and turning them over when you do. Serve with plenty of napkins!

Yield: 3 to 4 servings

Assuming 4, each will have: 637 calories; 50 g fat; 37 g protein; 8 g carbohydrate; 1 g dietary fiber; 7 g usable carbs—and that's if you use up all the sauce.

⊚ General Mike's Finger-Lickin' Ribs

General Mike is another combatant from the tongue-in-cheek army of Protein Uber Alles. Our tester, Ray, said that this was enough sauce for a large package of country ribs, with some left over. Also said it tasted good!

> 1 ½ cups (375 g) spicy brown mustard
> ¼ cup (60 ml) soy sauce
> ¼ cup (60 ml) wine vinegar
> 6 packets Splenda, or 12 teaspoons granulated Splenda
> 1 tablespoon (10 g) crushed garlic
> Pepper to taste
> 1 slab pork spareribs, about 7 pounds (3.2 kg)
>   or country-style ribs or really any pork ribs

Mix together everything but the ribs, and coat ribs with the resulting sauce.

Start both burners of your grill on high. Once they are well heated, place the ribs on the grill, close the lid, and sear for about 10 minutes. After 10 minutes, flip over the ribs and cook for an additional 5 to 10 minutes, depending on how much you want them charred.

Turn off one side of your grill and move all the ribs to that side, leaving the other side/burner on high. About every 15 minutes check on the progress of the ribs, turn them end-to-end, and recoat them with the mustard sauce as necessary. Typically within 20 to 30 minutes the ribs will be done.

Feel free to use this sauce on chicken, as well!

Yield: 8 servings

Each with: 755 calories; 62 g fat; 46 g protein; 5 g carbohydrate; 1 g dietary fiber; 4 g usable carbs—that carb count holds only if you eat all of the sauce.

◎ Grandma Angelica's Catsurra

Suzanne Dove sends this recipe, which she says has been in her family for years! Aren't those the best?

3–4 pounds (1.4–1.9 kg) boneless country-style pork ribs
1 large onion, sliced
2 tablespoons (30 ml) olive oil
2–3 (480–720 ml) cups water
1 cup (240 ml) chicken broth
1/4 teaspoon pepper
1/4 teaspoon seasoned salt
1/2 teaspoon salt
1 tablespoon allpice
1/4 teaspoon oregano
1/4 teaspoon basil
1 clove garlic, chopped
1–2 carrots, sliced
1–2 stalks celery, sliced
1–1 1/2 heads cabbage
1/2 cup (120 ml) dry red wine

Cut ribs into large pieces. In a Dutch oven or large, heavy-bottomed pot, brown the pork and onion in olive oil. When the pork is brown, add water and chicken broth. Add spices, cover, and simmer on medium-low for 1/2 hour.

Add carrots and celery and continue to cook another 1/2 hour to 1 hour.

Cut the cabbage into wedges, or chop coarsely, and add, along with the wine. (The wine is optional, more carbs but gives a little better flavor.) Cook until the cabbage is done, about 20 to 30 minutes.

I put the allspice on the table so guests can add more to their bowl. (I always do.)

Yield: Makes 5 to 7 servings

Assuming 5, each will have: 276 calories; 17 g fat; 18 g protein; 8 g carbohydrate; 2 g dietary fiber; 6 g usable carbs.

Pork and Provolone with White Wine and Mushrooms

I confess, I came up with this to get rid of extra pork, smoked provolone, and mushrooms I had kicking around my fridge—and it got top marks from my husband! Easily worth making again, and then some.

> 2 pounds (1 kg) boneless pork loin, in 4 slices about ³/₄"
>   (1.875 cm) thick
> 6 ounces (170 g) sliced smoked provolone cheese
> 1 tablespoon (15 ml) olive oil
> 1 tablespoon (15 g) butter
> ¹/₂ medium onion, chopped
> 4 cloves garlic, crushed
> 2 cups (200) sliced mushrooms
> 1 cup (240 ml) dry white wine
> 1 teaspoon chicken bouillon concentrate

You'll need four pieces of pork loin that are roughly the same shape. One piece at a time, put the pork in a heavy zipper-lock bag, and using any heavy blunt instrument that comes to hand—I use a 3-pound dumbbell—pound your pork out till it's between ¹/₄" (6.25 mm) and ¹/₂" (1.25 cm) thick.

Sandwich the sliced smoked provolone between the pounded pieces of pork, using 3 ounces (85 g) in each of two "pork and cheese sandwiches." Heat the oil and butter in your big, heavy skillet, over medium-high heat, and lay the pork-and-cheese sandwiches in it. Sauté for about 5 minutes per side, or until golden, turning carefully.

When the pork-and-cheese sandwiches are browned on both sides, add the onion, garlic, and mushrooms to the skillet, scattering them around the pork.
Mix the wine and chicken bouillon concentrate together, and pour around the pork. Cover, turn burner to low, and simmer for 20 minutes.

When time's up, lift the pork-and-cheese sandwiches out with a spatula, put them on a platter, and cover with a lid to keep warm. Now turn up the burner under the skillet, and let the sauce boil hard for about 5 minutes—you want just ¹/₂ cup or so of liquid left amongst the mushrooms and onions. Thicken this a trifle with your guar or xanthan shaker if you like, but it's not essential by any means. Scrape the mushrooms, onions, and sauce over the meat and cheese, and cut in portions to serve.

Yield: 6 servings

Each with: 396 calories; 21 g fat; 39 g protein; 4 g carbohydrate; trace dietary fiber; 4 g usable carbs.

⊚ Albondigas

I didn't know whether to put these tasty Mexican meatballs in the pork chapter or the beef chapter! They're great by themselves, or you can serve them over cauli-rice.

1 pound (455 g) ground pork
1 pound (455 g) ground beef
1 cup (120 g) shredded zucchini
¼ cup (40 g) finely minced onion
2 eggs
½ teaspoon oregano
½ teaspoon pepper
½ teaspoon cumin
1 teaspoon salt or Vege-Sal
14 ½ ounces (411 g) canned diced tomatoes
2 chipotle chiles canned in adobo (or less or more, to taste)
¾ cup (180 ml) chicken broth

In a big mixing bowl, combine the two meats. Add the zucchini and the onion to the meat, along with the eggs. Measure in the seasonings. Using clean hands, smoosh everything together until it's all very well combined—in particular, you shouldn't be able to tell where one meat ends and the other begins. Form into meatballs a little smaller than a walnut. Put on a plate, and set in the fridge.

Put the tomatoes in your blender—don't drain them first. Add the chipotles, and then blend the whole thing till smooth. Dump this combination into your big, heavy skillet, and put it over a medium-high flame. When it comes to a boil, turn the burner down and let the sauce simmer for 5 minutes. Stir in the chicken broth, and bring the sauce back to a simmer.

Add the meatballs, and bring to a simmer a third time. Cover the skillet, and let the whole thing simmer for 45 to 50 minutes, then serve.

Yield: 8 servings

Each with: 364 calories; 28 g fat; 22 g protein; 5 g carbohydrate; 1 g dietary fiber; 4 g usable carbs.

Sara Emmert's "The Last Pork Chop Recipe You'll Ever Need"

6 pork chops (bone-in or boneless, makes no difference)
4–8 tablespoons (60–120 ml) soy sauce
1–2 teaspoons celery salt
1–2 teaspoons garlic powder

Lay the chops out on a plate or platter. Dowse them in soy sauce—I'd say about a tablespoon or so per chop, per side. Liberally sprinkle with celery salt—don't be afraid here. Add a pinch of the garlic powder, and flip to repeat seasonings on the other side of the chop. Broil or grill until done, a guesstimate of 5 minutes per side. Sara prefers them broiled. Baste several times with the leftover sauce from the plate so that they don't dry out.

Note: Our tester, Ray, added ¼ cup (60 ml) of lemon juice to this, with good results.

Each chop will have: 248 calories; 15 g fat; 24 g protein; 3 g carbohydrate; trace dietary fiber.

⊚ Lemon-Ginger Pork Chops

1 pound (455 g) pork chops, 1" (2.5 cm) thick
1 tablespoon grated ginger root
1 tablespoon (15 ml) olive oil
1 tablespoon (15 ml) soy sauce
1 tablespoon (15 ml)dry sherry
1 1/2 teaspoons lemon juice
1 tablespoon (15 ml) water
1/2 clove garlic, crushed
1/4 teaspoon toasted sesame oil
1/4 teaspoon Splenda
1 scallion, sliced, including the crisp part of the green shoot

In your large, heavy skillet, over medium-high heat, brown the pork chops on both sides in the olive oil. Mix together everything else but the scallion, and pour into the skillet. Turn the chops to coat both sides. Cover the pan, turn the burner to low, and let the chops simmer for 30 to 40 minutes. Spoon pan juices over chops and top with a little sliced scallion to serve.

Yield: 3 to 4 servings

Assuming 3, each will have: 289 calories; 20 g fat; 24 g protein; 1 g carbohydrate; trace dietary fiber; 1 g usable carb.

Dorothy Markuske's Pork Chops in Cream Sauce Topped with Seasoned Goat Cheese

Here's a seriously gourmet recipe. Our tester, Diana, gave this a 10!

Salt and pepper
4 pork chops, boneless
1 tablespoon (15 ml) olive oil
2–3 tablespoons (30–45 g) butter
1 shallot, chopped
2 cloves garlic, chopped
5 mushrooms, sliced
3 tablespoons (45 ml) sherry
1 tablespoon (4 g) fresh oregano, chopped
1 tablespoon (2.5 g) fresh thyme, chopped
1 teaspoon fresh rosemary, chopped fine
1 cup (240 ml) heavy cream
8 ounces (225 g) goat cheese
1 clove garlic, chopped fine
1 teaspoon fresh oregano, chopped
1 teaspoon fresh thyme, chopped

Salt and pepper both sides of pork chops. In your big, heavy skillet, brown pork chops in oil over medium heat 3 to 4 minutes each side. Remove chops and keep warm.

Pour the oil out of the pan. Melt the butter in the same pan, then sauté the shallot, then 2 cloves garlic, until soft—about 1 minute. Add the mushrooms, plus a little salt and pepper. Cook until mushrooms start to get color and soften, about 2 to 3 minutes.

Add sherry and one tablespoon each oregano, thyme, and rosemary, and stir around, scraping the bottom of the pan to dissolve the brown bits. Bring the mixture to a boil and reduce sherry, about 1 minute. Stir in cream, mixing well.

Add pork chops and any drippings back into the cream sauce. Cover and simmer until pork chops are cooked, 3 to 5 minutes.

In a small bowl mix goat cheese, 1 clove garlic, 1 teaspoon oregano, and 1 teaspoon thyme.

Divide goat cheese between the pork chops, topping them. Cover again and continue to simmer until cheese is warm. Serve by drizzling cream sauce over chops and garnish with sprig of thyme, rosemary, and oregano.

Note: Dorothy suggests you could also make this with boneless, skinless chicken breasts.

Yield: 4 servings

Each with: 751 calories; 60 g fat; 42 g protein; 6 g carbohydrate; 1 g dietary fiber; 5 g usable carbs.

Diane Kingsbury's Spicy Chops

This recipe is so good, our tester, Julie, has made it three times since testing!

> 4 boneless pork chops, 1/2" (1.25 cm) thick
> 1/4 cup (60 ml) lime juice
> 1 tablespoon (7 g) chili powder
> 1 tablespoon (15 ml) olive oil
> 1 teaspoon ground cumin
> 1 teaspoon ground cinnamon
> 1/2 teaspoon hot pepper sauce
> 1/4 teaspoon salt
> 2 cloves garlic, minced

Trim chops and place them in a shallow dish. Make the marinade by combining in a small bowl the lime juice, chili powder, olive oil, cumin, cinnamon, hot pepper sauce, salt, and garlic. Pour over chops and cover. Marinate in the refrigerator at least 6 hours, turning the chops over occasionally. Drain chops and discard the marinade.

Preheat charcoal grill and grill the chops for 10 to 12 minutes until done (160°F [75°C] degrees internal temperature) and juices run clear, turning once halfway through grilling.

Tester's note: Julie says this works well in the broiler or in your electric tabletop grill as well. She also says you can slice up the meat and wrap it in low-carb tortillas for a fajita-like version.

Yield: 4 servings

Each chop will give you: 196 calories; 10 g fat; 22 g protein; 4 g carbohydrate; 1 g dietary fiber; 3 g usable carbs.

◎ Jeannie Aromi's Pernil

5–6 pound (2.3–2.7 kg) pork shoulder roast
2 tablespoons (30 ml) olive oil
1 tablespoon (15 ml) vinegar (any kind will do)
4 cloves of garlic, sliced lengthwise into about 3–4 pieces per clove
1 teaspoon dried oregano

Preheat your oven to 425°F (220°C).

Place meat skin-side up in a shallow roasting pan. With a knife, make deep vertical slits in the meat, avoiding the bone, each about 1" (2.5 cm) to 2" (5 cm) deep. Drizzle the oil over the meat and rub it all over with your hands. Repeat with the vinegar, followed by the oregano. Put a piece of garlic vertically into each slit as deeply as you can. It's OK if some ends stick out; they will get brown and crispy and delicious.

Place the pan in the middle of the oven. Put a second pan with an inch of water in it on the rack below the meat. Roast at 425°F (220°C) for 15 minutes, then lower temperature to 325°F (170°C) and roast for 30 minutes per pound. Check the water pan now and then to see if it needs a refill. Serve the crackling skin along with the meat (talk about pork rinds!). Enjoy.

Jeannie's note: "This recipe is for a traditional Puerto Rican dish called pernil, which is basically a very garlicky roast fresh ham. I learned how to make this from my late mother-in-law, for my husband. It's traditionally served with rice and beans, which I make for the rest of my family, while I usually have un-Puerto Rican sauerkraut with mine!"

Yield: A 6-pound (2.7 kg) roast will feed 10

Each serving will have: 508 calories; 39 g fat; 35 g protein; 1 g carbohydrate; trace dietary fiber.

◎ Jill Boelsma's Pork Loin Roast

Here's an easy slow-cooker recipe. Our tester, Julie, says she'd pay big money in a restaurant for a pork roast this tender and juicy!

>   4 pounds (1.9 kg) pork loin roast
>   2 cups (480 ml) (approximately) heavy cream
>   1/2 cup (120 ml) water
>   Salt and pepper to taste
>   Guar or xanthan, optional

Place loin in slow cooker fat-side up and add about 1/2" (1.25 cm) of heavy cream to the bottom of the pot. Add about 1/2 cup (120 ml) of water, a liberal grinding of pepper, and salt to taste. Put on lid, set pot on low, and go out and have a life. (If you are home and can keep an eye on it, set lid ajar so that some evaporation takes place and turn the roast every once in a while. If all of the liquid evaporates, add more cream and water.) Figure on giving it 7 to 8 hours.

Roast should be very tender when prodded with a fork after 6 to 8 hours of crocking. Remove roast and skim off fat if there is an abundance of it. Blend "gravy" with a whisk or hand blender. May be thickened with guar or xanthan, but that's not always necessary, depending upon how much evaporation has taken place. Slice roast and pour creamy light brown gravy over meat. Ohmygod! Yum.

Yield: Assuming 8 servings

Each will have: 296 calories; 19 g fat; 29 g protein; 1 g carbohydrate; trace dietary fiber.

Mary Beth Wilson's Pork Tenderloin Medallions in Garlic Cream Reduction

2 pork tenderloins (about 1 lb)

Salt and pepper to taste

1 pinch dry mustard

12 (yes 12) large garlic cloves, minced

1 teaspoon butter

1 teaspoon vegetable oil

¾ cup (180 ml) white wine

1 ½ teaspoons fresh rosemary, finely chopped (I keep my sprigs whole and take them out of the sauce before serving)

¾ cup (180 ml) heavy cream

1 whole sprig rosemary, for garnish

Slice tenderloins into thin medallions; flatten with the palm of your hand. Sprinkle with salt, pepper, and mustard and fry in oil and butter until browned, about 4 minutes per side. Place on ovensafe plate and keep warm. Sauté garlic in small amount of butter and oil until very lightly browned. Add wine and rosemary and cook on medium-high heat until reduced by half. Add cream and cook until thickened and slightly reduced. Pour over medallions to serve.

Mary Beth's note: "This sauce works well with all meats and even fish (use about 3 pounds (1.4 kg) of fish to make the sauce quality come out right). It is a very elegant dish with little effort. Serve with green beans."

Yield: Assuming 4 servings

Each will have: 353 calories; 23 g fat; 25 g protein; 5 g carbohydrate; trace dietary fiber.

Jill Boelsma's "Breaded" Pork Tenderloin

1 pork tenderloin (not pork loin)

1/2 cup (25 g) pork rind crumbs (page 452)

1 slice low-carb bread, made into fresh crumbs

1/4 cup (40 g) grated Parmesan cheese

Salt and pepper to taste

2 eggs, beaten

1/4 cup (30 g) low-carb bake mix

Olive, canola, or peanut oil

Remove silver skin from pork tenderloin and slice into 1"- to 2"- (2.5 to 5 cm) thick rounds (or you can have the nice meat guys at the grocery store do this for you!). Place each round in a zipper-lock bag, one at a time, and using any heavy, blunt instrument that comes to hand, pound out to 1/4" (6.25 mm) thickness.

Combine pork rinds, bread crumbs, cheese, salt, and pepper. Beat your eggs in a shallow bowl, and put your bake mix on a plate. Roll each piece of pork in the bake mix, dip in the egg wash, and coat with pork rind/bread crumbs/cheese mix. Allow to rest on a wire rack for 10 to 15 minutes.

Heat 1/4" (6.25 mm) of oil in skillet over medium-high heat and fry pork 2 or 3 cutlets at a time until deep golden brown on each side. Drain on paper towels and keep in warm oven until all medallions are cooked.

Yield: If this serves 3 ...

Each serving will have: 508 calories; 30 g fat; 53 g protein; 4 g carbohydrate; 2 g dietary fiber; 2 g usable carbs.

◎ Ham Kedgeree

Oh, boy, are you going to thank me for this recipe the Monday after Easter. This quick and tasty skillet supper, based on a traditional dish from the British occupation of India, will help you use up both leftover ham and hard-boiled eggs! It's good enough that you may find yourself buying precooked ham and boiling up some eggs at other times of year.

1/2 head cauliflower
3 tablespoons (45 g) butter
1 tablespoon (7 g) curry powder
3 tablespoons (30 g) minced onion
2 cups (220 g) ham, cut in 1/2" (1.25 cm) cubes
4 hard-boiled eggs, coarsely chopped
1/4 cup (60 ml) heavy cream
Salt and pepper
1/4 cup (15 g) chopped fresh parsley

Run the cauliflower through the shredding blade of your food processor. Put it in a microwaveable casserole with a lid, add a couple of tablespoons of water, cover, and microwave on high for 6 minutes.

Melt the butter in your large, heavy skillet over low heat, and add the curry powder and onion. Sauté them together for 2 to 3 minutes. Add everything else, stir gently but thoroughly (gently so that you don't completely pulverize the hunks of egg yolk), heat through, and serve.

Yield: 4 servings

Each with: 340 calories; 27 g fat; 19 g protein; 6 g carbohydrate; 1 g dietary fiber; 5 g usable carbs.

◎ Orange-Maple Ham Slice

If you're alert, you'll figure out that this recipe is, er, derivative of the recipe for Ham Glaze elsewhere in this book. Ham slices are much quicker, though! (We're not talking about deli-sliced ham, here, by the way. We're talking about a big, oval slice of ham, like a steak. Look with the hams in the meat case.)

1 tablespoon (15 ml) sugar-free pancake syrup

1 1/2 teaspoons lemon juice

3 drops orange extract

1/2 teaspoon brown mustard

1 tablespoon (15 g) butter

1 pound (455 g) ham slice

Mix together the sugar-free pancake syrup, lemon juice, orange extract, and mustard. Melt the butter in your big, heavy skillet, and cook the ham slice in it, browning on both sides—it should take no more than 5 minutes per side or so. Now remove the ham steak to a platter, and pour the sauce into the skillet. Stir it around, scraping up the browned bits—add a tablespoon or so of water if you think you need it. Put the ham slice back in the pan, turning it to coat both sides, and give it another minute or so, then serve.

Yield: 3 to 4 servings

Assuming 3, each will have: 382 calories; 30 g fat; 26 g protein; trace carbohydrate; trace dietary fiber, so an even smaller trace of usable carb, though this doesn't include the polyols in the sugar-free pancake syrup.

Winter Night Sausage Bake

This one-dish meal is serious down-home comfort food. Feel free to make it with turkey sausage, if you prefer.

> 1 1-pound (455 g) roll pork sausage
> 1 apple
> 1 medium onion
> 1 1/2 teaspoons chicken bouillon granules
> 1 cup (240 g) water
> Guar or xanthan
> Salt and pepper to taste
> 1 batch The Ultimate Fauxtatoes (page 136)

Preheat oven to 350°F (180°C).

Slice your pound of pork sausage into patties. Put 'em in your big, heavy skillet over medium heat. You're going to cook them until they're browned on both sides.

In the meanwhile, slice the apple and the onion thin, and have them standing by.

When the sausage patties are cooked, lay them in an 8" x 8" (20 x 20 cm) baking dish you've sprayed with nonstick cooking spray. Now put the apple and onion slices in the skillet, and sauté them in the sausage grease until they're tender and turning golden. Spread the apples and onions on top of the sausage.

Put the chicken bouillon concentrate and the water in the skillet, and stir it around, scraping up any tasty brown stuff stuck to the skillet. Thicken the whole thing to a not-too-thick gravy consistency with your guar or xanthan shaker, salt and pepper to taste, and pour this gravy over the sausage, apple, and onion.

Now spread your Ultimate Fauxtatoes in an even layer over the whole thing. Bake for 20 minutes, and serve.

Yield: 4 to 5 servings

Assuming 4, each will have: 642 calories; 51 g fat; 24 g protein; 22 g carbohydrate; 9 g dietary fiber; 13 g usable carbs.

◎ Celia Volk's Portobello Mushroom Pizza

Here's a great pizza substitute. Our tester, Ray Stevens, says this is surprisingly easy for something that seems so fancy.

> 2 large portobello mushrooms, washed
> ¼–½ cup (60–120 g) stewed tomatoes, Italian recipe, chopped up (find the lowest-carb brand you can!)
> ¼ pound (115 g) bulk Italian sausage, cooked, crumbled, and drained
> ¼ cup (25 g) chopped black olives
> 8–10 pepperoni slices
> ¼–½ cup (30–60 g) shredded mozzarella cheese

Preheat oven to 350°F (180°C).

Destem the mushrooms, placing them gill-side up on a baking sheet. Put half of the stewed tomatoes on each mushroom. Add the sausage, olives, pepperoni (or your choice of pizza toppings), and even the sliced mushroom stems if you like. Top with the mozzarella cheese.

Bake for 20 to 30 minutes, or until cheese begins to brown.

Yield: Makes 2 pizzas

Each having: 491 calories; 39 g fat; 24 g protein; 12 g carbohydrate; 3 g dietary fiber; 9 g usable carbs.

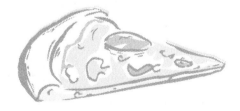

◎ Tom Budlong's Italian Sausage and Peppers

Add a green salad with Italian dressing, and there's dinner.

> 1 package fresh sweet Italian sausages. (Usually about five links
>   —this recipe can be easily adapted for a different quantity.)
> 1–2 tablespoons (15–30 ml) olive oil
> 1 half each green, red, and yellow bell peppers
>   (or any mix of your choice), sliced into thin strips
> 1 small onion, sliced into strips
> 1 cup (100 g) fresh button or brown mushrooms, sliced
> 3 cloves fresh garlic (or to taste), roughly chopped
> 1 cup (225 g) no-sugar-added spaghetti sauce
> Italian seasoning
> Salt
> Freshly ground black pepper
> Optional—If you can find it in your supermarket, Tom finds that
>   a few grindings of dried porcini mushrooms adds additional flavor.

In a nonstick skillet or using a light coating of olive oil, brown the sausages on both sides and set aside. In the same skillet, add some olive oil and sauté the peppers, onions, mushrooms, and garlic over low heat until soft.

Add the spaghetti sauce and season to taste with Italian seasoning, salt, pepper, and optional porcini mushrooms. Return the sausages to the skillet, and simmer over very low heat, stirring occasionally until the sausages are done through. This dish actually improves the longer it cooks and is even better when reheated another day.

Yield: About 4 servings

Each with: 479 calories; 40 g fat; 18 g protein; 13 g carbohydrate; 3 g dietary fiber; 10 g usable carbs.

◎ Susan Higgs's Lemon-Rosemary Lamb Chops

Our tester, Julie, who calls this "wonderful, easy, and delicious," says this should be on the menu of every restaurant that has a low-carb menu!

Marinade:

- 16 ounces (455 gm) sour cream
- Zest and juice of 1 lemon (fresh is fantastic)
- Fresh rosemary (strip the leaves off 4-6 stalks)
- 3 cloves garlic, minced
- 1 medium onion, finely chopped
- ¼ cup olive oil
- 15 precut lamb rib chops, almost ½" (1.25 cm) thick

Combine everything but the lamb chops, and mix really, really well.

Coat the chops really well in the mixture and drop them in a zipper-lock bag. Once all are coated and in the bag, pour the leftover marinade in on top of them. Seal and marinate for 24 to 48 hours.

Heat up your electric tabletop grill. Once hot, pull the chops out of the marinade and cook 4 to 6 at a time, depending upon the size of your grill. Give them 8 minutes without lifting the lid, then check for doneness. Susan says grilling for 8 minutes gave her a nice medium-ish doneness, but cook to your taste. Keep the ones that are done warm while you grill the rest.

Susan's note: Susan suggests a cucumber/onion vinegar salad and green beans as sides with this, and who am I to argue?

Yield: Makes 10 servings

Each with: 593 calories; 50 g fat; 30 g protein; 6 g carbohydrate; trace dietary fiber.

◎ Susan Higgs' Lamb Florentine

I adore lamb, but a whole leg, or even a half, is awfully big for my two-person household. Susan comes to the rescue with this recipe for using up leftover roast lamb! Our tester, Julie McIntosh, says, "It tastes like it's a ton of trouble, it looks fancy, and it's easy. Everyone loved it, including my husband who doesn't even like spinach as a general rule. This Susan Higgs person is a genius!" I can but concur.

> 1–2 pounds (455 g–1 kg) cooked lamb, cut into bite-sized pieces
> 3–4 10-ounce (280 g) packages frozen chopped spinach, thawed and drained
> 1/3 cup butter
> 3 tablespoons (45 g) mayonnaise
> 5 tablespoons (50 g) grated Parmesan cheese
> 3 tablespoons (45 ml) dry sherry
> Salt and pepper to taste
> 1/2 cup (75 g) shredded Parmesan cheese

Preheat oven to 350°F (180°C).

Mix all ingredients together, then put in a 2-quart casserole dish or a 9" x 13" (22.5 x 32.5 cm) pan. Cover (use foil if your pan doesn't have a lid) and bake for 30 minutes.

Remove cover, sprinkle the top with shredded Parmesan cheese, and bake until cheese is brown (about 10 to 15 minutes).

Yield: Serves 4 to 6

Assuming 5 servings, each will have: 558 calories; 46 g fat; 29 g protein; 8 g carbohydrate; 5 g dietary fiber; 3 g usable carbs.

◎ Fiery Indian Lamb and Cauliflower

This is a fairly authentic Indian dish, and it is quite hot! Feel free to halve the red pepper if you like it milder.

> 1 pound (455 g) lean lamb
> 4 cloves garlic, crushed
> 2 teaspoons grated gingerroot
> 2 teaspoons red pepper flakes
> 1 1/2 teaspoons ground cumin
> 2 teaspoons pepper
> 2 tablespoons (30 g) butter
> 1 tablespoon (15 ml) olive oil
> 1 medium onion, chopped
> 1/2 cup (115 g) plain yogurt
> 1/2 head cauliflower, in small florets
> Salt to taste

Trim your lamb well, and cut it into 1/2" (1.25 cm) to 1" (2.5 cm) cubes. Put it in a mixing bowl, and add the spices. Stir to coat all the lamb cubes evenly, and let the lamb sit in this dry marinade for at least 15 minutes.

Melt the butter in your large, heavy skillet over medium-low heat, and add the olive oil. Now add the onion, and sauté until it's translucent and turning golden. Stir in the yogurt until smooth. Now add the lamb cubes, and stir to coat. Let this cook on low heat until the lamb cubes are no longer pink, and all excess water has cooked off the yogurt.

Now add 1 cup (240 ml) water and let the lamb simmer until the liquid is reduced by half, and the lamb cubes are quite tender. Stir in the cauliflower, cover, and let the whole thing simmer for 15 minutes, or until the cauliflower is tender. Uncover, simmer another 5 minutes to boil off extra liquid, and salt to taste. Serve.

Yield: 3 to 4 servings

Assuming 3, each will have: 440 calories; 34 g fat; 24 g protein; 9 g carbohydrate; 2 g dietary fiber; 7 g usable carbs.

Greek Meatza

A good recipe deserves a variation! Here's my new, Greek-style version of meat-crust pizza.

> 2 pounds (1 kg) ground lamb
> 1/2 medium onion, minced
> 4 cloves garlic, crushed
> 1 1/2 teaspoons dried oregano
> 1 teaspoon salt
> 1/2 cup (115 g) pizza sauce (Ragu makes one with no sugar, but read the label!)
> 10 ounces (280 g) frozen chopped spinach, thawed and very well-drained
> 1/3 cup (35 g) sliced black olives
> 1/2 cup (120 g) canned diced tomatoes, drained
> 2 cups (240 g) shredded Monterey Jack cheese
> 1 cup (120 g) crumbled feta cheese

Plunk the first five ingredients in a large mixing bowl, and using clean hands, moosh everything together really well. Pat out into an even layer in a 9" x 13" (22.5 x 32.5 cm) pan, and bake at 350°F (180°C) for 20 minutes. Pour off the grease.

Spread the pizza sauce over the meat layer. Spread the spinach evenly over the sauce, top that with the olives and tomatoes. Spread the two cheeses over that. Turn your broiler to low, and broil about 4" (10 cm) from the heat for about 6 to 8 minutes, or until browned and bubbly.

Yield: 8 servings

Each with: 510 calories; 40 g fat; 30 g protein; 7 g carbohydrate; 2 g dietary fiber; 5 g usable carbs.

◉ Irish Stew

I came up with this for St. Patrick's Day, and it's amazing. The Ketatoes mix gives it a true potato flavor, while keeping the carb count remarkably low. This takes time, but not that much work—so make it on a day when you're hanging around the house getting chores done.

2 large turnips, cut in ½" (1.25 cm) cubes
½ head cauliflower, cut in ½" (1.25 cm) cubes or chunks
3 medium onions, sliced
½ cup (25 g) Ketatoes mix
2 pounds (1 kg) leg of lamb, cut in 1" (2.5 cm) cubes
Salt and pepper
Water to cover
½ teaspoon chicken bouillon concentrate
½ teaspoon beef bouillon concentrate
Guar or xanthan

You'll need your meat and vegetables all cut up before you do anything else; make sure your lamb cubes are well trimmed of all fat. Spray a Dutch oven or large, heavy soup kettle with nonstick cooking spray.

Now, put a layer of mixed turnip and cauliflower in the bottom of your pot. Add a layer of onion. Scatter 2 tablespoons of the Ketotatoes mix over that, then put in a layer of cubed lamb. Salt and pepper the lamb. Now repeat the layers two more times, at which point you should be out of meat and veggies.

Pour cold water over everything to just barely cover. Put a lid on the pot, and set it over the lowest possible flame. Let it simmer for 2 hours.

Take the lid off, and stir in the bouillon concentrate. Now, continue to simmer over lowest heat, uncovered, for another 2 hours or so—you're cooking down the gravy a little.

Finally, using your whisk and your guar or xanthan shaker, thicken up the gravy to taste, and also salt and pepper to taste, then serve.

Yield: 8 servings

Each with: 234 calories; 7 g fat; 29 g protein; 13 g carbohydrate; 5 g dietary fiber; 8 g usable carbs.

About Lamb Steaks

Everyone's heard of lamb chops, but I prefer lamb steaks. I buy a whole leg of lamb, and ask the nice meat guy behind the counter to cut two smallish roasts off either end (a perfect size for my 2-person household) and slice the rest into steaks between $1/2$" (1.25 cm) and 3/4" (1.875 cm) thick. These are meatier than lamb chops, and generally less expensive, as well. Here are some things to do with lamb steaks—but I suspect they'd all work with chops, as well.

◎ Five-Spice Lamb Steak

    8 ounces (225 g) lamb leg steak
    1 tablespoon (15 g) oil
    1 teaspoon grated gingerroot
    1 clove garlic, crushed
    2 tablespoons (30 ml) dry sherry
    1 teaspoon five-spice powder
    $1/2$ teaspoon Splenda
    1 teaspoon soy sauce

Slash the edges of your lamb steak to keep it from curling. In your big, heavy skillet, over medium heat, start pan-frying the lamb steak in the oil. You'll want to give it about 6 minutes per side.

While that's happening, mix together everything else. When the lamb steak is cooked on both sides, pour this mixture into the skillet. Turn the steak over once or twice to coat, and let it cook just another minute or two. Serve with the pan liquid scraped over it.

Yield: 1 to 2 servings

Assuming 1, each will have: 576 calories; 44 g fat; 33 g protein; 2 g carbohydrate; trace dietary fiber; 2 g usable carbs.

◎ Lamb Steak with Walnut Sauce

8 ounces (225 g) lamb leg steak
Salt and pepper
1 tablespoon (15 ml) olive oil
2 tablespoons (20 g) minced onion
2 tablespoons (15 g) chopped walnuts
1 clove garlic
2 tablespoons (8 g) chopped parsley
1/4 teaspoon dried oregano
1/4 teaspoon ground rosemary
2 tablespoons (30 ml) lemon juice

Preheat your electric tabletop grill. Rub the steak with a little olive oil, and salt and pepper both sides lightly. When the grill is hot, put the steak on, and set a timer for 5 to 6 minutes.

In a small, heavy skillet, over medium-low heat, heat the olive oil and sauté the onion, walnuts, and garlic until the onion is soft. Stir in the parsley, oregano, and rosemary, and cook another couple of minutes, until the parsley is wilted. Stir in the lemon juice, and let it simmer for a minute or so.

By now your lamb steak is done. Pull it out, throw it on a plate, and spoon the walnut sauce over it. Serve.

Yield: 1 to 2 servings

Assuming 1, each will have: 651 calories; 53 g fat; 37 g protein; 8 g carbohydrate; 2 g dietary fiber; 6 g usable carbs.

Orange-Rosemary Lamb Steak

8 ounces (225 g) lamb leg steak
1 tablespoon (15 ml) olive oil
1 1/2 teaspoons butter
2 tablespoons (30 ml) lemon juice
1/4 teaspoon orange extract
1 teaspoon Splenda
1/2 teaspoon ground rosemary

Slash the edges of your lamb steak to keep it from curling.

Put your big, heavy skillet over medium heat, and add the olive oil and butter, swirling them together as the butter melts. Add the lamb steak, and give it about 5 to 6 minutes per side. Remove to serving plate.

While the lamb steak is cooking, stir together the lemon juice, orange extract, and Splenda. When you've removed the steak from the skillet, add the lemon juice mixture, and stir it around, scraping up the browned bits from the bottom of the skillet. Stir in the rosemary, and let the whole thing simmer for a moment or two. Pour this sauce over the lamb steak, and serve.

Yield: 1 to 2 servings

Assuming 1, each will have: 593 calories; 50 g fat; 32 g protein; 3 g carbohydrate; trace dietary fiber; 3 g usable carbs.

Balsamic-Mint Lamb Steak

8 ounces (225 g) lamb leg steak
2 tablespoons (30 ml) olive oil
¼ teaspoon beef bouillon concentrate
1 tablespoon (15 ml) boiling water
1 tablespoon (15 ml) balsamic vinegar
1 teaspoon chopped fresh mint

Slash the edges of your lamb steak to keep it from curling. Then heat the olive oil over medium-high heat in your big, heavy skillet, and start the steak sautéing. You'll want to give it 5 to 7 minutes per side.

Meanwhile, dissolve the bouillon concentrate in the water, and stir in the balsamic vinegar.

When your steak is done to your liking, remove it to a serving plate, and pour the bouillion-vinegar mixture into it. Stir it around to dissolve the yummy brown stuff stuck to the skillet, then stir in the mint. Pour this sauce over the steak, and serve.

Yield: 1 serving

655 calories; 58 g fat; 32 g protein; 1 g carbohydrate; trace dietary fiber; 1 g usable carb.

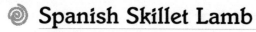 Spanish Skillet Lamb

This authentically Spanish skillet dish is quick, easy, and tasty.

> 16 ounces (455 g) lamb leg (cutting up a lamb steak or two is good)
> 4 tablespoons (40 g) chopped onion
> 2 tablespoons (30 ml) olive oil
> 2 cloves garlic, crushed
> 2 teaspoons paprika
> 2 tablespoons (30 ml) lemon juice

Cut the lamb into strips—make sure it's well trimmed of fat. In your big, heavy skillet, over high heat, start sautéing the lamb and onion in the olive oil. When the lamb is getting browned all over, stir in the garlic, paprika, and lemon juice.

Turn burner to medium-low, cover, and let the whole thing simmer for about 15 minutes—check once or twice to make sure your pan hasn't gone dry, and add just a little water if it's threatening to. Serve over cauli-rice if you like, but this is just fine the way it is.

Yield: 2 to 3 servings

Assuming 3, each will have: 369 calories; 30 g fat; 22 g protein; 4 g carbohydrate; 1 g dietary fiber; 3 g usable carbs.

Spice-Rubbed Leg of Lamb with Apricot-Chipotle Glaze

A whole leg of lamb will feed a crowd! If you don't have a crowd, feel free to ask the nice meat guys to cut your leg of lamb in half. Keep the tapered shank end for your roast and make half the rub and glaze. Have the broader end sliced 1/2" (1.25 cm) thick for lamb steaks. I've never been charged for this service!

> 1/4 cup (30 g) paprika
> 1 tablespoon (7 g) ground cumin
> 1 tablespoon (7 g) ground cinnamon
> 1 tablespoon (7 g) ground coriander
> 2 teaspoons garlic powder
> 1 teaspoon salt or Vege-Sal
> 1 teaspoon pepper
> 2 tablespoons (3 g) Splenda
> Leg of lamb, about 8 pounds (3.6 kg)
> Apricot-Chipotle Glaze (page 439)

Combine all the spices with the Splenda, and stir well. Sprinkle liberally over your leg of lamb, coating the whole surface. Roast at 325°F (170°C) for 30 minutes per pound of lamb.

About 1/2 hour before cooking time is up, start basting with the Apricot-Chipotle Glaze. Baste two or three times before the cooking time is through. Remove lamb from oven, and allow to rest for 10 to 15 minutes before carving. Serve with remaining Apricot-Chipotle Glaze.

Yield: 15 to 16 servings, so invite a crowd

Assuming 15, each will have: 499 calories; 37 g fat; 35 g protein; 6 g carbohydrate; 1 g dietary fiber; 5 g usable carbs.

chapter eleven

Main Dish Salads

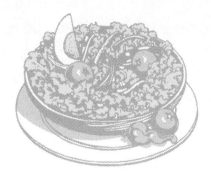

More and more, I rely on main dish salads. I can't think of anything tastier or more nutritious. Most main dish salads are fairly quick and easy, too, especially when you consider that you don't need another darned thing with them—no side dishes to mess around with.

So here is a huge variety of main dish salads of every description, and I hope you enjoy them all! Certainly they'll take you way beyond the ubiquitous chicken Caesar salad. (I mean, they're good, but haven't they been a little, well, overdone, of late?)

We start with chicken salads, which come in two basic varieties: those that call for you to grill a boneless, skinless chicken breast, and those that call for leftover cooked chicken. This latter variety is a fine reason to always cook a few extra pieces of chicken when you're roasting some for supper. But if you don't have cold cooked chicken on hand, you can quickly cook one of those boneless, skinless breasts, or, in a pinch, use canned chunk chicken, though it's definitely a distant third choice. You can also use cold leftover turkey, a good thing to keep in mind the weekend after Thanksgiving!

Artichoke Chicken Salad

½ cup (150 g) canned artichoke hearts, sliced

2 cups (220 g) diced cooked chicken

⅓ cup (75 g) canned water chestnuts, diced or sliced

¼ cup (25 g) stuffed olives, sliced

1 tablespoon (15 ml) soy sauce

¼ cup (60 ml) Italian salad dressing, homemade or bottled

¾ cup (90 g) diced celery

1 tablespoon (15 g) butter

½ cup (60 g) pecans, chopped

Combine everything but the butter and pecans in a medium-sized mixing bowl, and toss well.

In a medium-sized heavy skillet, over medium heat, melt the butter and add the pecans. Let them toast, stirring often, for 5 or 6 minutes. Add to the salad, and toss.

Serve on a bed of lettuce, if you like.

Yield: 3 servings

Each with: 614 calories; 49 g fat; 31 g protein; 12 g carbohydrate; 3 g dietary fiber; 9 g usable carbs.

Caribbean Grilled Chicken Salad

1 1/2 pounds (680 g) boneless, skinless chicken breast
3 tablespoons (45 ml) Teriyaki Sauce (page 531)
4 cups (80 g) iceberg lettuce, chopped
4 cups (80 g) leaf lettuce, chopped
1 1/2 cups (115 g) red cabbage, chopped
1/3 cup (80 g) canned pineapple chunks in juice, diced small
Honey-Lime-Mustard Dressing (page 212)
1/2 cup (130 g) salsa

Put the chicken and the Teriyaki Sauce in a zipper-lock bag. Seal the bag, pressing out the air as you go, and throw it in the fridge for at least an hour or two, and all day won't hurt a bit.

Okay, mealtime's rolling around. First, plug in your electric tabletop grill. Then assemble your greens (and your red!) in a big salad bowl. Cut the pineapple into little bitty chunks—that measurement is after cutting it up, by the way—and throw that in, too.

Your grill is hot! Pull the chicken out of the fridge, drain the Teriyaki Sauce into a little bowl, and throw the chicken on the grill. Set your oven timer for 3 minutes.

Meanwhile, toss the salad with the Honey-Lime-Mustard dressing. When the timer goes off, open the grill, baste the chicken with the Teriyaki Sauce you reserved, turning it over to get both sides. Close the grill and set the timer for another 2 minutes.

Pile your salad on four serving plates. When the timer goes off, pull the chicken out and put it on your cutting board. Slice it up and divide it between the four salads. Top each serving with 2 tablespoons (30 g) of salsa and serve.

Yield: 4 servings

Each with: 326 calories; 12 g fat; 41 g protein; 13 g carbohydrate; 4 g dietary fiber; 9 g usable carbs.

Ginger-Almond Chicken Salad

1 1/2 pounds boneless, skinless chicken breast

1/4 cup (60 ml) Teriyaki Sauce (page 527)

6 cups (120 g) iceberg lettuce, chopped

6 cups (120 g) red leaf lettuce, chopped

2 cups (150 g) shredded red cabbage

2 cups (150 g) shredded cabbage (use bagged cole slaw mix, if you like)

1/2 cup (60 g) shredded carrot

8 scallions, sliced, including the crisp part of the green shoot

1 tablespoon (15 g) butter

2/3 cup (80 g) slivered almonds

1 cup (240 ml) Ginger Salad Dressing (page 211)

Marinate the chicken breasts in the Teriyaki Sauce for at least 30 minutes, and all day won't hurt a bit.

When mealtime rolls around, plug in your electric tabletop grill to preheat. While that's happening, start assembling your vegetables in a big ol' salad bowl.

Okay, the grill's hot. Throw your chicken breasts in, and set your oven timer for 3 minutes.

Melt the butter in a medium skillet, and start sautéing the almonds in it. You want them just barely golden.

While the chicken and almonds are cooking, pour on the dressing, and toss the salad.

The timer went off! Go baste the chicken on both sides with the Teriyaki Sauce it marinated in, and close the grill again. Run back to the stove and reset the timer for another 2 to 3 minutes. Stir the almonds while you're there!

Whew! Okay, chicken's done, almonds are golden. First take the almonds off the heat so they don't burn. Now remove your chicken from the grill, to your cutting board.

Pile the salad on four serving plates. Slice the chicken breasts, and divide between the four salads. Top each with almonds, and serve.

Yield: 4 servings

Each with: 613 calories; 39 g fat; 48 g protein; 21 g carbohydrate; 8 g dietary fiber; 13 g usable carbs.

⊚ Asian Chicken Salad

Michael Barber is the executive sous chef at the Hyatt Regency DFW and he very kindly sent me this recipe. Low-carb options like this one can be found on low-carb menus at Hyatts across the nation.

> 3 cups (60 g) shredded Napa cabbage
> 1 cup (75 g) shredded red cabbage
> ¼ cup (30 g) red peppers, julienned
> ¼ cup (35 g) carrot, julienned
> 1 tablespoon (6 g) sliced green onions
> 2 cooked chicken breast halves, without skin
> ½ cup (120 ml) Spicy Peanut Dressing (page 216)
> 1 sprig cilantro

Thinly slice chicken breast on a bias. Place all ingredients except cilantro leaves in a mixing bowl and toss. Garnish with cilantro leaves.

Yield: Makes 2 servings

Each with: 508 calories; 34 g fat; 35 g protein; 18 g carbohydrate; 6 g dietary fiber; 12 g usable carbs.

⊚ Chicken Chili Cheese Salad

You got your chicken, you got your vegetables, you got your cheese. Pretty nutritious, you think? All that, and it tastes good, too. Feel free to make this with leftover turkey or ham, if you prefer. Or, for that matter, with canned chunk chicken, should you not have any cold cooked chicken in the house.

½ head cauliflower
1 cup (120 g) diced celery
½ red bell pepper, diced
⅓ cup (55 g) diced red onion
¼ cup (30 g) diced green chilies
4 ounces (115 g) Monterey Jack cheese, cut into ¼" (6.25 mm) cubes
1 ½ cups (165 g) diced cooked chicken
⅓ cup (80 g) mayonnaise
½ teaspoon ground cumin
1 teaspoon chili powder
½ teaspoon dried oregano
1 tablespoon (15 ml) white vinegar
1 ½ teaspoons lime juice
2 ounces (55 g) sliced black olives, drained

First, chop your cauliflower into ½" (1.25 cm) chunks. Throw it in a microwaveable casserole with a lid, add a couple of tablespoons of water, cover, and nuke it on high for 7 minutes.

While that's cooking, assemble your other vegetables, your cheese, and your chicken in a big darned mixing bowl.

As soon as the microwave beeps, pull out your cauliflower, uncover it, and drain it. Let it sit and cool for a few minutes, though—you don't want to melt your cheese. While you're waiting for the cauliflower to cool, measure your mayonnaise, cumin, chili powder, oregano, vinegar, and lime juice. Stir everything together.

Okay, cauliflower cooled a bit? Dump it in with the chicken, cheese, and veggies, and stir everything round. Dump in the olives, pour on the dressing, and toss to coat. You can eat this right away, if you like, or chill it for a few hours. This is nice served on a bed of lettuce, but you could serve it stuffed into tomatoes, too.

Yield: 3 to 4 servings

Each with: 462 calories; 39 g fat; 24 g protein; 7 g carbohydrate; 2 g dietary fiber; 5 g usable carbs.

Jerk Chicken Salad

1 cup (110 g) diced cooked chicken

4 scallions, sliced, including the crisp part of the green shoot

1 stalk celery, diced

2 tablespoons (30 g) mayonnaise

1 teaspoon spicy brown mustard

1/2 teaspoon sugar-free imitation honey

1 teaspoon lime juice

1/2 teaspoon jerk seasoning, purchased or homemade

1/4 cup (50 g) diced peaches (I used frozen unsweetened peaches, but use fresh if you've got 'em)

Put your chicken, scallions, and celery in a mixing bowl. Whisk together the mayo, mustard, sugar-free imitation honey, lime juice, and jerk seasoning; pour it over the chicken; and toss. Add the peach dice, toss again, then serve, on lettuce if you like.

Yield: 2 servings

Each with: 407 calories; 29 g fat; 22 g protein; 6 g carbohydrate; 2 g dietary fiber; 4 g usable carbs.

Oriental Chicken, "Rice," and Walnut Salad Wrapped in Lettuce

1/2 head cauliflower
1 tablespoon (15 g) butter
1/2 cup (60 g) walnuts, chopped
4 teaspoons soy sauce, divided
2 cups (220 g) diced cooked chicken
2 tablespoons (30 ml) rice vinegar
2 tablespoons (30 ml) oil
3 teaspoons grated gingerroot
Salt
20 lettuce leaves

First run your cauliflower through the shredding blade of your food processor. Put it in a microwaveable casserole with a lid, add a couple of tablespoons of water, cover, and nuke it on high for 6 minutes. When the microwave beeps, uncover your cauliflower right away! You don't want white mush.

While that's happening, melt the butter in a medium skillet, and add the walnuts. Stir over medium heat for a few minutes, until they're getting crisp. Stir in 2 teaspoons of the soy sauce and sauté for another minute, to evaporate the soy sauce a bit. Remove from heat.

Put the diced chicken, walnuts, and cauli-rice in a big mixing bowl. Stir together the rice vinegar, oil, grated gingerroot, and the other 2 teaspoons of soy sauce. Pour over the chicken and cauliflower, and toss well. Salt to taste.

Serve the salad mounded on 4 plates, with lettuce leaves on the side. Wrap the salad up in the leaves to eat.

Yield: 4 servings

Each with: 437 calories; 36 g fat; 26 g protein; 5 g carbohydrate; 2 g dietary fiber; 3 g usable carbs.

Chinese Chicken Salad

2 quarts (1.9 L) torn lettuce, loosely packed

1 cup (75 g) shredded cabbage (use bagged cole slaw mix if you like)

2 tablespoons (25 g) canned water chestnuts, diced

2 tablespoons (15 g) shredded carrot

3 scallions, sliced, including the crisp part of the green shoot

1 tablespoon (7 g) sesame seeds

1/4 cup (30 g) slivered almonds

1/2 tablespoon (7 g) butter

1 batch Soy and Sesame Dressing (page 207)

1 1/2 cups (165 g) cooked diced chicken

3 slices bacon, cooked and drained

In a big salad bowl combine the lettuce, cabbage, water chestnuts, carrots, and scallions. Set aside.

In a medium skillet, over medium heat, stir the sesame seeds and almonds in the butter until the almonds are just barely golden. Remove from heat and set aside.

We're on the home stretch. Pour the dressing over the vegetables, and toss well. Add the almonds and sesame seeds, and toss again. Pile the salad on three plates, and top each serving with 1/3 of the chicken. Crumble a strip of bacon over each serving, and serve.

Yield: 3 servings

Each with: 505 calories; 38 g fat; 29 g protein; 14 g carbohydrate; 5 g dietary fiber; 9 g usable carbs.

Tex-Mex Chicken Salad

$1/2$ head cauliflower

1 cup (120 g)

$1/2$ red bell pepper, diced

$1/3$ cup (55 g) diced red onion

$1/4$ cup (30 g) canned green chiles

4 ounces (115 g) Monterey Jack cheese, cut in $1/4$" (6.25 mm) cubes

$1/4$ cup (25 g) sliced black olives

1 cup (110 g)diced cooked chicken

$1/3$ cup (80 g) mayonnaise

$1/2$ teaspoon ground cumin

$1/2$ teaspoon dried oregano

1 teaspoon chili powder

1 tablespoon (15 ml) white wine vinegar

1 $1/2$ teaspoons lime juice

$1/3$ cup (20 g) chopped fresh cilantro

Chop the cauliflower, including the stem, into $1/2$" (1.25 cm) bits. Put them in a microwaveable casserole with a lid, add a couple of tablespoons of water, cover, and nuke it on high for 7 minutes.

Assemble all your other veggies, not to mention the cheese and the chicken, in a big mixing bowl.

When the cauliflower comes out, uncover it and let it sit to cool for at least 5 minutes, and more won't hurt—you don't want it to melt your chunks of cheese. When the cauliflower has cooled a bit, drain it and add it to the other stuff.

Meanwhile, mix together the mayo, cumin, oregano, chili powder, white wine vinegar, and lime juice. Pour over the assembled vegetables and protein, and toss well. Add the cilantro and toss again. Chill it if you have time, but it's pretty darned good even if it's still slightly warm!

Yield: 3 servings

Each with: 526 calories; 45 g fat; 25 g protein; 9 g carbohydrate; 3 g dietary fiber; 6 g usable carbs.

Cobb Salad

Cobb salad is currently very trendy. Here's how to make your own.

> 4 cups (80 g) romaine lettuce, chopped
> 2 ounces (55 g) deli turkey breast
> or 2 ounces (55 g) cooked chicken
> 1 hard-boiled egg
> 1/2 small tomato
> 1/2 California avocado
> 2 ounces (55 g) crumbled blue cheese
> 3 slices bacon, cooked and drained
> Cobb Salad Dressing (page 213) or another dressing of your choice

This is very simple: Arrange the lettuce in a bed on a plate—or a couple of plates, if you're going to call this two servings. Cut the turkey or chicken into strips or cubes; slice the egg, tomato, and avocado.

Arrange the various ingredients in stripes or in spoke fashion on the bed or beds of lettuce. Top with the Cobb Dressing or another dressing of your choice. That's it!

Yield: 1 huge serving, or 2 smaller ones

Assuming 1 serving, it will have: 647 calories; 47 g fat; 44 g protein; 16 g carbohydrate; 9 g dietary fiber; 7 g usable carbs.

◎ Thai Cobb Salad

Hey, a classic salad deserves a variation!

12 ounces (340 g) boneless, skinless chicken breast

2 tablespoons (30 ml) Teriyaki Sauce (page 531)

6 cups (120 g) torn mixed greens (I used romaine, leaf lettuce, and iceberg)

1/2 cup (30 g) chopped cilantro

1/2 cup (120 ml) Ginger Salad Dressing (page 211)

1/2 teaspoon red pepper flakes (optional)

1/2 California avocado

1/3 cup (40 g) shredded carrot

1/4 cup (30 g) chopped peanuts

4 scallions, sliced, including the crisp part of the green shoot

1 cup (100 g) diced cucumber

Put the chicken in a zipper-lock bag with the Teriyaki Sauce. Seal the bag, pressing out the air as you go, and turn the bag a few times to coat. Let the chicken marinate for at least 1/2 hour, and longer would be nice.

When time comes to actually make your salad, pull out your marinated chicken and pour the marinade off into a small bowl. Heat your electric tabletop grill.

While the grill is heating, put your greens in a big salad bowl with the cilantro, add the Ginger Salad Dressing and red pepper flakes, and toss well.

Okay, the grill is hot. Throw in the chicken, and set your oven timer for 3 minutes.

While the chicken is cooking, slice your avocado.

When the timer beeps, baste the chicken on both sides with the reserved marinade. Re-close the grill, and set the oven timer for 2 more minutes.

Pile the dressed greens on two serving plates. Arrange the various ingredients in stripes, or in spoke fashion, leaving room, of course, for a stripe or spoke of chicken.

When the timer beeps, pull out the chicken, throw it on your cutting board, and slice or cube it. Arrange it on the salads as well, and serve.

Yield: 2 to 3 servings

Assuming 2, each will have: 637 calories; 40 g fat; 50 g protein; 25 g carbohydrate; 12 g dietary fiber; 13 g usable carbs.

Mexican Chicken Salad

1 ½ cups (165 g) diced chicken

¼ cup (40 g) red onion, diced

½ green bell pepper, diced

½ medium tomato, diced

½ avocado, sliced

2 tablespoons (30 ml) olive oil

2 tablespoons (30 ml) cider vinegar

1 tablespoon (1.5 g) Splenda

½ teaspoon cumin

1 clove garlic, crushed

3 cups (60 g) romaine lettuce, broken up

⅓ cup (40 g) shredded Monterey Jack cheese

3 tablespoons (45 g) salsa

Put your chicken, onion, bell pepper, tomato, and avocado in a mixing bowl.

Whisk together the olive oil, vinegar, Splenda, cumin, and garlic. Pour over the salad, and toss.

Arrange beds of lettuce on three plates, scoop the chicken salad on top.
Now put two tablespoons of shredded Monterey Jack on each serving, top that with a tablespoon of salsa, and serve.

Yield: 3 servings

Each with: 461 calories; 35 g fat; 27 g protein; 10 g carbohydrate; 4 g dietary fiber; 6 g usable carbs.

◎ Pat Best's Deviled Chicken Salad

This is a real winner for pot-lucks and pitch-ins—or just make it for the family.

4 tablespoons (60 g) butter

½ cup (12 g) Splenda

¼ cup (60 g) spicy brown mustard

1 teaspoon salt

1 teaspoon curry

6 boneless chicken breasts, about 3 pounds (1.4 kg)

½ cup (60 g) finely chopped celery

⅓ cup (30 g) Gram's Gourmet Flax 'N Nut Crunchies Cinnamon flavor or ⅓ cup (40 g) chopped toasted almonds (but you don't get the sweet-spicy note that way!)

½ cup (120 g) mayonnaise

Preheat oven to 350°F (180°C).

Melt your butter in a saucepan. Add Splenda, mustard, salt, and curry powder, and stir until well combined.

Roll the boneless chicken in the butter mixture until coated. Arrange on a prepared pan. Bake for 30 to 40 minutes, or until just done. Let cool.

Chop the cooled chicken into bite-sized pieces. Toss with chopped celery and the Flax 'N Nut Crunchies or almonds. Gently stir in the mayonnaise until just moist. Add more mayonnaise if necessary.

Chill at least 1 hour, but overnight is fine, too.

Depending on serving sizes, this will serve 6 to 8. Recipe doubles easily. You can vary the presentation by serving this on a bed of lettuce, in hollowed-out tomatoes, or by rolling it in a low-carb tortilla!

Yield: Assuming 8 servings

Each will have: 381 calories; 31 g fat; 25 g protein; 2 g carbohydrate; 1 g dietary fiber; 1 g usable carb.

Susan Higgs's Chicken Salad Surprise

Our tester, Julie, pronounced this "marvelous!"

Salad:

 3 cups (330 g) cooked chicken, diced
 3 stalks celery, finely diced or sliced
 1 medium apple, unpeeled and diced
 ½ cup (60 g) slivered almonds, toasted
 1 small onion, finely diced

Dressing:

 ⅓ cup (80 g) mayonnaise
 1 teaspoon lemon juice
 ½ teaspoon salt
 ½ teaspoon white pepper
 2 teaspoons curry powder
 1 tablespoon (15 ml) dry sherry

Put the chicken, celery, apple, almonds, and onion in a bowl. Mix mayo, lemon juice, pepper, salt, curry, and dry sherry in a separate bowl, adjusting amounts to taste as needed. Stir dressing into the chicken and veggies. Serve on top of crisp lettuce leaves, which can be rolled up, burrito style, for eating.

Susan's note: "I love to roll this up in crisp lettuce leaves and serve it for lunch. With a side of tomato-basil soup, you have a fantastic lunch!"

Yield: 4 to 5 servings

Assuming 5, each will have: 370 calories; 24 g fat; 30 g protein; 11 g carbohydrate; 3 g dietary fiber; 8 g usable carbs.

Teresa Egger's Calcutta Chicken and "Rice" Salad

Note that the cauli-rice remains uncooked in this recipe—easy!

   3 cups (450 g) cauliflower "rice" (shredded cauliflower)
   2 cups (220 g) cooked chicken
   1 cup (200 g) crushed pineapple
   1 cup (120 g) sliced celery (I sometimes use bell peppers, any color)
   1 cup (240 g) mayonnaise
   ¼ cup (80 g) sugar-free peach or apricot preserves
   ¾ teaspoon curry powder (I add a full teaspoon—I like curry powder)
   Salt and pepper to taste
   1 cup (120 g) shredded cheese (Try cheddar or Monterey Jack)

Combine uncooked cauli-rice, chicken, pineapple, celery, and bell pepper, if desired. Toss together.

Blend together remaining ingredients except cheese. Stir this dressing into the chicken mixture. Serve on salad greens, garnished with shredded cheese.
(If you prefer, you can stir the cheese into the salad.)

Yield: 6 servings

Each with: 475 calories; 40 g fat; 21 g protein; 14 g carbohydrate; 2 g dietary fiber; 12 g usable carbs.

Avocado, Egg, and Blue Cheese Salad

A very unusual egg salad! Avocados are not only delicious and low carb, but they're the best source of potassium on the planet!

> 1 stalk celery, diced
> 2 scallions, sliced, including the crisp part of the green shoot
> 1/2 avocado, diced
> 3 hard-boiled eggs, chopped
> 1/4 cup (30 g) crumbled blue cheese
> 3 tablespoons (45 ml) vinaigrette dressing
>   (I like Paul Newman's Olive Oil and Vinegar)

This is very simple. Just combine vegetables, eggs, and cheese in a mixing bowl. Add the dressing, and toss. Serve on a bed of lettuce.

Yield: 2 servings

Each with: 370 calories; 32 g fat; 14 g protein; 7 g carbohydrate; 2 g dietary fiber; 5 g usable carbs.

Grandma Mel's Egg and Olive Salad

Pamela Merritt sends this salad for olive lovers!

> 6 hard-boiled eggs
> 1/2 cup (50 g) green olives (more to taste)
> 1/3 cup (80 g) mayonnaise
> 1/8 teaspoon Cajun seasoning
> Dash salt and pepper

Shell eggs and coarsely chop with knife—you want big chunks. Then slice up the olives, and mix with the eggs and seasonings. After refrigerating the salad at least two hours, you can put it on cucumber slices, where it is particularly good, or use as any egg salad.

Yield: Assuming 4 servings

Each has: 357 calories; 34 g fat; 13 g protein; 3 g carbohydrate; 1 g dietary fiber; 2 g usable carbs.

Cajun Steak Caesar Salad

Had enough chicken Caesar salads? Try this!

> 1 tablespoon (7 g) Cajun seasoning, homemade or purchased
> 12 ounces (340 g) sirloin steak, trimmed
> 1 ½ quarts (1.4 L) romaine lettuce, broken up
> ⅛ red onion, sliced paper thin
> ½ cup (75 g) grated Romano cheese
> ¼ cup (60 ml) bottled Caesar salad dressing (I like Paul Newman's)
> ½ teaspoon Tabasco sauce

Sprinkle the Cajun seasoning on both sides of the steak, and put the steak in to broil as close to your broiler as you can. Assuming it's 1" (2.5 cm) thick, you'll want to give it about 5 minutes 30 seconds per side—I set my oven timer so I don't overcook—but cook it to your liking.

While the steak is broiling, put the lettuce in your salad bowl.

Spray a microwaveable plate with nonstick cooking spray, and spread the Romano on it. Put it in the microwave for 1 minute on high.

Stir the salad dressing and the Tabasco sauce together. Pour over the romaine, and toss.

Okay, your steak should be done now. Pull it out, and slice it thin across the grain. Pile the lettuce on two serving plates, add the thinly sliced red onion, and top with the sliced steak.

Pull the cheese out of the microwave—it will be a crisp sheet. Crumble the crisp cheese over the two salads, and serve.

Yield: 2 servings

Each with: 634 calories; 46 g fat; 44 g protein; 11 g carbohydrate; 4 g dietary fiber; 7 g usable carbs.

◉ Tracy Lohr's Quick Taco Salad

3 cups (60 g) iceberg or romaine lettuce (bagged salad works great)

4–8 ounces (115–225 g) ground beef, or veggie burger, thawed if necessary

1 1.25-ounce (35 g) packet taco seasoning or 2 teaspoons homemade (page 531)

Any low-carb toppings you wish. Choose from:

Avocado, sliced or diced

Hot sauce

Olives

Shredded Jack or cheddar cheese

Sour cream

Kidney beans or black beans (if you're on South Beach, these are "legal")

Diced onions or sliced scallions

Tomatoes

Salsa, ranch dressing, or a combination of the two

Make a bed of lettuce on a serving plate.

Put the beef or veggie patty in a skillet on medium-high heat and add 2 tablespoons of water and 2 teaspoons of taco seasoning. Stir and chop the burger and spices. Continue stirring, chopping, and cooking till either the beef is done or the veggie patty has absorbed the water. Taste and adjust seasoning. Remove from heat.

Dump the meat/veggie patty mixture on top of the lettuce. Top that with your favorite taco fixings.

If you want more than one serving, adjust the amount of meat/veggie patty and the amount of taco seasoning and water.

Yield: Serves 1

Carb count will vary with toppings, but using 8 ounces (225 g) of ground beef, 1 scallion, 1 tablespoon (15 g) salsa, and 2 tablespoons (30 ml) ranch dressing, you're looking at: 897 calories; 77 g fat; 42 g protein; 10 g carbohydrate; 4 g dietary fiber; 6 g usable carbs.

Ham and Cheese Salad

When I tried this recipe, I didn't eat much else till it was gone!!

> 1/2 head cauliflower
> 8 ounces (225 g) cooked ham, cut in 1/4" (6.25 mm) cubes
> 8 ounces (225 g) Swiss cheese, cut in 1/4" (6.25 mm) cubes
> 1/4 cup (40 g) finely diced red onion
> 3/4 cup (75 g) chopped dill pickle
> 3/4 cup (60 g) snow pea pods, cut in 1/2" (1.25 cm) pieces
> 1/3 cup (80 g) mayonnaise
> 1 tablespoon (15 g) brown mustard
> 1 tablespoon (15 ml) white wine vinegar
> 1 teaspoon dried tarragon

First chop your cauliflower into 1/2" (1.25 cm) chunks—include the stem. Put it in a microwaveable casserole with a lid, add a couple of tablespoons of water, and cover. Nuke it on high for 7 minutes.

Use the time while your cauliflower is cooking to put your ham, cheese, onion, and pickle in a big mixing bowl.

Then pinch the ends off of your snow pea pods, and pull off any strings. Cut into 1/2" (1.25 cm) pieces, and put those in a microwaveable bowl. Add a tablespoon of water and cover. When the cauliflower is done, pull it out of the microwave and uncover immediately—both to stop the cooking and to let it cool.

Put your snow peas in the microwave, and nuke them on high for just 1 minute. When they're done, uncover immediately, drain them, and add them to the mixing bowl.

While your cauliflower is cooling, measure the mayo, mustard, vinegar, and tarragon into a small bowl and stir together well.

When the cauliflower is cool enough to not melt the cheese, drain it and add it to the mixing bowl. Add the dressing, and toss to coat. This is good right away, but it's better if you let it sit in the fridge for at least a few hours, to let the flavors blend.

Yield: 4 servings

Each with: 472 calories; 38 g fat; 28 g protein; 8 g carbohydrate; 1 g dietary fiber; 7 g usable carb.

Indy Airport Tuna Salad

This salad is the reason I hope my flights out of Indianapolis leave out of Concourse C! I loved it from the start, and it was a snap to duplicate.

    1 quart (.95 L) romaine lettuce, broken up
    1 hard-boiled egg, chopped
    ¾ cup (40 g) diced red onion
    6 ounces (170 g) canned tuna, drained
    2 tablespoons (30 ml) balsamic vinaigrette (I like Paul Newman's)

Put everything in a big salad bowl and toss. That's it!

Yield: 1 serving

Each with: 462 calories; 23 g fat; 54 g protein; 10 g carbohydrate; 5 g dietary fiber; 5 g usable carb.

Tuna Salad with Mustard-Mayo and Olives

    6 ounces (170 g) canned tuna in water, drained
    1 hard-boiled egg, chopped
    1 stalk celery, diced
    6 dill pickle slices, chopped
    6 kalamata olives, pitted and chopped (just press down on them
       to pit them!)
    3 tablespoons (45 g) mayonnaise
    2 teaspoons brown mustard
    3 tablespoons (30 g) minced red onion

Pretty darned simple: Just assemble everything in a mixing bowl, and stir well. Serve on a bed of lettuce, if you like.

Yield: 2 servings

Each with: 332 calories; 24 g fat; 26 g protein; 4 g carbohydrate; 1 g dietary fiber; 3 g usable carb.

◉ Submarine Salad

Here's a salad with everything you'd find in a great submarine sandwich—except the bread! If your grocery store deli doesn't have some of these cold cuts, substitute your favorites. Except bologna. One slice of bologna, and you've lost your East Coast sub shop accent.

- 2 quarts (1.9 L) shredded lettuce, loosely packed
- 1 ounce (30 g) prosciutto or boiled ham
- 1 ounce (30 g) capacolla
- 1 ounce (30 g) mortadella
- 1 ounce (30 g) Genoa salami
- 1 ounce (30 g) provolone cheese (smoked provolone if you can get it!)
- 1 ounce (30 g) mozzarella cheese
- 1/8 medium red onion, sliced paper-thin
- 3 tablespoons (21 g) roasted red pepper, diced
- 4 fresh basil leaves, minced
- 1/2 small tomato, sliced in thin wedges
- 2 tablespoons (30 ml) olive oil
- 1/2 clove garlic, crushed
- 1 tablespoon (15 ml) red wine vinegar
- 1 dash pepper
- 1 dash salt

Make a bed of lettuce on each of two serving plates.

Slice the meats and cheeses into strips. Arrange artistically on the beds of lettuce. Top that with the onion, diced red pepper, and chopped fresh basil. Add the tomato wedges, too. Now mix together the oil, garlic, vinegar, pepper, and salt, and drizzle over the salads, then serve.

Yield: 2 servings

Each with: 377 calories; 29 g fat; 18 g protein; 13 g carbohydrate; 5 g dietary fiber; 8 g usable carbs.

Shrimp and Avocado Salad

Here's a cool summer night's dinner that will take all of 10 minutes to assemble, yet impress the heck out of any guests who might happen to have wandered in—or just the family.

> 2 pounds (1 kg) shrimp, cooked and shelled
> 1 California avocado
> 10 scallions, sliced thin
> ⅔ cup (160 ml) bottled vinaigrette dressing
> (I like Paul Newman's Olive Oil and Vinegar)
> 1 head romaine lettuce

This is very simple if you buy your shrimp already shelled and cooked. I like to use little bitty shrimp for this, but feel free to use middle-sized shrimp, if that's what you have on hand.

Put the shrimp in a big mixing bowl. Peel and seed your avocado, and dice it, somewhere between ¼" (6.25 mm) and ½" (1.25 cm) big. Put that in the bowl, too. Slice your scallions, including the crisp part of the green, and throw them in the bowl as well.

Pour on the dressing, and gently stir the whole thing up to coat all the ingredients. Let that sit for a few minutes while you break or cut up the lettuce. Arrange it in beds on 6 serving plates.

Now stir the shrimp salad one last time, to get up any dressing that's settled to the bottom of the bowl, and spoon it out onto the beds of lettuce. Serve immediately.

Yield: 6 servings

Each with: 352 calories; 21 g fat; 35 g protein; 8 g carbohydrate; 4 g dietary fiber; 4 g usable carbs.

Eleanor Monfett's Cheddar Broccoli Salad

Our tester, Ray, calls this recipe "great stuff."

>   6 cups (1.05 kg) fresh broccoli florets
>   6 ounces (170 g) shredded cheddar
>   1/3 cup (55 g) chopped onion
>   1 1/2 cups (360 g) mayonnaise
>   1/2–3/4 cup (12-18 g) Splenda
>   3 tablespoons (45 ml) red wine vinegar or cider vinegar
>   12 bacon strips, cooked and crumbled

In a large bowl, combine the broccoli, cheese, and onion. Combine the mayonnaise, Splenda, and vinegar; pour over broccoli mixture and toss to coat. Refrigerate for at least 4 hours. Just before serving, stir in the bacon.

Yield: 8 servings

Each with: 455 calories; 47 g fat; 10 g protein; 4 g carbohydrate; 2 g dietary fiber; 2 g usable carbs.

chapter twelve

Soups

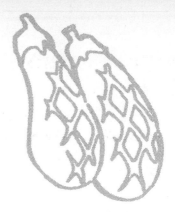

Used to canned soups? Many of them are distressingly carb-y, with rice, noodles, cornstarch, potatoes, and other stuff we don't want. Furthermore, a surprising number of them have added sugar or corn syrup, and often they have other noxious additives.

Yet few things soothe and satisfy like a bowl of soup. So make a pot! You've got a remarkable variety here to choose from: Simple soups; complex soups; hearty down-home soups; elegant, sophisticated soups; soups from all over the world—we've got it all!

Note: You'll find that packaged broth comes in two sizes: quarts and 14.5-ounce (411 g) cans. Why this should be, I have no idea. But in any of these recipes, if you substitute two 14.5-ounce (411 g) cans for a quart of broth, no harm will come to your soup. You'll just get a slightly lesser volume. You may make up the difference with water, if you really want to, but I don't see why you'd bother.

◉ Tuscan Soup

This Italian-style soup somehow manages to be delicate and substantial at the same time. Really addictive.

> 16 ounces (455 g) hot Italian sausage links
> 2 quarts (1.9 L) chicken broth
> 1 cup (240 ml) heavy cream
> 1/2 head cauliflower, sliced 1/4" (6.25 mm) thick
> 6 cups (120 g) chopped kale
> 1/2 teaspoon red pepper flakes
> 2 cloves garlic, crushed

First sauté the sausage until done. Remove from your skillet, and let it cool a little while you . . .

Start heating the chicken broth and cream in a big, heavy-bottomed saucepan, over medium heat. Add both the vegetables to the soup.

Okay, your sausage is cool enough to handle! Slice it on the diagonal, about 1/2" (1.25 cm) thick. I like to cut each slice in half, too, to make more bites of sausage, but that's not essential. Put the sliced sausage in the soup, too.

Stir in the red pepper flakes and the garlic. Turn the burner to lowest heat, and let the whole thing simmer for an hour, stirring now and then.

Yield: 6 servings

Each with 487 calories; 41 g fat; 20 g protein; 10 g carbohydrate; 2 g dietary fiber; 8 g usable carbs.

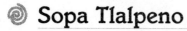 Sopa Tlalpeno

This simple Mexican soup takes no more than 20 to 25 minutes!

1 ½ quarts (1.4 L) chicken broth
1 pound (455 g) boneless, skinless chicken breast
1 chipotle chile canned in adobo
1 California avocado
4 scallions, sliced
Salt and pepper
¾ cup (90 g) shredded Monterey Jack cheese

Pour the chicken broth into a large, heavy-bottomed saucepan, reserving ½ cup (120 ml), and place it over medium-high heat. While it's heating, cut your chicken breast in thin strips or small cubes, then add it to the broth. Let the whole thing simmer for 10 to 15 minutes, or until the chicken is white clear through.

Put the reserved chicken broth in your blender with the chipotle, and blend until the chipotle is pureed. Pour this mixture into the soup, and stir.

Split the avocado in half, remove the seed, peel it, and cut it into ½" (1.25 cm) chunks. Add to the soup, along with the scallions, and salt and pepper to taste.

Ladle the soup into bowls, and top each serving with shredded cheese.

Yield: 6 servings

Each with: 235 calories; 13 g fat; 26 g protein; 4 g carbohydrate; 2 g dietary fiber; 2 g usable carbs.

☻ Thai Chicken Soup

You can have this light but filling soup done in a big half an hour!

 1 quart (.95 L) chicken broth
 1 pound (455 g) boneless, skinless chicken breast
 1 tablespoon (15 ml) lemon juice
 1 tablespoon (15 ml) lime juice
 2 tablespoons (20 g) grated gingerroot
 1/2 cup (120 ml) coconut milk
 8 scallions
 2 teaspoons chili paste
 1 teaspoon fish sauce (nuoc mam or nam pla)
 3 tablespoons chopped fresh cilantro

In a big, heavy saucepan, start heating the chicken broth while you cut the chicken breast into small cubes or thin strips. Throw your cut-up chicken into the pot, along with the lemon juice, lime juice, and ginger. Let the whole thing simmer for 20 minutes.

Stir in the coconut milk and scallions, and let it cook another 10 minutes or so.

Stir in the chili garlic paste and fish sauce. Ladle into bowls, top each serving with chopped cilantro, and serve.

Yield: 3 to 4 servings

Assuming 4, each will have: 260 calories; 12 g fat; 32 g protein; 6 g carbohydrate; 2 g dietary fiber; 4 g usable carbs.

☻ Chinese Soup with Bok Choy and Mushrooms

 1 quart (.95 L) chicken broth
 2 tablespoons (20 g) grated gingerroot
 2 teaspoons soy sauce
 1 cup (100 g) sliced mushrooms
 8 ounces (225 g) boneless pork loin, cut in thin 1/2" (1.25 cm) strips
 1 1/2 cups (115 g) bok choy, sliced thin, leaves and stems both
 1 egg

In a large saucepan, over medium-high heat, combine the chicken broth, gingerroot, and soy sauce. Let them simmer together for 5 minutes.

Now add the mushrooms and pork. Let the soup simmer for another 15 minutes.

Stir in the bok choy, and let the soup simmer for another 5 to 10 minutes.

Beat the egg. Now pour it in a thin stream over the surface of the simmering soup, let it sit for 10 seconds, then stir with the tines of a fork. Serve.

Yield: 4 servings

Each with: 130 calories; 5 g fat; 17 g protein; 3 g carbohydrate; 1 g dietary fiber; 2 g usable carbs.

◎ Cathy Kayne's Chinese Beef Soup

Our tester, Pat Lacy, said this was easy and took only 30 minutes—you've gotta love that.

> 1 pound (455 g) ground beef
> ½ pound (225 g) mushrooms, chopped
> ½ onion, chopped
> 1 whole bok choy, stem chopped, leaves shredded
> 1 15-ounce (420 g) can black soy beans rinsed and drained
> 2 14.5-ounce (405 ml) cans chicken stock
> Soy sauce, garlic, pepper to taste

Stir-fry beef, mushrooms, and onion until cooked. Add bok choy and stir. When bok choy is almost done, add beans and broth. Add soy and spices to taste. Heat through and serve.

You could substitute chicken for the beef, or make it just with veggies. So easy and quick!

Yield: Makes 6 servings

Each with: 256 calories; 20 g fat; 14 g protein; 3 g carbohydrate; 1 g dietary fiber; 2 g usable carbs.

◎ Tee's Taco Soup

Ray says of this, "The result is something to be proud of!"

> 1 onion, chopped
> Olive oil for sautéing
> 2 cloves garlic
> 2 pounds (1 kg) lean ground beef (chuck or round)
> 3–4 teaspoons chili powder
> ½ teaspoon cumin
> Salt and pepper to taste
> 1 15-ounce (420 g) can tomato sauce
> ½ head cauliflower, shredded (optional, nice ricelike texture)
> 1 pound cheddar cheese, or American, sliced
> 1 small can green chiles
> 15 ounces (420 g) black beans, cooked, optional
> 2–3 tablespoons (30–45 g) jalapeno salsa (or minced jalapenos)
> 1 16-ounce (455 g) container sour cream

In your soup kettle or a big, heavy bottomed saucepan, sauté the onion in olive oil. When it's translucent, add the garlic and sauté briefly. Add in the beef and cook and crumble till completely browned. (Tee used a good ground chuck or round, so she didn't drain the meat—that way she could keep the flavorful juices in the pan.)

Add chili powder, cumin, and salt and pepper. Then add your tomato sauce and stir it all up. Add the cauliflower and let it cook for just a few minutes, if it's used.

Add the cheese 1 slice at a time so it melts nicely, using a low heat and stirring constantly. Then add the green chilies, beans (if using), and jalapeno salsa; let it get nice and hot, then add the sour cream and stir again.

Yield: 12 servings

Each with: 404 calories; 32 g fat; 21 g protein; 9 g carbohydrate; 3 g dietary fiber; 6 g usable carbs.

Broccoli Blue Cheese Soup

I'd never had soup made with blue cheese before, but this is amazing. It certainly appealed to my blue-cheese-fan husband!

 1 cup (160 g) chopped onion
 2 tablespoons (30 g) butter
 1 turnip, peeled and diced
 1 ½ quarts (1.4 L) chicken broth
 1 pound (455 g) frozen broccoli, thawed
 1 cup (240 ml) Carb Countdown Dairy Beverage
 ¼ cup (60 ml) heavy cream
 1 cup (120 g) crumbled blue cheese

In a large saucepan, sauté the onion in the butter over medium-low heat—you don't want it to brown.

When the onion's soft and translucent, add the turnip and the chicken broth to the pot. Bring to a simmer, and let the whole thing simmer over medium-low heat for 20 to 30 minutes.

Add the thawed broccoli, and let simmer for another 20 minutes.

Scoop the vegetables out with a slotted spoon, and place them in your blender. Add a ladleful of the broth, and run the blender until the vegetables are finely pureed. Return to pot.

Stir in the Carb Countdown, the heavy cream, and the blue cheese. Simmer for another 5 to 10 minutes, stirring occasionally, and serve.

Yield: 6 servings

Each with: 243 calories; 17 g fat; 14 g protein; 9 g carbohydrate; 3 g dietary fiber; 6 g usable carbs.

◎ Cheesy Cauliflower Soup

This was originally a potato-cheese soup, but it sure is good this way!

- 4 cups (600 g) cauliflower, diced small
- 1 tablespoon finely chopped onion
- 2 tablespoons (20 g) finely chopped celery
- 1 tablespoon (7 g) grated carrot
- 3 cups (720 ml)chicken broth
- 1 teaspoon salt
- 2 teaspoons white vinegar
- 1 ½ cups (360 ml) Carb Countdown Dairy Beverage or half-and-half
- 1 ½ cups (180 g) shredded cheddar cheese
- Guar or xanthan
- 2 slices bacon, cooked and drained
- 1 tablespoon minced green onion

Put the cauliflower, onion, celery, and carrot in a large, heavy-bottomed saucepan. Add the chicken broth, salt, and vinegar; bring up to a simmer; and let cook for 30 to 45 minutes.

Stir in the Carb Countdown or half-and-half, then whisk in the cheese a little at a time, giving each addition time to melt before adding more. Thicken it a little with your guar or xanthan shaker if you think it needs it.

Serve, and top each serving with a little crumbled bacon and minced green onion (though it's wonderful without them!).

Yield: 5 servings

Each with: 235 calories; 16 g fat; 17 g protein; 7 g carbohydrate; 2 g dietary fiber; 5 g usable carbs.

Cheesy Onion Soup

1 quart (.95 L) beef broth
1 medium onion
$\frac{1}{2}$ cup (120 ml) heavy cream
$\frac{1}{2}$ cup (120 ml) Carb Countdown Dairy Beverage
1 $\frac{1}{2}$ cups (180 g) shredded sharp cheddar cheese
Guar or xanthan
Salt and pepper to taste

Pour your beef broth into a large saucepan, and start it heating over a medium-high flame. Slice your onion paper thin, and add it to the broth. When the broth starts to boil, turn the heat to low, and let the whole thing simmer for 1 hour. If you like, you can do this ahead of time: turn off the burner and let the whole thing cool, and do the rest later. If you do this, bring the broth up to heat again before proceeding.

Gently stir in the cream and the Carb Countdown Dairy Beverage. Now stir in your cheese, a bit at a time, until it's all melted in. Thicken a little if you want with your guar or xanthan shaker, but stir with a ladle or spoon instead of a whisk—you don't want to break up the strands of onion. Salt and pepper to taste, and serve.

Yield: 4 servings

Each with: 359 calories; 26 g fat; 24 g protein; 8 g carbohydrate; trace dietary fiber; 8 g usable carbs.

Swiss Cheese and Broccoli Soup

2 tablespoons (20 g) minced onion

1 tablespoon (15 g) butter

14 ounces (400 ml) chicken broth

10 ounces (280 g) frozen chopped broccoli, thawed

1 cup (240 ml) Carb Countdown Dairy Beverage

1/2 cup (120 ml) heavy cream

1 1/2 cups (180 g) shredded Swiss cheese

Guar or xanthan

In a large, heavy-bottomed saucepan, sauté the onion in the butter until it's translucent. Add the chicken broth and the broccoli, and simmer for 20 to 30 minutes, until the broccoli is quite tender.

Stir in the Carb Countdown and cream. Bring back up to a simmer. Now stir in the cheese, a little at a time, letting each batch melt before you add some more. When all the cheese is melted in, thicken a little with your guar or xanthan shaker, if you think it needs it, and serve.

Yield: 4 servings

Each with: 356 calories; 28 g fat; 20 g protein; 7 g carbohydrate; 2 g dietary fiber; 5 g usable carbs.

◎ Sheryl McKenney's Easy Cheese Soup

Our tester, Ray, really liked this soup. He didn't have seasoning blend on hand, so he just chopped an onion, some celery, and some peppers, and said it worked great.

1 can chicken broth (full fat)

1 cup (175 g) frozen seasoning vegetables
  (chopped onion, celery, green and red pepper)

½ teaspoon. white pepper

1 pint (570 ml) heavy cream

1 teaspoon thickener
  (guar, xanthan, or ThickenThin Not Starch, by Expert Foods)

1 8-ounce (225 g) package shredded cheese
  (Sheryl used 4-cheese blend, Ray used pepper Jack)

1 cup (150 g) shredded Parmesan cheese

In large saucepan heat chicken broth and seasoning vegetables on medium to medium-high, and simmer until vegetables are tender. Add white pepper and stir in heavy cream and thickener. When it is simmering, add cheeses and stir until melted and bubbling. Remove from heat and serve.

Yield: About 4 servings

Each with: 717 calories; 68 g fat; 24 g protein; 5 g carbohydrate; trace dietary fiber; 5 g usable carbs.

Cherie Johnson's Cheeseburger Soup

A favorite fast food meal in a bowl!

> 1 pound (455 g) ground beef
> ¾ cup (90 g) chopped celery
> ¼ cup (35 g) chopped carrot
> ¾ cup (120 g) chopped onion
> 1 teaspoon dried basil
> 1 teaspoon dried parsley
> ½ teaspoon xanthan gum
> 3 cups (720 ml) chicken broth
> 1 ½ cup (360 ml) cream or half-and-half
> 2 cups (240 g) shredded cheddar cheese
> ¼ cup (60 g) sour cream

Brown the hamburger and celery, carrot and onion together in a large pot. Drain the grease.

Stir in basil and parsley. In a blender, blend together the xanthan gum and the chicken broth. Add to beef and veggie mixture. Bring to a boil, then reduce heat and simmer 10 to 15 minutes.

Add cream and cheese and stir until cheese is melted. Add sour cream and heat through. Do not boil.

Dana's note: As with my cheese soups, if you find this a little thin, feel free to use the ol' guar or xanthan shaker.

Yield: Makes 4 very generous servings

Each with: 878 calories; 75 g fat; 40 g protein; 10 g carbohydrate; 1 g dietary fiber; 9 g usable carbs.

Melissa Miller's Ham and Broccoli Cheese Soup

This recipe put our tester, Ray, in mind of the soups he's eaten in Amish restaurants. You could use leftover ham or go buy a chunk of cooked ham or a couple of smoked ham hocks at the grocery store, if you like.

1 1/2 pounds cooked ham, preferably on the bone
1/2 cup (40 g) dried mushrooms
1/2 large bag frozen broccoli (approximately 3 cups [675 g])
12 ounces (340 g) grated cheddar cheese
Salt and pepper to taste

Place ham in your slow cooker and cover with water—if you're using leftover ham, you can just plunk the whole ham bone in there. Add the dried mushrooms and other spices/seasonings as desired. Cook on low overnight or until ham falls off bone.

Carefully remove meat from liquid, making sure to remove all the bone pieces from the meat. Chop meat and set aside.

Place remaining liquid from the slow cooker into large saucepan (I used a Dutch oven) and bring to a low boil. Add broccoli and cook until broccoli is tender but not mushy. Add cheese, stirring until melted. Add meat and stir till mixed in well.

Carefully ladle out 2 to 3 cups (475–710 ml) of the liquid/vegetable/meat mixture and place in your blender. Puree until smooth and add back into the rest of the soup. Stir to blend. If you have a hand blender, you can simply do this step right in the pot, instead.

Salt and pepper to taste. Serve with a side salad and low-carb rolls (if desired).

Melissa's note: "I found this made a very hearty soup, and by pureeing part of it, it allowed me to thicken the soup without adding any thickener. It sure satisfied my craving for a thick hearty soup on a cold winter day."

Tester's note: Ray found he couldn't fit a whole ham bone in his slow cooker. If you have a smaller slow cooker, consider cutting the meat off the bone before putting it in, or using the remains of a half-ham, instead. If you can simmer the ham on the bone, though, do—it makes for great flavor. Also, Ray couldn't find dried mushrooms, so he used fresh, and said they worked out great.

Yield: 8 servings

Each will have: 343 calories; 23 g fat; 27 g protein; 6 g carbohydrate; 2 g dietary fiber; 4 g usable carbs.

Tee's Crockpot Jambalaya

Here's a great, flexible jambalaya recipe. Asked if he would make this again, Ray, our tester, answered with a hearty, "Oh, yeah! I already plan to!"

    2 6.5-ounce (180 g) cans minced clams
    1/2 cup (120 ml) wine (red or white)
    14 ounces (400 g) tomato sauce
    14 ounces (400 g) canned diced tomatoes
    1 onion, diced
    2 cloves garlic, minced
    2 teaspoons Better than Bullion chicken base
    1 bay leaf
    3 teaspoons Tee's Cajun Seasoning (page 451)
    1/3 cup (55 g) brown rice (optional)
    1 pound (455 g) chorizo sausage links, diced
    1/2 pound (225 g) ham steak, diced
    1 pound (455 g) skinless chicken pieces
    1 small package okra, frozen
    1 pound (455 g) shrimp
    1/4 cup (60 ml) heavy cream

Put liquid of clams in a fairly large slow cooker (save clams for the very end). Add next 9 ingredients. Add half of the chorizo and half of the ham. Top with chicken pieces. Sprinkle chicken with a little extra seasoning. Add the other half of ham and chorizo. Let cook till tender (about 5 or 6 hours on low). If there is too much liquid, let it cook for 1/2 hour to 1 hour without the lid, on high. It can be thickened with guar or xanthan if needed. Add okra in the last hour or two if possible, if frozen. It can disintegrate if cooked too long unless fresh. If shrimp is not cooked, add about 1/2 hour before serving. If it is cooked, add at the very end. Then add the clams and cream and let heat. Remove bay leaf before serving.

Tee's note: "This recipe is great for using up leftovers. I've used leftover pork roast instead of chicken (not barbeque pork, but my Puerto Rican roast pork!); you could use leftover chicken or turkey, you can use whatever sausage or ham you would like, any leftover fish or seafood would be great added in at the end. I've also used bacon or pancetta for flavoring instead of ham, and I've used andouille instead of chorizo sausage. Kielbasa would be fine also. A very versatile recipe."

Yield: 15 servings

Each will have: 324 calories; 18 g fat; 27 g protein; 11 g carbohydrate; 2 g dietary fiber; 9 g usable carbs.

◉ Holly Holder's Cheesy Chipotle Soup

I wish I'd thought of this recipe. I adore chipotle peppers. If you haven't tried them, they're smoked jalapenos, and you buy them in little bitty cans in the Mexican food section of big grocery stores. They add a terrific smokey-hot flavor to all sorts of things. If you want this a little cooler, you could use just one, I suppose. Me, I like to breathe fire!

> 2 pounds (1 kg) ground beef
> ½ cup (80 g) chopped onion
> 2 cloves garlic, minced
> 2 cups (240 g) zucchini, sliced
> 1 4-ounce (115 g) can mushrooms, undrained
> 4 cups (960 ml) beef stock (homemade or canned)
> 1 14.5-ounce (411 g) can diced tomatoes with green chilies, undrained
> 2 chipotle peppers in adobo sauce, chopped
> ½ pound (225 g) Velveeta, cubed or sliced
>   or ½ pound (225 g) cheddar cheese, shredded

Brown ground beef, onion, and garlic together and drain. Add all other ingredients except Velveeta or cheddar. Simmer 30 minutes. Add the cheese and simmer until it melts.

Yield: This makes almost a gallon of soup!

Making it 10 servings, and using the Velveeta, each will have: 417 calories; 33 g fat; 23 g protein; 8 g carbohydrate; 1 g dietary fiber; 7 g usable carbs. If you use cheddar, the carb count will be considerably lower.

◎ Chicken and Andouille Gumbo

This chunky, vegetable-rich soup is spicy and filling! I've replaced the traditional gumbo file (powdered sassafras leaves) thickener with guar or xanthan, because I figure you'll have one of these in the house anyway.

    2 tablespoons (30 g) butter
    2 cloves garlic, crushed
    ¾ cup (120 g) chopped onion
    ½ cup (60 g) diced celery
    10 ounces (280 g) frozen sliced okra, thawed
    1 pound (455 g) boneless, skinless chicken breast,
        cut in ½" (1.25 cm) cubes
    1 quart (.95 L) chicken broth
    1 14 ½-ounce (411 g) can diced tomatoes
    1 tablespoon (4 g) chopped fresh parsley
    1 teaspoon dried thyme
    1 bay leaf
    ½ teaspoon cayenne
    ¼ teaspoon pepper
    1 pound (455 g) andouille sausage links
    2 tablespoons (30 ml) Worcestershire sauce
    1 tablespoon (15 ml) lemon juice
    Tabasco sauce to taste
    Guar or xanthan

Melt the butter in a big soup kettle, over medium-low heat, and add the garlic, onion, and celery. Sauté them together for 5 minutes or so, until the onion is just starting to soften.

Add the thawed sliced okra and the cubes of chicken, and continue to sauté until the chicken is white all over. Add the chicken broth, the can of diced tomatoes, parsley, thyme, bay leaf, cayenne, and pepper, bring the whole thing up to a simmer, turn the burner down, and simmer for an hour.

When the hour's up, put your andouille links in a skillet, over medium-high heat. Brown them all over—prick the casings all over with a fork as you do this. When the sausages are browned, remove them from the skillet, to your cutting board, and slice ½" (1.25 cm) thick. You can leave the slices round, or cut each round in half, which is what I do—depends on how big a bite of sausage you want! Add the sausage slices to the pot. Ladle a little of the broth into the skillet, stir it around to dissolve the nice brown crusty stuff, and pour it back into the pot.

Add the Worcestershire sauce and lemon juice to the soup, and stir it up. Let the whole thing simmer for another 15 minutes or so. Now check—is the level of heat right for your tongue? Or do you want it hotter? If so, stir in a little Tabasco. Thicken the broth just a tad with your guar or xanthan shaker, remove bay leaf, and serve.

Now, you get to decide how you want to serve your gumbo. You can serve it as is, of course, and it will be nice as can be. But the traditional way to serve gumbo is ladled over rice, and you certainly may serve yours over cauli-rice. And here in my hometown of Bloomington, Indiana, there is a popular restaurant that serves its "gumbo of the day" Hoosier-style—over mashed potatoes. So you could have your gumbo over a scoop of Ultimate Fauxtatoes!

Yield: 6 servings

Each with: 513 calories; 38 g fat; 31 g protein; 13 g carbohydrate; 2 g dietary fiber; 11 g usable carbs. Analysis does not include any cauli-rice or fauxtatoes you may serve with your gumbo.

⊚ UnPotato and Sausage Soup

Talk about comfort food! This is creamy and filling, with a good, rich potato flavor. Just the thing for a stormy winter night.

> 1 pound (455 g) Polish sausage
>
> 2 tablespoons (30 g) butter
>
> 3/4 cup (120 g) chopped onion
>
> 4 cups (600 g) cauliflower, diced
>
> 1/2 cup (60 g) shredded carrot
>
> 1 small green pepper, diced
>
> 3 cups (720 ml) water
>
> 1 teaspoon salt or Vege-Sal
>
> 1/2 teaspoon pepper
>
> 3 cups (720 ml) Carb Countdown Dairy Beverage
>
> 1/2 cup (25 g) Ketatoes mix
>
> Guar or xanthan

Slice your sausage into rounds. Melt 1 tablespoon (15 g) of the butter in your big skillet, over medium heat, and start frying the sausage slices in it—you're just browning them a little. You can skip this step if you're in a hurry, but I think it adds a bit of flavor.

In a big, heavy-bottomed saucepan, melt the rest of the butter and start sautéing the onion over medium-low heat.

When the onions are turning golden, throw in the other veggies. Pour in 2 cups (480 ml) of the water. When the sausage slices are browned on both sides, add them to the pot. Pour the third cup (240 ml) of water into the skillet, and scrape the bottom with your spatula, to get all the good brown flavor stuck to the skillet. Pour this into the saucepan, too. Add the salt and pepper. Bring everything to a simmer, and let it cook for 30 minutes.

When the cauliflower is soft, stir in the Carb Countdown Dairy Beverage, then whisk in the Ketatoes mix. Thicken your soup a little more with your guar or xanthan shaker, if you like, and bring it back to the simmer, then serve.

Yield: 6 servings

Each with: 454 calories; 31 g fat; 25 g protein; 19 g carbohydrate; 8 g dietary fiber; 11 g usable carbs.

Sopa De Frijoles Negros

This is a really-truly bean soup! The high-carb but flavorful black beans are diluted with the low-carb black soy beans. Add plenty of seasonings, and you've got a great south-of-the-border soup.

2 15-ounce (420 g) cans Eden brand black soy beans

1 15-ounce (420 g) can black beans

1 14 1/2 ounce (411 ml) can chicken broth

1 tablespoon (15 ml) olive oil

1/2 cup (80 g) chopped onion

4 cloves garlic, crushed

1 cup (130 g) salsa

2 tablespoons (30 ml) lime juice

1 tablespoon (7 g) ground cumin

1/2 teaspoon red pepper flakes

1/2 teaspoon salt or Vege-Sal

1/2 cup (115 g) plain yogurt

1/4 cup (15 g) chopped cilantro

Put half of the beans and half of the chicken broth in your blender or in your food processor with the S-blade in place. Run the machine until the beans are pureed. Dump into a bowl that holds at least 2 quarts, and puree the other half of the beans and the other half of the chicken broth. Add that to the first batch.

Heat the olive oil in a heavy-bottomed saucepan, over medium-low heat, and add the onion. Sauté until the onion is turning translucent. Add the bean puree and the garlic. Now stir in the salsa, lime juice, cumin, red pepper flakes, and salt or Vege-Sal. Turn the burner up a bit until the soup is heated through, then turn it back down to the lowest setting, and let your soup simmer for 30 to 45 minutes. Serve with a dollop of plain yogurt (or sour cream, if you prefer) and a sprinkling of chopped cilantro.

Yield: 6 servings

Each with: 255 calories; 11 g fat; 18 g protein; 25 g carbohydrate; 13 g dietary fiber, 13 g usable carbs. (This is obviously not an Induction dish, but for comparison, I analyzed a standard black bean soup recipe. It had 43 grams of carbohydrate and 10 grams of fiber per serving, for a usable carb count of 33 grams, or about 2 and half times as much. Less protein, too.)

Pat Best's Hearty Black Soy Bean Soup

Bean soups are a favorite, but sadly most beans are high carb. Here's a bean soup made with the traditional ham, but with low-carb black soy beans.

　　1 large onion, finely chopped
　　3 cloves garlic, minced
　　1 smoked ham bone, pork knuckle, or ham hock
　　4 15-ounce (420 g) cans black soy beans (I use Eden's)
　　2 14 1/2-ounce (411 g) cans chicken broth
　　2 tablespoons (30 ml) red wine vinegar
　　Salt and pepper to taste
　　1 pound (455 g) boiled ham chunks

Garnish:
　　Chopped raw onion
　　Sour cream
　　Chopped boiled eggs

In a large pot, sauté onion and garlic until onion is soft, but not brown or burnt. Add all remaining ingredients except for the boiled ham chucks to the pot, cover, and simmer on low heat for 1 hour and 45 minutes to 2 hours. Remove the ham bone, ham hock, or the pork knuckle. With a potato masher, mash the beans to make a think soup consistency. If soup is too thick, add additional chicken broth until you reach the desired consistency. Add the boiled ham chunks and continue to simmer, covered, for 15 to 20 minutes longer or until ready to eat. Serve with garnishes. Freezes well!

Tester's note: Linda Fund said she couldn't find Eden canned black soy beans, so she used uncooked black beans instead, and just cooked them longer—and it worked fine.

Yield: Serves 8 to 10 people

Assuming 10, each serving has: 385 calories; 23 g fat; 31 g protein; 15 g carbohydrate; 9 g dietary fiber; 6 g usable carbs.

◎ Pat Best's Hearty Black Soy Bean Soup, the Short-Cooking Version

Our tester, Barbo, raved, "God this is good stuff. Hats off to Pat Best!!"

1 large onion, finely chopped
⅓ pound (140 g) boiled ham chunks (find boiled ham in the deli case)
2 cloves garlic, minced
2 15-ounce (420 g) cans Eden black soy beans
1 14 ½-ounce (411 g) can chicken broth
1 tablespoon (15 ml) red wine vinegar
Salt and pepper to taste

Garnish:

Chopped raw onion
Sour cream
Chopped boiled eggs

In a 3-quart (2.9 L) microwave-safe casserole with a lid, combine onion, ham chunks, and garlic. Cover and microwave, on high, for 5 minutes, stirring once.

Meanwhile, place 1 can of the black soy beans in a blender or food processor and blend until smooth. Add blended beans and all other ingredients to the garlic/ham/onion mixture in the microwave-safe casserole, cover, and microwave on high for 8 to 10 minutes, stirring twice, until heated through. Add salt and pepper to taste. Thin soup, if too thick, with additional chicken broth. Serve hot with garnishes and a healthy side salad!

Tester's note: Barbo suggests using this microwave-and-blender method to make chili, too.

Yield: Serves 4

Each serving: 462 calories; 29 g fat; 32 g protein; 21 g carbohydrate; 12 g dietary fiber; 9 g usable carbs.

Lisa Bousson's
Fantastic Creamy Broccoli Soup

Our tester, Ray, loved this soup. Since this doesn't have a ton of protein,
I recommend you serve this as a first course, rather than a main course.

    4 slices bacon
    4 green onions, diced (green part, too)
    3 cups (525 g) chopped fresh or frozen broccoli
    2 cups (480 ml) chicken broth
    1 cup (100 g) sliced mushrooms
    Salt to taste
    Pepper to taste
    ½ teaspoon guar or xanthan
    2 cups (480 ml) heavy cream

Fry bacon till crisp, drain. Pour off all but 2 tablespoons of drippings; add onion
and sauté until tender. Add bacon, broccoli, broth, mushrooms, salt, and pepper.
Bring to boil and simmer until broccoli is tender. Whiz guar or xanthan with cream
in blender to get rid of lumps, then add to the broccoli mix. Reduce heat to low
and cook until thickened and reduced to desired thickness.

Yield: About 6 appetizer-sized servings

Each with: 327 calories; 32 g fat; 6 g protein; 6 g carbohydrate; 1 g dietary fiber;
5 g usable carbs.

◎ M. E. Grundman's Salad Soup

This is more a rule than a recipe. I know this sounds odd, but our tester, Barbo Gold, said she'd make this again, and experiment with different sorts of salads, so give it a try!

Put any leftover salad in blender. Add chicken (or beef) stock and run blender until contents are pureed. Pour into another container. Contents may look rather odd, depending on what was in the salad, but the next step makes it work! Add whipping cream to taste. The cream makes it all work. Serve hot or cold. Adjust amount of stock and cream according to the volume of leftover salad.

Last time, I used leftover spinach salad with a curry vinagrette, pecans, onions, crisp bacon, and yellow raisins, added beef stock and wondered at the outcome. Before the cream, it looked like pond scum, but after the cream it was a divine cold soup! The little bits of pecan and raisin and bacon were wonderful.

I'm afraid that this was impossible to analyze, because we don't know what salad you'll be using, or how much. However, we can tell you that 1 cup (240 ml) of chicken or beef broth has about 1 gram of carbohydrate in it, and 1/2 cup (120 ml) heavy cream has 3 grams. Go from there!

Cathy Kayne's
Spicy Garlic Ginger Beef Soup

Here's a soup for you lovers of Asian cuisine. Julie says, "Lots of work, but interesting and very spicy!" You'll note this is low calorie as well as low carb.

Oil for stir-frying
1 pound (455 g) cube steaks, diced
½ red onion, diced
1 bell pepper, diced
3 ribs celery, diced
1–2 teaspoons minced garlic
½ teaspoon chili garlic paste (more if you like it really hot)
1 teaspoon diced fresh gingerroot
2 teaspoons soy sauce (or more, to taste)
4 cups (960 ml) chicken or beef broth, or 2 cups of each
2 cups (300 g) diced cooked turnips
3–4 cups (60–80 g) fresh spinach leaves
Salt and pepper to taste
Chinese five-spice powder

Put a tablespoon of oil in a wok or stockpot over high heat, and stir-fry cube steak with the red onion, diced bell pepper, and diced celery. After a few minutes of stir-frying, mix in the garlic, chili garlic paste, and ginger. Add soy sauce, and continue stir-frying.

When the meat is cooked, add 4 cups (.95 L) of broth of your choice (Cathy used ½ chicken and ½ beef). Simmer for 10 minutes. Add cooked diced turnips and 3 cups fresh spinach leaves. Add salt and pepper and Chinese five-spice powder to taste. Simmer until leaves are wilted.

Very spicy due to the chili paste and garlic, but warming! The next day the turnips have a great spicy flavor! The Chinese five-spice adds a nice cinnamon flavor, too.

Dana's note: About those turnips: I would peel and dice them raw, then put them in a microwaveable casserole with a tablespoon or two of water, and nuke them on high until tender — 10–12 minutes or so.

Yield: About 6 servings

Each with: 199 calories; 10 g fat; 17 g protein; 8 g carbohydrate; 3 g dietary fiber; 5 g usable carbs.

◎ Curried Pumpkin Soup

This is high enough in carbohydrate, and low enough in protein, that you should think of it as a first course, rather than a main course—and the yield for this recipe reflects that. But what a great starter for Thanksgiving dinner!

¼ cup (40 g) minced onion
1 clove garlic
1 tablespoon (15 g) butter
1 quart (.95 L) chicken broth
1 ½ cups (240 g) canned pumpkin
½ cup (120 ml) Carb Countdown Dairy Beverage
2 teaspoons curry powder
Salt and pepper to taste

In a large, heavy-bottomed saucepan, over medium-low heat, sauté the onion and garlic in the butter until just softened. Add the chicken broth, and simmer for a half an hour.

Stir in the canned pumpkin, Carb Countdown Dairy Beverage, and curry powder. Bring back to a simmer, and simmer gently for another 15 minutes. Salt and pepper to taste, then serve.

Yield: 6 servings

Each with: 80 calories; 4 g fat; 5 g protein; 7 g carbohydrate; 2 g dietary fiber; 5 g usable carbs.

Marilyn Olshansky's Pumpkin-Coconut Bisque

An unusual, amazing soup—our tester, Doris Courtney, gave this a 10! Sure to impress dinner guests.

    2 tablespoons (30 g) butter
    ⅔ cup (110 g) chopped onion
    3 garlic cloves, minced
    1 29-ounce (810 g) can pumpkin
    2 14 ½-ounce (411 ml) cans chicken broth
    2 packets Splenda, or 4 teaspoons granulated Splenda
    ½ teaspoon (rounded) ground allspice
    ½ teaspoon dried, crushed red pepper
    1 13 ½-ounce (380 ml) can coconut milk

Melt butter in large, heavy pot over medium heat. Sauté the onion and garlic until golden, about 10 minutes. Add the pumpkin, broth, Splenda, allspice, and pepper. Bring to a boil and reduce the heat. Simmer covered, about 30 minutes, to blend the flavors.

Puree the soup with an hand-held blender or in a blender or food processor.

Return the soup to the pot and bring to a simmer. Stir in the coconut milk and season to taste with salt and pepper.

Tester's note: Doris says to tell you this freezes well.

Yield: Makes 8 servings

Each with: 179 calories; 14 g fat; 4 g protein; 12 g carbohydrate; 3 g dietary fiber; 9 g usable carbs.

⊚ Mary Anne Ward's Sausage Soup with Kale

This soup is a hearty one-dish meal.

    1 tablespoon (15 ml) olive oil
    1 small onion, diced
    1 small green bell pepper, diced
    2 ribs of celery, diced
    1 pound (455 g) sausage cut into bite-sized pieces
        (chorizo is good—try making it yourself)
    2 cloves garlic, diced fine
    1 teaspoon red chili flakes
    6–8 cups (120–160 g) kale, cut into 1" (2.5 cm) strips
    1 quart (.95 L) turkey stock (or chicken broth)
    Salt and pepper to taste
    Sour cream

Heat the oil in a 1-quart (.95 L) saucepan over medium-high heat. Sauté the onion, bell pepper, and celery for about 2 minutes.

Add the sausage and cook till it starts to brown around the edges. Add the garlic and chili flakes and cook for 2 minutes more, stirring constantly. Add the kale and stir another couple of minutes. Add the stock and bring to a boil, then reduce to a simmer for 20 minutes. Check seasoning and adjust with salt and pepper.

Add a generous dollop of sour cream to each bowl as it is served.

Dana's note: The kale is the biggest source of carbs in this recipe, so I would actually recommend the 6 cup (120 g) measurement. That's what the analysis is based on.

Yield: At 10 servings

Each will have: 313 calories; 24 g fat; 14 g protein; 10 g carbohydrate; 2 g dietary fiber; 8 g usable carbs.

Chunky Cream of Chicken and Portobello Soup

Elegant!

> 4 tablespoons (60 g) butter
> 1 cup (160 g) chopped onion
> 2 stalks celery, diced
> 1 large carrot, shredded
> 2 cups (200 g) portobello mushrooms, cut in matchstick strips
> 2 quarts (1.9 L) chicken broth
> 2 bay leaves
> 1 pound (455 g) boneless, skinless chicken breast
> ½ cup (120 ml) heavy cream
> Salt and pepper
> Guar or xanthan

Melt the butter in a large, heavy-bottomed saucepan, and add the vegetables. Sauté until the onion is translucent and the mushrooms change color. Add the chicken broth and the bay leaves, bring to a simmer, and let cook on low for 30 minutes.

Scoop out about half of the broth and vegetables into your blender, and puree. Return to the pan. Stir in the diced chicken breast, and let simmer for another 20 minutes. Stir in the cream and salt and pepper to taste, and thicken just a little with your guar or xanthan shaker. Remove bay leaves, and serve.

Yield: 6 servings

Each with: 318 calories; 19 g fat; 26 g protein; 11 g carbohydrate; 2 g dietary fiber; 9 g usable carbs.

Karen Sonderman's
Cream of Chicken Mushroom Soup

It's best to plan to make this soup over two days—one day you simmer the chicken to make broth, the next you finish the soup. Ray, who tested this, says it's perfect for a potluck or pitch-in, because it makes a huge vat of really tasty soup!

1 chicken, about 3 ½ pounds (1.6 kg), cut up

8 cups (1.9 L) water

2 chicken bouillon cubes

2 celery stalks, sliced

1 small onion, chopped

1 pound (455 g) sliced mushrooms

1 tablespoon (15 ml) lemon juice

½ stick butter

7 ounces (200 g) canned mushrooms

1 teaspoon guar

1 ½ pints (710 ml) heavy cream

Salt and pepper to taste

First, put the chicken in a big saucepan or soup kettle with 6 to 8 cups (1.4–1.9 L) water. Add the chicken boullion cubes, celery, and chopped onion. Simmer until chicken meat falls off bones.

Remove chicken from broth, skin, debone, and dice the meat. Meanwhile, chill the broth, so you can easily remove the grease from the top. Return the meat to the broth, and put your soup back on a burner. Bring it up to a simmer.

Add the mushrooms, lemon juice, and butter. Simmer until the mushrooms soften.

In your blender puree the canned mushrooms, drained, with 1 cup of the chicken broth and the guar. Stir this puree into the soup to thicken it. Stir in the cream; salt and pepper to taste.

Simmer briefly and serve.

Yield: Assuming 8 servings

Each will have: 535 calories; 49 g fat; 17 g protein; 8 g carbohydrate; 2 g dietary fiber; 6 g usable carbs.

Linda Blackburn's Cream of Chicken Soup

Our tester, Julie, really liked this, and says she'll make it again, both to eat and to use for making casseroles.

> 1 14 ½-ounce (405 ml) can chicken broth, low-sodium and fat-free
> ¼ cup (60 ml) heavy whipping cream
> Pepper
> 1 ½ teaspoons xanthan gum (more if you want it thicker)

Heat broth to boiling. Add whipping cream (you can use less if you want, or more), stir, and turn down heat to medium for about a minute. Add pepper to taste. Taste broth to make sure it has enough chicken flavor. If not, add chicken bouillon crystals until you get the flavor you like. Take and put in mixing bowl or blender. Add xanthan gum and blend if using a blender. Linda uses one of those handheld blenders and says it works very well. When adding xanthan gum, add just a little bit at a time until you get it as thick as you want it.

Yield: Makes 2 servings

Each with: 136 calories; 12 g fat; 5 g protein; 2 g carbohydrate; trace dietary fiber.

Debra Rodríguez's Crab Chowder

Our tester, Ray Stevens, says to give this one a gold star!

2 cups vegetable or chicken stock or broth

1 tablespoon (7 g) Old Bay seasoning blend
   (found near seafood department or on spice aisle)

1 1-pound (455 g) bag frozen cauliflower

1 cup water

2 ribs celery, chopped

1 medium yellow onion, chopped

1 small red bell pepper, seeded and diced

1 bay leaf, fresh or dried

2 tablespoons (30 g) butter

1 1/2 cups (360 ml) heavy cream

8 ounces (225 g) cooked lump crabmeat

1/4 teaspoon xanthan gum, or use your shaker (optional)

Tabasco sauce to taste

Salt and freshly ground black pepper

Bring chicken or vegetable broth to a boil in a large saucepan over medium to medium-high heat. Add the Old Bay seasoning and frozen califlower. Cover and cook until the cauliflower is soft (15–20 minutes). Using a potato masher or handheld blender, mash the cauliflower, leaving a few chunks.

Return the pan to the heat. Add the water, chopped celery, onion, red bell pepper, and bay leaf. Cover and let simmer for another 20 to 25 minutes or until the celery is tender.

Add butter, cream, and crabmeat. Whisk in xanthan gum (if desired). Add a few dashes of Tabasco (if desired) and adjust seasoning, if needed. Heat through, but do not boil! Remove bay leaf before serving.

Yield: Makes 4 generous servings

Each with: 475 calories; 40 g fat; 17 g protein; 13 g carbohydrate; 4 g dietary fiber; 9 g usable carbs.

Mexican Cabbage Soup

Great on a nasty, cold, rainy night! This is not hot, despite the chilies in the canned tomatoes—feel free to pass the hot sauce at the table if you want to spice it up. With all these vegetables, this is a complete meal, but if the family insists, you could add some corn tortillas for them.

> 1 quart beef broth (1 l)
> 14-ounce can diced tomatoes with green chilies (400 g)
> 1 pound ground round or other very lean ground beef (500 g)
> 1 tablespoon oil
> 1/2 cup chopped onion (50 g)
> 1 teaspoon minced garlic or 2 cloves garlic, crushed
> 1 teaspoon ground cumin
> 2 teaspoons oregano
> 2 cups bagged coleslaw mix (150 g)

In a large, microwaveable container combine the beef broth and canned tomatoes. Microwave on High for 8 to 10 minutes.

While the broth and tomatoes are heating through, start browning and crumbling the beef in the oil. Use a large soup kettle or heavy-bottomed saucepan. When the beef's about half browned, add the onion and garlic. Continue cooking until the beef is entirely browned. Add the cumin and oregano, and stir them in, then add the heated beef stock and tomatoes. Stir in the coleslaw mix and bring the whole thing to a simmer. Cook for another minute or so, and serve.

Yield: 4 servings, each with 9 grams of carbohydrates and 2 grams of fiber, for a total of 7 grams of usable carbs and 24 grams of protein.

Mary's Pepperoni Pizza Soup

Here's what our tester, Julie, said when asked if she'd make this soup again: "Oh ... My ... Gosh ... Yes! This is destined to become a low-carb favorite of mine. It truly does satisfy the pizza craving." Yippee!

> 1 tablespoon (15 ml) oil
> 1/2 cup (80 g) chopped onion
> 1 cup (100 g) sliced mushrooms
> 1 cup (120 g) chopped green bell pepper
> 1 14–15-ounce (400–420 g) can pizza sauce, no sugar added (Ragu makes one.)
> 1 14 1/2-ounce (411 ml) can chicken broth
> 1 cup (240 ml) water
> 1 teaspoon dried oregano
> 3 ounces (85 g) sliced pepperoni
> 1 cup (120 g) shredded mozzarella cheese

Heat the oil in large saucepan over medium heat. Add the onion, mushrooms, and bell pepper. Cook, stirring frequently, until tender, about 7 minutes.

Stir in pizza sauce, chicken broth, water, oregano, and pepperoni. Bring to a boil. Lower heat; simmer about 5 minutes. Ladle into soup bowls. Top with cheese just before serving.

Tester's note: Julie says, "I chose to use low-sodium chicken broth. The sauce and the pepperoni have a ton of sodium, no need to add more in the broth. Also, next time—and there will be many next times—I will add some zero-carb sausage and perhaps some thick-cut bacon. . . . Any zero-carb pizza meat would be wonderful in this."

Yield: Makes 4 generous servings, or 6 more modest ones

Assuming 4, each will have: 308 calories; 21 g fat; 16 g protein; 15 g carbohydrate; 4 g dietary fiber; 11 g usable carbs.

Jen Wardell's
Low-Carb Spinach Bisque Soup

Diana Lee tested this and rated it a 10!

2 tablespoons (20 g) finely diced onion

1 tablespoon (15 g) butter

1 10-ounce (280 g) package frozen chopped spinach

1 can (about 1 ¾ cups [420 ml]) chicken broth

1 cup (240 ml) half-and-half

1 cup (120 g) sharp cheddar cheese, shredded

4 ounces (115 g) cream cheese, cubed

¼ cup (40 g) Parmesan cheese, grated

Salt and pepper to taste

In a skillet, brown the onion in the butter. In a large saucepan, start the frozen spinach simmering in the broth. Add the browned onion to broth. When spinach is cooked (no longer frozen, and warmed through), add remaining ingredients. Heat through until cheeses melt.

Yield: 4 servings (4 cup servings or 3 bowl servings)

Each will have: 376 calories; 31 g fat; 17 g protein; 8 g carbohydrate; 2 g dietary fiber; 6 g usable carbs.

Amy Dungan's Broccoli, Ham, and Cheese Soup

Julie McIntosh, who tested this, calls it "great in all aspects"—including that her kids liked it!

    3 cups (600 g) steamed broccoli, chopped into bite-sized pieces
    4 ounces (115 g) cream cheese, softened
    ¾ cup (180 ml) heavy whipping cream
    1 ½ cups (360 ml) water
    1 chicken bouillon cube
    Pepper to taste
    ½ cup (150 g) sliced mushrooms
    ½ cup (55 g) chopped, cooked ham
    4 ounces (115 g) shredded cheddar cheese

First, of course, you'll steam your broccoli—you can steam a whole head and chop it up, or you can buy frozen broccoli cuts and use 3 cups (600 g) of them.

Combine 1 cup of the broccoli, the cream cheese, heavy cream, and ¼ cup water in your food processor, with the S-blade in place. Process until smooth. Transfer mixture to a large saucepan. Add bouillon, pepper, the rest of the broccoli, the mushrooms, the ham, and the rest of the water. Simmer over medium heat until the mushrooms are soft. Add cheddar and stir until melted, then serve.

Amy's note: "We like to add a little more cheese to ours. Sometimes we go overboard on the ham and mushrooms, too! If you do this, be sure to add to the carb count. This is also really good with cooked bacon in it."

Yield: Makes 6 servings

Each with: 279 calories; 25 g fat; 10 g protein; 4 g carbohydrate; 1 g dietary fiber; 3 g usable carbs.

chapter thirteen

Sauces, Seasonings, and Other Incidental Stuff

More and more low-carbohydrate condiments, sauces, and seasonings are hitting the market every day, but it's still fun to come up with your own, and it certainly gives you a wider variety to choose from. For more sauces, seasonings, and condiments, see chapter 15, the "Bonus Chapter"—I've included a bunch of recipes from other books that you'll need to make recipes in this book!

Apricot-Chipotle Glaze

I invented this for my Easter leg of lamb, but there's no reason you can't use it on pork and chicken, too—anywhere you want a hit of sweet-and-hot flavor.

> 1/2 cup (80 g) minced red onion
> 1/4 cup (60 ml) canola oil
> 4 cloves garlic, crushed
> 1/2 cup (120 ml) red wine vinegar
> 1/2 cup (160 g) low-sugar apricot preserves
> 2 chipotle chiles canned in adobo
> 5 tablespoons (7.5 g) Splenda
> 2 tablespoons (30 ml) lemon juice

In a saucepan, sauté the onion in the oil until it's soft. Add the garlic and vinegar, and whisk in the preserves. Bring to a simmer, and let cook for 5 minutes or so.

Let it cool for a few minutes, then pour the glaze into your blender, and add the chipotles, Splenda, and lemon juice. Whirl until the chipotles are ground up. Use to baste meat or poultry that's roasting or grilling.

Yield: 12 to 14 servings

Assuming 14, each will have: 52 calories; 4 g fat; trace protein; 4 g carbohydrate; trace dietary fiber; 4 g usable carbs.

⊚ Maple-Orange Ham Glaze

It's common to glaze a roasting ham with brown sugar, honey, or the like—but we all know what that does to the carb count! Here's a glaze that'll impress your family and friends, while leaving your diet intact.

> 1/2 cup (120 ml) sugar-free pancake syrup
> 1/4 cup (60 ml) lemon juice
> 1 teaspoon Splenda
> 1/4 teaspoon orange extract
> 1 tablespoon (15 g) brown mustard
> 1 tablespoon (15 g) butter

Simply combine everything in a small saucepan over low heat, and simmer for five minutes. Use to baste a ham during the last hour of roasting time. You can also use this to glaze a ham steak, for a much quicker supper!

Yield: Enough for a good-sized ham

The whole batch has: 133 calories; 13 g fat; 2 g protein; 6 g carbohydrate; trace dietary fiber; 6 g usable carbs. Carb count does not include the polyols in the sugar-free pancake syrup.

⊚ Easy Orange Salsa

> 1/2 cup (130 g) salsa
> 1/4 teaspoon orange extract
> 2 teaspoons Splenda

Just measure everything into a bowl, stir, and serve.

Yield: 4 servings of 2 tablespoons

Each with: 9 calories; trace fat; trace protein; 2 g carbohydrate; 1 g dietary fiber; 1 g usable carb.

◎ Simple No-Sugar Pickle Relish

24 ounces (680 g) sour pickle spears
1 cup (160 g) chopped onion
⅓ cup (8 g) Splenda
½ teaspoon celery seed
½ teaspoon mustard seed
2 tablespoons (30 ml) cider vinegar
Guar or xanthan

Open your jar of pickle spears, and pour off the liquid into a nonreactive saucepan. Throw the chopped onion into the pickle liquid, and stir in the Splenda, celery seed, and mustard seed. Bring to a simmer, turn to low, and let the whole thing simmer for 20 to 30 minutes.

In the meanwhile, cut your pickle spears into 3 to 4 chunks each, and throw 'em into your food processor with the S-blade in place.

When the onions are done simmering, pour the contents of the saucepan into the food processor. Add the 2 tablespoons of cider vinegar. Pulse the food processor until everything's chopped to about the consistency of commercial pickle relish. Thicken it up a bit with a little guar or xanthan, to make up for the lack of syrupiness, and pour the whole thing back into the pickle jar. Store in the fridge, and use as you would commercial pickle relish.

Yield: 3 cups, or 24 servings of 2 tablespoons

Each with: 6 calories; trace fat (13.0% calories from fat); trace protein; 1 g carbohydrate; trace dietary fiber; 1 g usable carbs.

◎ Major Grey's Chutney

Major Grey's chutney is not a brand, but a type, and it's the most popular kind of chutney in the United States—maybe in the world. But I'm afraid it's usually loaded with sugar. This version isn't, of course! I also substituted peaches for the mangoes you usually find in Major Grey's chutney—peaches are a whole lot easier to find. Go ahead and use frozen unsweetened peach slices in this. It'll save you lots of time and trouble, and since you're going to cook them, the difference in texture won't matter in the end.

> 2 pounds (1 kg) peach slices
> 1/3 cup (45 g) paper-thin ginger root slices
> 1 1/2 cups (38 g) Splenda
> 3 cloves garlic
> 1 teaspoon red pepper flakes
> 1 teaspoon cloves
> 1 1/2 cups (360 ml) cider vinegar
> Guar or xanthan

Put everything in a large, nonreactive saucepan, and stir to combine. Bring to a boil, turn the burner to low, and simmer for 1 1/2 to 2 hours. Thicken a bit with guar or xanthan if you like, and store in an airtight container in the fridge.

Yield: 1 quart (.95 L), or 32 servings of 2 tablespoons

Each with: 15 calories; trace fat; trace protein; 4 g carbohydrate; 1 g dietary fiber; 3 g usable carbs.

Pat Best's Gingered Cranberry Sauce

Keep in mind that the crystallized ginger does contain some sugar; you could use fresh gingerroot and extra Splenda to taste, if you like.

> 2 cups (480 ml) water
> 2 cups (50 g) Splenda
> 1/3 cup (75 g) crystallized ginger
> 1 12-ounce (340 g) bag fresh cranberries, rinsed

In a medium saucepan bring the water to a boil. Add the Splenda, ginger, and cranberries, reducing the heat to a simmer for 10 minutes. Cool completely and store in the refrigerator for up to one week.

Pat's note: "Can be made without ginger and will still taste delicious. We like it with chicken as well as with our turkey over the holidays."

Tester's note: Barbo Gold suggests a variation: Omit the ginger and add 1/2 to 1 teaspoon vanilla extract and the grated zest of 1 orange.

Yield: Serves 12 to 15 people

Assuming 12, per serving: 30 calories; trace fat; trace protein; 8 g carbohydrate; 1 g dietary fiber; 7 g usable carbs.

Jen Wardell's Low-Carb Cocktail Weenie Sauce

Remember the sauce for cocktail weenies and meatballs made with chili sauce and grape jelly your mom used to make? Our tester, Ray, says, "Grab some toothpicks and have a party!"

> 1 cup (240 g) low-carb ketchup
>   (preferably Dana's No-Sugar Ketchup, page 528)
> 1/4–1/3 cup (60–80 ml) sugar-free raspberry or grape flavoring syrup

Mix the ketchup and the syrup in a large skillet. Cook with meatballs or small hot dogs, small sausages, or cut-up regular-size hot dogs or sausages.

Jen's note: "I use this with 2 pounds [1 kg] of meat."

In one whole batch: 181 calories; 1 g fat; 7 g protein; 47 g carbohydrate; 8 g dietary fiber; 39 g usable carbs.

◎ Linda Wagner's
Any Way You Want It BBQ Sauce

This barbecue sauce lends itself to variation, hence the name. Our tester, Julie, said she really liked the flexibility, and that she'd choose this over the commercial low-carb barbecue sauces if it were sold at her grocery store.

8 ounces (225 g) tomato sauce

3 tablespoons (45 ml) vinegar

1 teaspoon molasses

1 tablespoon (15 ml) Worcestershire sauce

¼ teaspoon liquid smoke

2 ½ tablespoons (3.75 g) Splenda

1 teaspoon salt

½ tablespoon (3 g) paprika

1 teaspoon dry mustard

1 teaspoon chili powder

1 teaspoon minced dried onion

¼ teaspoon black pepper

½ teaspoon cloves

Combine tomato sauce, vinegar, molasses, Worcestershire sauce, and liquid smoke in a medium-sized saucepan, to help prevent splatters. Combine the Splenda and spices, mixing well, and add them, along with the dried onion, to the tomato sauce mixture. Simmer for 10 to 15 minutes, stirring often. This can be served hot as a dipping sauce or as a traditional BBQ sauce, or it can be poured over chicken, beef, or pork and baked until meat is tender. Without the liquid smoke and molasses, it can double for ketchup, and by adding an extra 1 teaspoon of chili powder and 1 teaspoon of ground cumin, you can give meats a Southwestern flare. If you like a spicier sauce, add cayenne to your taste.

Yield: 1 ¼ cups (300 g), or 10 servings of 2 tablespoons

Each with: 13 calories; trace fat; trace protein; 3 g carbohydrate; trace dietary fiber; 3 g usable carbs.

Nancy Harrigan's Coconut Ginger Sauce

This exotic sauce can be used for Nancy Harrigan's Spinach Balls (page 75) or to bake seafood or chicken.

> 14 ounces (400 ml) coconut milk
> 1 tablespoon (10 g) dried minced onion
> 1/4 teaspoon garlic powder
> 1 tablespoon (6 g) ground ginger
> 1/3 cup (80 ml) coconut oil or melted butter

Simply mix all ingredients together.

Yield: About 8 servings

Each with: 197 calories; 21 g fat; 1 g protein; 4 g carbohydrate; 1 g dietary fiber; 3 g usable carbs.

Marco Polo Marinade

This marinade is named after its combined Italian and Chinese influences. It's wonderful for steak, but try it on chicken, too! Also good on vegetables.

> 1 cup (240 ml) bottled Italian salad dressing
> 1/4 cup (60 ml) soy sauce
> 2 teaspoons grated ginger root
> 2 tablespoons (3 g) Splenda
> 4 drops blackstrap molasses

Just measure everything and stir it together, then use to marinate or season whatever you like!

Yield: 1 1/4 cups (300 ml), or 5 servings of 1/4 cup

228 calories; 23 g fat; 1 g protein; 6 g carbohydrate; trace dietary fiber; 6 g usable carbs. However, you can drop this lower by using a seriously low-carb Italian dressing—and anyway, since you use this as a marinade, you're unlikely to consume anything like 1/4 cup (60 ml) of this at a time.

Chipotle Mayonnaise

This is a great dip for asparagus, artichokes, broccoli—whatever you've got!

½ cup (120 g) mayonnaise
1 chipotle chile canned in adobo

This is way too good for how little work it takes: Put the mayonnaise and the chipotle in your food processor, with the S-blade in place. Add a teaspoon of the adobo sauce the chipotle was canned in. Now, run the food processor until it's smooth. That's it. This will keep for at least a week in a snap-top container in the fridge—if you manage not to eat it all, that is.

Yield: 4 servings of two tablespoons (30 g)

Each with: 197 calories; 23 g fat; 1 g protein; trace carbohydrate; trace dietary fiber; no usable carb.

Mustard-Horseradish Dipping Sauce

I came up with this to dip some stuffed mushrooms in, but it's very versatile.

½ cup (120 g) mayonnaise
2 teaspoons spicy brown mustard
1 teaspoon prepared horseradish
½ teaspoon Splenda
1 teaspoon white vinegar

Simply mix everything together. Good for dipping most anything! Chicken bites, veggies, whatever you've got.

Yield: About 6 servings

Each with: 134 calories; 16 g fat; trace protein; trace carbohydrate; trace dietary fiber; no usable carb.

Chili Lime Mayo

¼ cup (60 g) mayonnaise
2 teaspoons lime juice
¼ teaspoon chili paste
2 teaspoons minced cilantro

Just stir everything together, and serve over anything Asian or Mexican.

Yield: 4 servings of 1 tablespoon (15 g)

Each with: 100 calories; 12 g fat; trace protein; trace carbohydrate; trace dietary fiber; 0 g usable carb.

Curried Mock Hollandaise

Oh, man, this is the bomb with artichokes or asparagus! This is a variation of the Hollandaise for Sissies recipe (page 532).

4 egg yolks
1 cup (230 g) sour cream
1 tablespoon (15 ml) lemon juice
½ teaspoon salt or Vege-Sal
1 teaspoon curry powder
2 cloves garlic, crushed

You'll need either a double boiler or a heat diffuser for this—it needs very gentle heat. If you're using a double boiler, you want the water in the bottom hot, but not boiling. If you're using a heat diffuser, use the lowest possible heat under the diffuser.

Put all the ingredients in a heavy-bottomed saucepan or the top of a double boiler. Whisk everything together well, let it heat through, and serve with vegetables.

Yield: 6 servings

Each with: 125 calories; 11 g fat; 3 g protein; 3 g carbohydrate; trace dietary fiber; 3 g usable carbs.

Adobo Seasoning

Adobo is a popular seasoning in Latin America and the Caribbean. It's available at many grocery stores, in the spice aisle or the international aisle, but if you can't find it, it sure is easy to make.

> 10 teaspoons (30 g) garlic powder
> 5 teaspoons dried oregano
> 5 teaspoons pepper
> 2 ½ teaspoons paprika
> 5 teaspoons (30 g) salt

Simply measure everything into a bowl, stir, and store in a lidded shaker jar.

Yield: A little over ½ cup (70 g), or about 48 servings of ½ teaspoon

Each with: 3 calories; trace fat; trace protein; 1 g carbohydrate; trace dietary fiber; 1 g usable carb.

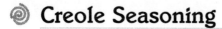 # Creole Seasoning

Creole seasoning is great when you want to add a hit of spicy-hot flavor to pork, chicken, seafood—or just about anything, actually. You can buy it premade, but you know how food manufacturers are—you have to keep an eye out for added sugar. It's easy to stir some up on your own.

    2 tablespoons (30 g) salt
    3 teaspoons garlic powder
    3 teaspoons onion powder
    3 teaspoons paprika
    3 teaspoons dried thyme
    2 teaspoons cayenne pepper
    1 1/2 teaspoons pepper
    1 1/2 teaspoons dried oregano
    2 bay leaves
    1/2 teaspoon chili powder

Put everything in your food processor or blender, crumbling the bay leaf as you put it in. Run until the bay leaf is pulverized, and everything is evenly mixed. Pour into a lidded shaker jar for storage.

Yield: 1/2 cup (70 g) or 48 servings of 1/2 teaspoon

2 calories; trace fat; trace protein; 1 g carbohydrate; trace dietary fiber; 1 g usable carb.

◎ New Orleans Gold

Hot and spicy New Orleans seasoning! Good on chicken, steak, pork, seafood-heck, anything but ice cream.

2 1/2 tablespoons (17 g) paprika
1 tablespoon (18 g) salt
2 tablespoons (18 g) garlic powder
1 tablespoon (6 g) pepper
1 tablespoon (9 g) onion powder
1 tablespoon (6 g) cayenne
1 tablespoon (3 g) dried oregano
1 tablespoon (3 g) dried thyme
1 1/2 teaspoons dried basil
1 1/2 teaspoons celery seed

Combine the ingredients in a food processor with the S-blade attachment, and run for thirty seconds.

Yield: 54 servings of 1 teaspoon

Each with: 4 calories; trace fat; trace protein; 1 g carbohydrate; trace dietary fiber; 1 g usable carb.

◎ Lorraine Achey's Parmesan-Dill Seasoning Mix

Use this easy sprinkle-on seasoning to dress up chicken or fish.

1 tablespoon (5 g) Parmesan cheese
1 tablespoon (2 g) dill weed
1 tablespoon (9 g) onion powder
1 tablespoon (4 g) parsley flakes
1/2 teaspoon salt
1/8–1/4 teaspoon black pepper

Mix all ingredients and store in airtight container. Use to season egg, chicken, or tuna salad. Or Lorraine's favorite, Dilled Almonds (page 67)!

Yield: Roughly ¼ cup (40 g), or 12 servings of 1 teaspoon apiece

Per teaspoon: 5 calories; trace fat; trace protein; 1 g carbohydrate; trace dietary fiber; 1 g usable carb.

◎ Tee's Cajun Seasoning Mix

Our tester, Julie, says this is as good or better than any commercial Cajun seasoning she's tried.

> 2 tablespoons (14 g) paprika
> 2 tablespoons (12 g) cayenne
> 1 tablespoon (9 g) onion flakes or onion powder
> 2 tablespoons (12 g) black pepper
> 2 tablespoons (6 g) oregano
> 2 tablespoons (5 g) basil
> 1 tablespoon (3 g) thyme
> 2 tablespoons (18 g) garlic powder
> 1 tablespoon (7 g) chili powder
> 1 tablespoon (7 g)cumin

Just measure everything into a bowl, stir together well, and store in a lidded shaker jar.

Yield: 1 cup (145 g) or 48 teaspoons

Each teaspoon will have: 18 calories; 1 g fat; 1 g protein; 4 g carbohydrates; 1 g fiber; 3 g usable carbs.

Italian Seasoned Crumbs

Use the way you would packaged Italian seasoned crumbs—to "fill" meatballs or "bread" chicken or chops. To get pork rind crumbs, just run a bag of pork rinds through your food processor.

1 cup (50 g) pork rind crumbs
1/2 teaspoon dried parsley
1/2 teaspoon dried oregano
1/4 teaspoon garlic powder
1/4 teaspoon onion powder
1/4 teaspoon Splenda

Yield: Makes 1 cup (55 g), or 8 servings of 2 tablespoons

Each with: 65 calories; 4 g fat (9.9% calories from fat); 7 g protein; trace carbohydrate; trace dietary fiber; so call it 0 usable carb.

chapter fourteen

Cookies, Cakes, Pies, and Other Sweets

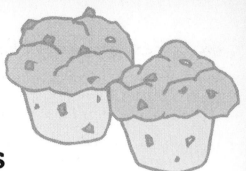

As I've mentioned numerous times before, my feelings about low-carbohydrate desserts and other sweets are mixed—on the one hand, anything that helps people walk away from sugar is a good thing, but on the other hand, it would be ideal for us to all get over the idea that we just have to have something sweet on a daily basis.

I'm as guilty as anyone—it's a rare day that I don't eat a little sugar-free dark chocolate. However, except when I'm developing recipes for y'all, I don't actually cook desserts much, for a very simple reason: If they're in the house, I eat them. If they're not, I don't miss them. So I'll make a dessert for a special occasion, or if I have a brilliant inspiration I just have to try out, and when it's gone, it's gone, and I'm not likely to make another for weeks, maybe months.

So these desserts are offered in hopes that they will help you wean yourself away from your sugar habit, and that they'll eventually become what a "treat" was meant to be: not a staple of the diet, eaten once or twice or even three times a day, but something pleasant that happens infrequently enough to really seem special.

You'll notice that many of these desserts, especially the baked goods, call for polyol. I haven't specified, in most of these, whether you should use maltitol, erythritol, sorbitol, Diabetisweet (isomalt), or some other version of polyol sweetener. This is because, with the notable exception of chocolate sauce, I haven't found much of a difference in how these sweeteners behave in cooking. I prefer erythritol for general use, because it is the least absorbable of the polyols and causes the least, uh, social offensiveness and gastric upset. But use what you can get; if it's a granular polyol sweetener, it should be fine.

◎ Chewy Oatmeal Cookies

Oh, boy! These are oatmeal cookies like the ones from your childhood.

⅓ cup (50 g) raisins

⅓ cup (80 ml) boiling water

½ cup (120 ml) coconut oil

1 egg

½ cup (100 g) polyol

1 cup (25 g) Splenda

1 tablespoon (20 g) blackstrap molasses

1 cup (120 g) vanilla whey protein powder

1 ¼ cups (155 g) almond meal

1 cup (100 g) rolled oats

2 teaspoons baking soda

1 teaspoon salt

¾ teaspoon cinnamon

½ cup (60 g) chopped pecans

Preheat oven to 275°F (140°C). (Yes, just 275°!)

Put the raisins in a bowl, and pour the boiling water over them. Let them sit while you . . .

Use your electric mixer to beat the coconut oil, egg, polyol sweetener, Splenda, and blackstrap together until smooth and well blended.

Okay, the raisins have been sitting in the hot water for five minutes—dump the raisins and water, both, into your blender or food processor, and run until you have a coarse puree. Add this to the batter, and mix in well.

In another bowl, combine the vanilla whey, almond meal, rolled oats, baking soda, salt, and cinnamon. Stir together, until ingredients are evenly distributed. Now, beat this mixture into the wet ingredients, adding about a third of the dry ingredients at a time. When all the dry ingredients are incorporated, mix in the chopped pecans.

I scooped this with a cookie scoop—like an ice cream scoop, only smaller; it holds 2 tablespoons of dough. So if you want to get about the same number of cookies I did (and about the same size) scoop the dough 2 tablespoonsful at a time. Put on cookie sheets you've sprayed with nonstick cooking spray, and keep in mind they'll spread—I fit about 10 cookies per sheet.

Bake for 18 minutes, or until just getting golden around the edges. Don't overbake or they won't be chewy! Cool on wire racks.

Yield: 35 nice big cookies

Each with: 100 calories; 6 g fat; 8 g protein; 5 g carbohydrate; 1 g dietary fiber; 4 g usable carbs. Carb count does not include polyol sweetener.

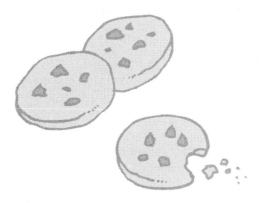

◎ Gingersnaps

Crisp and gingery-cinnamony, these cookies are nothing short of extraordinary.

¼ cup (60 g) butter
½ cup (120 ml) coconut oil
1 cup (25 g) Splenda
¼ cup (50 g) polyol
1 tablespoon (20 g) blackstrap molasses
1 egg
1 cup (125 g) almond meal
1 cup (120 g) vanilla whey protein powder
¼ cup (25 g) gluten
2 teaspoons baking soda
½ teaspoon salt
1 teaspoon ground ginger
2 teaspoons cinnamon
½ teaspoon ground cloves

Using your electric mixer, beat the butter, coconut oil, Splenda, polyol sweetener, blackstrap, and egg together until mixture is creamy and fluffy.

Beat in the almond meal, vanilla whey protein powder, and gluten, then the baking soda, salt, and spices.

Dough will be fairly soft, but cohesive. Spoon by the scant tablespoon onto ungreased cookie sheets, shaping a bit with the fingers to make little balls. Flatten balls slightly with the back of your spoon or fingers. Keep in mind when placing cookies on sheets that they will spread some—I find that 10 per sheet is about right.

Bake at 350°F (180°C) for about 7 to 9 minutes, or until just getting golden around the edges. Cool on wire racks, and store in an airtight container.

Yield: About 42 cookies

Each with: 76 calories; 5 g fat; 7 g protein; 2 g carbohydrate; trace dietary fiber; 2 g usable carbs. Carb count does not include polyol sweetener.

Chocolate Walnut Balls

This is a reworking of a recipe from *500 Low-Carb Recipes*—I kept the flavor and got rid of the hard-to-find soy powder and stevia-FOS blend. These are also a tad less crumbly, something readers had complained about. These make great Christmas cookies!

½ cup (120 g) butter, at room temperature
2 ounces (55 g) cream cheese, at room temperature
¾ cup (18 g) Splenda
¼ cup (50 g) polyol
1 egg
½ cup (60 g) almond meal
¾ cup (90 g) vanilla whey protein powder
¼ cup (25 g) wheat gluten
¼ teaspoon salt
1 ½ teaspoons baking powder
2 ounces (55 g) bitter chocolate
½ cup (60 g) chopped walnuts

Using your electric mixer, beat the butter and cream cheese until soft and well combined. Add the Splenda and polyol sweetener, and beat until well combined and fluffy. Add the egg, and beat until incorporated—don't forget to scrape down the sides of the bowl often!

Measure the almond meal, vanilla whey, gluten, salt, and baking powder into another bowl. Stir together. Now, beat this mixture into the other mixture, adding it about a third at a time.

Turn off the mixer while you melt the chocolate, then turn it back on, and beat in the chocolate. Add the walnuts, and beat just long enough to mix them in.

Chill this dough for a few hours, to make it easier to handle. Then preheat your oven to 375°F (190°C), and using clean hands, roll dough into small balls and place on cookie sheets you've greased or sprayed with nonstick cooking spray. Bake for 8 to 10 minutes.

If you don't want to take time to chill the dough, you can make these as drop cookies, and they'll work fine, they just won't look quite as formal.

Yield: 40 cookies

Each with: 74 calories; 5 g fat; 6 g protein; 2 g carbohydrate; trace dietary fiber; 2 g usable carbs. Carb count does not include polyol sweetener.

Peanut Butter Cookies

Another reworked recipe from *500 Low-Carb Recipes*. The original cookies tasted perfect—just like my mom's—but a few readers complained they were too crumbly. They also used soy powder and stevia-FOS blend, which many people couldn't find. These cookies omit those ingredients and hold together nicely—while still being yummy!

½ cup (120 g) butter, softened
¼ cup (50 g) polyol
¾ cup (18 g) Splenda
1 tablespoon (20 g) blackstrap molasses
1 egg
½ teaspoon baking soda
½ teaspoon salt
½ teaspoon vanilla
1 cup (250 g) natural peanut butter
⅓ cup (40 g) almond meal
⅓ cup (40 g) vanilla whey protein powder
⅓ cup (35 g) wheat gluten
2 tablespoons (15 g) oat bran

Preheat oven to 375°F (190°C).

In a large mixing bowl, use your electric mixer to beat the butter with the polyol sweetener, Splenda, blackstrap, and egg for several minutes—you want everything very well combined. Scrape down the sides of the bowl often, with a rubber scraper, to ensure that everything is evenly mixed.

Now beat in the baking soda, the salt, and the vanilla. Add the peanut butter, and beat that in, too.

Finally, beat in the almond meal, the vanilla whey protein, the wheat gluten, and the oat bran, again, making sure everything is evenly combined.

Spray cookie sheets with nonstick cooking spray. Roll cookie dough into 1" (2.5 cm) balls and place on sheets. Using the back of a fork, flatten the balls gently, making crisscross markings. Bake for 10 to 12 minutes. Cool on wire racks.

Yield: 42 cookies

Each with: 78 calories; 6 g fat; 4 g protein; 2 g carbohydrate; 1 g dietary fiber; 1 g usable carb. Carb count does not include polyol sweetener.

◉ Chocolate Dips

The high-carb version of this cookie is part of my earliest memories—my mother makes them for Christmas every year, and they're a favorite with everyone. They really dress up a holiday cookie plate, too!

1 ⅓ cups (160 g) vanilla whey protein powder
1 cup (125 g) almond meal
2 tablespoons (15 g) gluten
½ teaspoon salt
½ cup (120 g) butter, softened
½ cup (120 ml) coconut oil
⅓ cup (8 g) Splenda
2 tablespoons (25 g) polyol
1 teaspoon vanilla
½ cup (50 g) oat bran
2 tablespoons (30 ml) water
Dipping Chocolate (page 519)

Preheat oven to 325°F (170°C).

In one bowl, combine the vanilla whey, almond meal, gluten, and salt, and stir together.

In another, use your electric mixer to beat the butter and coconut oil together. When they're combined, beat in the Splenda and polyol sweetener, until the mixture is creamy and fluffy. Beat in the vanilla.

Now beat in the vanilla whey/almond meal combination, adding it in two or three lots. Finally, beat in the oat bran, then the water.

You'll have a stiff, somewhat crumbly dough. Use clean hands to form little logs, about 1 ½" (3.75 cm) long and the diameter of a thumb (unless your fingers are huge!), pressing them together well. Bake on ungreased cookie sheets for 25 to 30 minutes. Cool before dipping.

Dip one end of each cookie in the chocolate. Place on waxed paper to cool.

Yield: At least 36

Assuming 36, each will have: 107 calories; 7 g fat; 9 g protein; 3 g carbohydrate; trace dietary fiber; 3 g usable carbs. Carb count does not include polyol sweetener.

◎ Nut Butter Balls

The high-carb version of this recipe has been around for decades, under various names, including Russian Teacakes, of all things. They're another cookie my mom has made every Christmas as far back as I can remember.

1 cup (125 g) almond meal

¾ cup (90 g) vanilla whey protein powder

2 tablespoons (15 g) wheat gluten

1 cup (240 g) butter, softened

⅓ cup (8 g) Splenda

2 tablespoons (25 g) polyol

½ teaspoon salt

1 teaspoon vanilla

1 ½ cups (225 g) pecans, finely chopped

6 ounces (170 g) sugar-free dark chocolate, finely chopped

First measure and stir together the almond meal, vanilla whey, and gluten. Have this standing by.

Using an electric mixter, beat the butter with the Splenda and polyol until very creamy and fluffy. Beat in the salt and vanilla.

Now beat in the almond meal/vanilla whey combo, about a third at a time. Finally, beat in the chopped pecans and chopped chocolate.

Chill the dough for at least a few hours.

Preheat oven to 350°F (180°C). Using clean hands, make balls about 1 ½" (3.75 cm) in diameter, and place on ungreased cookie sheets. Bake for 10 to 12 minutes. While still warm, sift just a little extra Splenda over the tops of the cookies, to make them look spiffy (if you wait till they cool, none of it will stick!).

Yield: Makes about 50 cookies

Each with: 84 calories; 7 g fat; 5 g protein; 2 g carbohydrate; trace dietary fiber; 2 g usable carbs. Carb count does not include polyol, either added or in the sugar-free chocolate.

⦿ Hermits

Hermits are an old-fashioned cookie with a chewy texture and a brown-sugar-spicy flavor.

> 1/2 cup (120 g) butter
> 3/4 cup (18 g) Splenda
> 1/4 cup (50 g) polyol
> 2 1/2 teaspoons blackstrap molasses
> 1 egg
> 1/2 cup (120 ml) buttermilk
> 3/4 cup (90 g) almond meal
> 1/4 cup (25 g) wheat gluten
> 1/3 cup (40 g) vanilla whey protein powder
> 3/4 teaspoon cinnamon
> 1/2 teaspoon ground cloves
> 1/4 teaspoon baking soda
> 1/3 cup (50 g) currants
> 1/4 cup (30 g) chopped pecans

Preheat oven to 350°F (180°C).

In a large mixing bowl, with your electric mixer, beat the butter until soft. Add the Splenda, polyol, and blackstrap, and beat until light and creamy.

Beat in the egg and the buttermilk, and turn off the mixer while you . . .

Measure the almond meal, gluten, vanilla whey, cinnamon, cloves, and baking soda into a bowl. Stir them together to distribute the ingredients.

Turn the mixer back on, and beat in the dry ingredients, in three or four additions, scraping down the sides of the bowl when needed. Now add the currants and pecans, and mix just enough to blend.

Drop the batter onto greased cookie sheets, keeping in mind that they spread. Bake for 12 to 15 minutes, or until just starting to darken around the edges. Cool on wire racks, and store in a tightly lidded container.

Note: I've used currants instead of the traditional raisins in the hermits because they're little, and therefore distribute more evenly through the dough—to me, they taste like raisins anyway. If your currants are sort of dry, put them in a small bowl and pour a little boiling water over them before you start, then drain them right before you add them. And if you can't get currants, you could use raisins, but I'd suggest snipping each one into two or three pieces before adding them, or you're likely to end up with just one or two raisins per cookie.

Yield: About 40 cookies

Each with: 57 calories; 4 g fat; 4 g protein; 2 g carbohydrate; 2 g usable carbs. Carb count does not include polyol sweetener

◎ Tee's Butter Pecan Bars

Our tester, Kay, says you can vary this, and cut the carb count a tad, by substituting one of the many Atkins syrups for the molasses—though, of course, then they wouldn't be so classically butter pecan flavored.

> 1 stick butter (use salted, not unsalted, butter)
> 1 tablespoon (20 g) molasses
> 1 cup (25 g) Splenda
> 2 eggs
> ½ teaspoon vanilla
> ¼ cup (30 g) almond meal
> ¼ cup (30 g) oat flour (or ½ cup (60 g) low-carb flour of choice)
> 1 cup (125 g) chopped pecans

Preheat oven to 325°F (170°C).

Melt the butter by putting it in a microwaveable bowl and nuking on 40 percent power for about a minute. Stir in the molasses, then the Splenda, eggs, and vanilla, and mix well. Stir in the almond meal and oat flour, then the pecans.

Pour batter into an 8" x 8" (20 x 20 cm) square pan greased with oil. Bake for 25 to 30 minutes.

Note: Can also be made in mini-muffin pans for Butter Pecan Cupcakes.

Yield: Makes 16 bars

Each with: 159 calories; 12 g fat; 3 g protein; 11 g carbohydrate; 1 g dietary fiber; 10 g usable carbs. Carb count does not include polyol sweetener.

◎ Amanda's Sugar Cookies

Sheri Dornhecker says this is an adaptation of a recipe from her grandmother, who was a famous baker in Klamath Falls, Oregon. Grandma Amanda used to make these for the state police for keeping an eye on her house when Grandpa was away working on the railroad. Sherri insists that you mix these by hand, not with an electric mixer.

> 1 ½ cups (38 g) Splenda
> 1 cup (240 ml) olive or canola or peanut oil
> 2 eggs
> 1 ½ cups (150 g) vital wheat gluten
>   (add 2 tablespoons for high altitude, says our Colorado tester)
> ½ cup (60 g) vanilla whey protein powder
> 1 teaspoon baking soda
> ½ teaspoon salt
> 1 teaspoon cream of tartar
> 2 teaspoons vanilla extract
> 2 teaspoons lemon extract

Stir together the Splenda and oil. Add eggs; mix again. In a separate bowl, combine the dry ingredients, and stir to distribute evenly. Add dry ingredients to wet, then stir in the vanilla and lemon extracts.

You can refrigerate the dough for a while, or just proceed and roll into 1" (2.5 cm) balls. Place them on cookie sheets, and press each ball with a fork several times, flattening down. Grandma Amanda sprinkled her sugar cookies with colored sugar; you can sprinkle yours with Splenda, cinnamon, or a combination of the two.

Bake at 350°F (180°C) for 8 to 10 minutes or until brown around the edges.

Note: Our testers say this dough seems oily, but the cookies are not oily when baked. One of them also tried this with orange extract, and termed the results "awesome."

Yield: If you get about 4 dozen cookies out of a batch . . .

Each cookie will have: 83 calories; 5 g fat; 8 g protein; 1 g carbohydrate; trace dietary fiber; 1 g usable carbs.

◉ Ray's Peanut Butter Cookies

My pal and recipe tester Ray Stevens came up with these, and he says they are good but a little crumbly. Actually, I kinda like my peanut butter cookies a little crumbly.

> ¼ cup (60 g) butter
> ¼ cup (60 ml) coconut oil
> ½ cup (125 g) natural peanut butter
> ½ cup (12 g) Splenda
> ½ cup (8 g) Brown Sugar Twin
> 1 cup (100 g) wheat gluten
> ½ cup (60 g) whey protein
> ¾ teaspoon baking soda
> ½ teaspoon baking powder
> 1 egg

Melt butter and mix with coconut oil. Add peanut butter. Stir to combine. Add remaining ingredients and mix well. Refrigerate the dough overnight.

Form into walnut-sized balls. Place on cookie sheet you've sprayed with nonstick cooking spray, and flatten with a fork. Keep the fork clean using hot water. (Allow for the cookies to double in size after flattening.)

Bake in a 350°F (180°C) oven till edges start to get brown (about 10 to 15 minutes). Allow to cool.

Yield: About 40 cookies, depending on size

Each with: 77 calories; 5 g fat; 8 g protein; 1 g carbohydrate; trace dietary fiber; 1 g usable carbs.

◉ Jan Tucker's Chocolate Shortbread Cookies

A recipe for rich chocolate cookies.

>2 cups (250 g) almond meal
>
>½ cup (120 g) Splenda
>
>½ cup (120 g) softened butter
>
>½ teaspoon salt (if using salted butter omit salt)
>
>1 teaspoon vanilla extract
>
>3 tablespoons cocoa powder

Preheat oven to 300°F (150°C). Combine all ingredients with your electric mixer. Form dough into walnut sized balls. Place on parchment covered cookie sheet. Press down lightly with fork. Bake for 40 minutes.

Note: Jan says that this was originally a recipe for Almond Shortbread, calling for 1 teaspoon almond extract instead of the cocoa powder. You can try it that way if you prefer!

Yield: Makes about 30 cookies

Each with: 66 calories; 5 g fat; 4 g protein; 3 g carbohydrate; trace dietary fiber; 3 g usable carbs.

⊚ Espresso Chocolate Chip Brownies

A friend posted the original version of this recipe—definitely not low carb—online. (Thanks, Robin!) I couldn't resist the challenge. They're wonderful!

1 cup (25 g) Splenda

1/2 cup (60 g) vanilla whey protein powder

1/4 cup (30 g) almond meal

1/2 cup (50 g) unsweetened cocoa powder

1 tablespoon (12 g) instant coffee crystals (regular or decaf, as you prefer)

1/2 teaspoon salt

1/2 cup (120 g; 1 stick) butter

2 large eggs

1/4 cup (60 ml) water

6 ounces (170 g) sugar-free chocolate chips or 6 ounces (170 g) sugar-free dark chocolate bars, chopped to chocolate-chip-size in the food processor

Preheat oven to 350°F (180°C).

Put Splenda, vanilla whey protein, almond meal, cocoa, instant coffee crystals, and salt in a food processor with the S-blade in place. Pulse to combine. Add the butter, and pulse until the butter is "cut in"—well combined with the dry ingredients. Turn out into a bowl. Mix in the eggs, one at a time, beating well with a whisk after each. Then beat in the water. Finally, stir in the chocolate chips or chopped-up chocolate bars. Spray an 8" x 8" (20 x 20 cm) pan with nonstick cooking spray, and spread batter evenly in the pan. Bake for 15 to 20 minutes—do not overbake! Cool, and cut into squares.

Yield: I made 25 small brownies from this—I like to have the option of having a little something, and if I want more, I can always have two.

If you do, indeed, make 25, each brownie will have 3 g carbohydrate and 1 g fiber, for a usable carb count of 2 g; 3 g protein.

Yield: If you prefer, you can make 16 bigger brownies

At 4 g carb each, and 1 g fiber, for a usable carb count of 3 g, with 4 g protein. Carb count does not include polyol sweetener in the sugar-free chocolate.

Dana's Brownies

2 ounces (55 g) bitter chocolate

8 ounces (225 g) butter

½ cup (100 g) polyol sweetener

½ cup (12 g) Splenda

2 eggs

½ cup (60 g) vanilla whey protein powder

1 pinch salt

In the top of a double boiler, or in a saucepan over a heat diffuser set on lowest possible heat, melt the chocolate and the butter together. Stir until they're well combined. Scrape this into a mixing bowl.

Add the polyol sweetener, and stir well, then stir in the Splenda. Next, beat in the eggs, one at a time. Stir in the vanilla whey protein powder and salt.

Pour into an 8" x 8" (20 x 20 cm) baking pan you've sprayed well with nonstick cooking spray. Bake in a preheated 350°F (180°C) oven for 15 to 20 minutes. Do not overbake! Cut into 12 bars, and let cool in the pan. Store in a tightly covered container in the refrigerator.

Yield: 12 servings

Each with: 208 calories; 19 g fat; 9 g protein; 2 g carbohydrate; 1 g dietary fiber; 1 g usable carb. Carb count does not include polyol sweetener.

Sarah Driver's Brownies

Here's another low-carb brownie recipe. C'mon, can you have too many brownie recipes? Our tester, Ray, said, "I wish most restaurants made brownies this good!" This version uses no polyol sweetener, so it's good for those who really can't tolerate them at all.

½ cup (120 g) butter

½ cup (50 g) cocoa powder

1 cup (25 g) Splenda

¼ cup (4 g) Brown Sugar Twin

2 beaten eggs

1 teaspoon vanilla

Dash of salt

¼ cup (30 g) almond meal

¼ cup (30 g) oat bran flour (run oat bran through your food processor or blender to make this)

½ teaspoon xanthan gum

2 tablespoons (30 ml) water

Preheat oven to 350°F (180°C). Melt butter, add cocoa, and blend. Stir in Splenda, Brown Sugar Twin, eggs, vanilla, and salt. Add meal and flour, xanthan gum, and water; mix well and spoon into a greased 8" x 4" (20 x 10 cm) loaf pan. Bake 23 to 25 minutes, cool. Yum.

Yield: Eight 2"-square brownies

Each with: 157 calories; 14 g fat; 5 g protein; 6 g carbohydrate; 2 g dietary fiber; 4 g usable carbs.

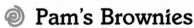 # Pam's Brownies

Pam Robles adapted this recipe from her favorite high-carb brownie recipe, and our tester loved them!

2 ounces (55 g) bitter chocolate
1 stick (112 g) butter
1 cup (25 g) granular Splenda
2 eggs
1 teaspoon vanilla extract
¼ cup (30 g) almond meal
¼ teaspoon salt
½–1 cup (60–125 g) chopped walnuts
   or pecans may be added if desired

Preheat oven to 350°F (180°C). Butter an 8" x 8" (20 x 20 cm) baking pan, and "flour" it with a little almond meal.

Melt the chocolate and butter together—you can do this in a saucepan over very low heat, or better, do it right in your mixing bowl, in your microwave. Using your electric mixer, beat in the Splenda, then the eggs, one at a time, beating well after each addition. Stir in the vanilla extract, then the almond meal and salt. Stir in the nuts, if using.

Pour mixture into pan, and bake at 20 to 25 min. Cool in pan. Cut into 2" (5 cm) squares and enjoy.

Yield: Makes 16 squares

Each with: 135 calories; 13 g fat; 4 g protein; 3 g carbohydrate; 1 g dietary fiber; 2 g usable carbs.

Black Forest Parfaits

This has too many carbs for you to want to eat it on a regular basis, but it's great for a company dinner or a holiday—really pretty, too.

> 1 4-serving-size package sugar-free instant chocolate pudding mix
> 2 cups (480 ml) Carb Countdown Dairy Beverage
> 1 cup (240 ml) heavy cream, chilled
> 1 tablespoon (10 g) sugar-free instant vanilla pudding mix
> 1 tablespoon (15 g) butter
> ½ cup (60 g) almond meal
> ½ cup (35 g) shredded coconut meat
> 2 tablespoons (30 g) cocoa
> 2 tablespoons (25 g) polyol
> 1 batch No-Sugar-Added Cherry Pie Filling (page 512)

Mix your sugar-free instant chocolate pudding mix with the Carb Countdown Dairy Beverage, and stir with a whisk for 2 minutes, or until thickened. Set aside.

Pour your chilled heavy cream into a deep mixing bowl. Add the tablespoon of sugar-free vanilla instant pudding mix, and using an electric mixer, whip until cream is stiff—do not overbeat, or you'll get sweetened vanilla butter! (Also do not try to do this step in a blender or food processor. It simply will not work.) Scoop out 1 ½ cups of the whipped cream, and add to the bowl with the chocolate pudding, and fold in with a rubber scraper.

In a medium skillet, melt the butter, and add the almond meal, coconut, cocoa powder, and polyol sweetener. Stir over medium heat for about five minutes, or until toasted. Remove from heat.

Okay, we're on the home stretch. Get out 6 pretty dessert dishes— preferably clear parfait glasses, so that everyone can see the layers. Spoon half of the chocolate mixture into the bottom of the dessert dishes, then top with half the chocolate crumbs, and half the cherry mixture. Repeat the layers, reserving just a couple of teaspoons of the crumbs. There should be just enough whipped cream left in the bowl to put a little dollop on top of each serving. Sprinkle the reserved little bit of crumbs on top of that, and chill for at least a few hours before serving.

Yield: 6 servings

Each with: 314 calories; 24 g fat; 10 g protein; 17 g carbohydrate; 2 g dietary fiber; 15 g usable carbs. Carb count does not include polyol sweetener.

Strawberry Cheese Pie

This is a killer company dessert! Feel free to use cream cheese instead, if you pre-fer—your carb count will remain about the same, though your calorie count will be higher.

> 8 ounces (225 g) Neufchatel cheese, softened (or regular or light cream cheese)
> 2 tablespoons (30 ml) heavy cream
> 1 tablespoon (1.5 g) Splenda
> 1/2 teaspoon vanilla extract
> Pie Crust, prebaked (page 132)
> 1 pound (455 g) frozen, unsweetened strawberries
> 1 cup (240 g) water
> 1/4 cup (6 g) Splenda
> 2 tablespoons (30 ml) lemon juice
> 2 teaspoons unflavored gelatin

Using your electric mixer, beat the Neufchatel cheese, heavy cream, the 1 tablespoon of Splenda, and the vanilla together until very smooth and fluffy. Smooth evenly over the bottom of your prebaked pie shell.

Put the strawberries, water, the 1/4 cup Splenda, and lemon juice in a nonreactive saucepan. Bring to a boil, then turn down to low, and let it simmer until the strawber-ries are soft.

Use a whisk to coarsely mash the strawberries. Now, stir with the whisk in a circle while you sprinkle the gelatin over the surface of the strawberry mixture, a little at a time. (You're trying to make sure that all the gelatin dissolves thoroughly, here, instead of leaving chewy little gelatin "seeds" in your finished pie.) Turn the burner off, and let the strawberry mixture cool until it's getting syrupy. Pour or spoon over the cream cheese layer, then put your pie in the fridge for at least several hours before serving.

Here's my confession: This actually makes a little too much strawberry mixture to fit in the pie shell, but I hate the idea of having a few leftover frozen strawberries just hanging around. So I pour the extra strawberry stuff into a custard cup, and chill it for a gelatin dessert. But if you prefer, you could use an ounce or two less cheese, instead, to make room for the extra strawberries.

Yield: 8 servings

Each with: 307 calories; 22 g fat; 20 g protein; 10 g carbohydrate; 2 g dietary fiber; 8 g usable carbs.

◎ Chocolate Raspberry Pie

This is fairly simple, but looks terribly elegant, what with the chocolate-brown crust and the deep pink filling. Yummy, too. It's best to make this for an occasion where it will all get eaten up. The leftovers will still taste great, but will look less and less impressive as days in the fridge go by.

> 1 package (4-serving size) sugar-free raspberry-flavored gelatin
> 1 tablespoon (15 ml) lemon juice
> 1 1/4 cups (300 ml) boiling water
> 1 pint (475 ml) no-sugar-added vanilla ice cream (I used Breyer's Carb Smart)
> Crisp Chocolate Crust (page 524)
> Maltitol-Splenda Chocolate Sauce (page 519)

In a large mixing bowl, combine the sugar-free raspberry gelatin with the lemon juice and boiling water. Stir until gelatin is completely dissolved. Now stir in the softened low-carb vanilla ice cream. Stick the bowl in the fridge for a few minutes until the mixture is thickened a bit, but not set, and pour into the Crisp Chocolate Crust. Chill for several hours, at least, and overnight is a good idea.

Serve with the Maltitol-Splenda Chocolate Sauce (page 515) or with Sugar-Free Chocolate Sauce (page 535).

Yield: 8 servings

Each with: 261 calories; 24 g fat; 8 g protein; 8 g carbohydrate; 4 g dietary fiber; 4 g usable carb. Carb count does not include the polyol sweetener in the ice cream or chocolate sauce.

◎ Brownie Mocha Fudge Pie

> 1 batch Dana's Brownies (page 467, but see instructions below)
> 4 teaspoons instant coffee granules, divided
> 2 cups (480 ml) heavy cream, divided, well chilled
> 3 tablespoons (30 g) sugar-free instant vanilla pudding mix, divided
> 1 1/2 cups (360 ml) Carb Countdown Dairy Beverage or 1 1/2 cups (360 ml) half-and-half
> 3 tablespoons (45 ml) Mockahlua (page 540)
> 2 4-serving-size packages sugar-free instant chocolate pudding mix

Make your brownies, adding 2 teaspoons of instant coffee granules. Instead of baking in an 8" x 8" (20 x 20 cm) pan, use a 10" (25 cm) pie plate you've sprayed well with nonstick cooking spray. Let your brownie crust cool thoroughly before starting on your filling.

Pour 1 cup of your heavy cream into a smallish, deep mixing bowl, and add 1 ½ tablespoons (15 g) of the sugar-free vanilla instant pudding powder. Using a whisk or an electric mixer, whip your cream until well thickened (but don't go overboard and make sweet vanilla butter!). Set this aside for a moment.

In another mixing bowl, dissolve 1 teaspoon of the instant coffee granules in the Carb Countdown Dairy Beverage, and stir in 2 tablespoons of the Mockahlua. Now add the sugar-free instant chocolate pudding mix, and beat with your electric mixer for a minute or two, until very smooth and thick. Add the whipped cream you made. Turn the mixer to its very lowest setting, and use to beat the whipped cream into the pudding mixture until everything is just combined. Spread this mixture over your brownie crust.

Okay, you need your cream-whipping bowl again—don't bother to wash it, though you'll want to wash your beaters. Pour the last tablespoon of Mockahlua and the last teaspoon of coffee granules into the bowl, and dissolve the coffee granules in the Mockahlua. Now add the second cup (240 ml) of heavy cream and the second 1 ½ tablespoons (15 g) of vanilla instant pudding powder. Whip until thickened—again, don't overbeat and get butter. Spread this coffee whipped cream over the pudding layer, and chill your pie well—at least a few hours.

Decorate with bitter chocolate shavings, if you like.

Yield: 12 servings

Each with: 378 calories; 35 g fat; 11 g protein; 8 g carbohydrate; 1 g dietary fiber; 7 g usable carbs. Analysis does not include polyol sweetener.

George Fairchild's Low-Carb Peanut Butter Pie

Small pinch of salt

1 cup (240 ml) whipping or heavy cream

1 8-ounce (225 g) package cream cheese

½ teaspoon vanilla

1 cup (25 g) Splenda

1 cup (250 g) natural peanut butter

1 prepared crust—try the Almond Crust (page 132)
    or the Pie Crust (page 132, prebaked)

First, whip your cream: In cold metal bowl add a small pinch of salt to 1 cup (240 ml) whipping or heavy cream and whip. To get the best results, place the bowl and beaters in a freezer for at least 1 hour before using.

Now, make your filling: With your electric mixer, blender, or in your food processor with the S-blade in place, combine the cream cheese, vanilla, Splenda, and peanut butter. Now gently fold into whipped cream until completely mixed. (Add the peanut butter mixture to the whipped cream, not vice versa.) Pour mixture into a low-carb pie shell and refrigerate for 2 hours.

Note: George says he also serves this filling in dessert dishes as a peanut butter mousse.

Yield: Assuming 10 servings (and no crust)

Each will have: 310 calories; 29 g fat; 7 g protein; 7 g carbohydrate; 1 g dietary fiber; 6 g usable carbs.

Maria Marshall's Low-Carb Chocolate Pecan Pie

This version of pecan pie includes chocolate, so you Kentuckians may want to substitute it for Derby Pie—but feel free to leave out the chocolate if you prefer your pecan pie plain.

> 3 eggs
> ½ cup (170 g) molasses-flavored sugar-free syrup sweetened with Splenda (Nature's Flavors makes one)
> 24 packets Splenda, or 1 cup (25 g) granulated Splenda
> 4 tablespoons (60 g) butter, melted
> 6 ounces (170 g) sugar-free chocolate chunks or chips
> 1 ½ cups (225 g) pecan halves, toasted and cooled
> 1 Pie Crust, unbaked (page 132)

Whisk eggs, then whisk in the Splenda syrup and Splenda. Blend in melted butter. Sprinkle chocolate and pecans over your favorite low-carb pie crust.

Pour filling over chocolate and pecans. Bake at 375°F (190°C) for 45 to 50 minutes.

Cool after removing from oven. Chill before serving. Cut with serrated knife.

Yield: 8 servings

Each with: 507 calories; 42 g fat; 20 g protein; 20 g carbohydrate; 4 g dietary fiber; 16 g usable carbs. Carb count does not include the polyol sweetener in the chocolate.

Chocolate Coconut Rum Balls

1/2 cup (130 g) almond butter (find this at your health food store)

3 ounces (38 g) cream cheese, softened

1/4 cup (60 ml) dark rum

1 tablespoon (7 g) cocoa powder

3/4 cup (53 g) shredded unsweetened coconut

Dipping Chocolate (see recipe page 518)

1/3 cup (8 g) Splenda

Beat the almond butter and cream cheese together until blended, then add the rum, Splenda, and cocoa powder. Then beat in 1/2 cup of the coconut.

Make your dipping chocolate, and using a fork, dip each ball. While the dipping chocolate is still soft, sprinkle the rest of the coconut over the balls. Store in the fridge.

Yield: Makes about 24 balls, each with: 65 calories; 6 g fat; 1 g protein; 2 g carbohydrate; trace dietary fiber; 2 grams usable carbs.

Jane's Pumpkin Pie

Deb Gajewski sends the decarbed version of the pumpkin pie she's been making for thirty years! She says, "Even people who don't like pumpkin pie will love this." She also says that orange zest is the secret ingredient!

Crust:

1 1/2 tablespoons (25 g) butter, softened

1/4 cup (30 g) ground pecans

Filling:

2 teaspoons low-carb baking mix

⅓ cup (8 g) Splenda

¼ cup (30 g) stevia

8 ounces (225 g) cream cheese, at room temperature (Philly preferred)

1 15-ounce (420 g) can pumpkin

1 teaspoon cinnamon

¼ teaspoon ginger

¼ teaspoon allspice

1 teaspoon vanilla

1 teaspoon orange zest

3 eggs, extra large

Sour Cream mixture: Mix together well

1 cup (230 g) sour cream

2 teaspoons Splenda

½ teaspoon vanilla

Grease 9" (22.5 cm) pie pan or springform pan with softened butter. Pour ground pecans into pan and shake to distribute evenly over bottom and sides of pan.

In a large bowl, mix together baking mix, sweeteners, and cream cheese. Add in pumpkin and spices. Add vanilla and orange zest. Add in eggs one at a time, mixing only enough to incorporate. Pour into prepared pie pan or springform pan. Bake at 350°F (180°C) for 55 minutes.

Top immediately with sour cream mixture.

Cool and refrigerate at least 4 hours or overnight before serving.

Note: Deb specified "Stevia Ultimate," but our tester couldn't find it, so she used regular white, powdered stevia extract and says the pie came out fine. So, if you can't find the "Ultimate," don't sweat it.

Yield: Makes 8 servings

Each with: 254 calories; 22 g fat; 7 g protein; 9 g carbohydrate; 2 g dietary fiber; 7 g usable carbs.

◎ Carol Tessman's Raspberry Pie

Our tester, Julie, loved this pie and said it couldn't be easier to make.

Crust:

> 1 ¼ cups (155 g) almond meal
> ¼ cup (6 g) Splenda
> ⅓ cup (80 g) butter, melted

Combine all ingredients, and press evenly over the bottom and up sides of a deep-dish 9" (22.5 cm) pie plate. Prick crust with fork. Bake in a 350°F (180°C) oven 10 to 12 minutes until crust starts to brown. Let cool.

Filling:

> 1 cup (240 ml) heavy whipping cream
> ½ teaspoon vanilla
> ½ cup (12 g) Splenda
> ⅔ cup (160 ml) boiling water
> 1 small (0.3 ounce; 9 g) box sugar-free raspberry gelatin
> 8 ice cubes
> ½ pint (125 g) fresh raspberries (optional)

Beat the cream, vanilla, and Splenda together until soft peaks form; set aside.

Add boiling water to gelatin; stir until gelatin is dissolved. Add 8 ice cubes, and stir until ice is melted and gelatin starts to thicken.

Fold into the whipped topping to combine. If desired, add ½ pint fresh raspberries. Pour into prepared crust and refrigerate at least 2 hours before serving

Yield: Serves 6 to 8

Assuming 8 servings, each will have: 259 calories; 22 g fat; 10 g protein; 7 g carbohydrate; 0 g dietary fiber; 7 g usable carbs.

◎ Grandma's Peach Cobbler

Well, except Grandma's was a lot higher-carb than this! This is a charming, old-fashioned dessert.

> 4 cups (800 g) sliced peaches
> 1/4 cup (6 g) Splenda
> 1/4 cup (50 g) polyol
> 1 tablespoon (15 ml) lemon juice
> 8 tablespoons (120 g) butter, divided
> 1/2 cup (60 g) almond meal
> 1/2 cup (60 g) vanilla whey protein powder
> 2 1/2 teaspoons baking powder
> 1 tablespoon (1.5 g) Splenda
> 1 teaspoon salt
> 1/2 cup (120 ml) heavy cream

Preheat oven to 375°F (190°C). Spray an 8" x 8" (20 x 20 cm) baking pan with nonstick cooking spray.

In a mixing bowl, combine the sliced peaches (I use unsweetened frozen peach slices—saves lots of time and trouble, and since they're going to be cooked, it makes no difference in the final texture), 1/4 cup (6 g) Splenda, polyol, and lemon juice. Toss everything together, and spread evenly in the pan. Dot with 2 tablespoons (30 g) of the butter.

In another mixing bowl (or heck, go ahead and use the same one if you like), combine the almond meal, vanilla whey, baking powder, the 1 tablespoon of Splenda, and the salt. Stir together to evenly distribute ingredients.

Melt the remaining 6 tablespoons (90 g) of butter. Measure the cream, and stir the butter into it. Pour into the dry ingredients, and mix with a few swift strokes of your whisk or a spoon—you just want to stir enough to ensure that there are no pockets of dry ingredients lurking.

Spread the batter evenly over the peaches, and bake for 30 minutes or until the crust is crisp and evenly golden brown. Serve warm.

Yield: 9 servings

Each with: 250 calories; 17 g fat; 14 g protein; 13 g carbohydrate; 2 g dietary fiber; 11 g usable carbs. Carb count does not include polyol sweetener.

Grandma's Blueberry Cobbler

Bet you would have thought of this!

4 cups (580 g) fresh blueberries or 4 cups (620 g) unsweetened frozen blueberries

¼ cup (6 g) Splenda

¼ cup (50 g) polyol

1 tablespoon (15 ml) lemon juice

8 tablespoons (120 g) butter, divided

½ cup (60 g) almond meal

½ cup (60 g) vanilla whey protein powder

2 ½ teaspoons baking powder

1 tablespoon (1.5 g) Splenda

1 teaspoon salt

½ cup (120 ml) heavy cream

Preheat oven to 375°F (190°C). Spray an 8" x 8" (20 x 20 cm) baking pan with nonstick cooking spray.

In a mixing bowl, combine the blueberries, ¼ cup (6 g) Splenda, polyol, and lemon juice. Toss everything together, and spread evenly in the pan. Dot with 2 tablespoons of the butter.

In another mixing bowl (or heck, go ahead and use the same one if you like), combine the almond meal, vanilla whey, baking powder, the 1 tablespoon (1.5 g) of Splenda, and the salt. Stir together to evenly distribute ingredients.

Melt the remaining 6 tablespoons of butter. Measure the cream, and stir the butter into it. Pour into the dry ingredients, and mix with a few swift strokes of your whisk or a spoon—you just want to stir enough to ensure that there are no pockets of dry ingredients lurking.

Spread the batter evenly over the blueberries, and bake for 30 minutes or until the crust is crisp and evenly golden brown. Serve warm.

Yield: 9 servings

Each with: 254 calories; 18 g fat; 13 g protein; 13 g carbohydrate; 2 g dietary fiber; 11 g usable carbs.

⊚ Grandma's Cherry Cobbler

I thought I was done with the whole cobbler thing, when Ray Stevens, one of my recipe testers, suggested a cherry version. Easier done than said!

2 batches No-Sugar-Added Cherry Pie Filling (page 512)
8 tablespoons (120 g) butter, divided
1/2 cup (60 g) almond meal
1/2 cup (60 g) vanilla whey protein powder
2 1/2 teaspoons baking powder
1 tablespoon (1.5 g) Splenda
1 teaspoon salt
1/2 cup (120 ml) heavy cream

Preheat oven to 375°F (190°C). Spray an 8" x 8" (20 x 20 cm) baking pan with nonstick cooking spray.

Spread your No-Sugar-Added Cherry Pie Filling in the prepared pan, and dot with 2 tablespoons of the butter.

In a mixing bowl, combine the almond meal, vanilla whey, baking powder, Splenda, and the salt. Stir together to evenly distribute ingredients.

Melt the remaining 6 tablespoons of butter. Measure the cream, and stir the butter into it. Pour into the dry ingredients, and mix with a few swift strokes of your whisk or a spoon—you just want to stir enough to ensure that there are no pockets of dry ingredients lurking.

Spread the batter evenly over the cherries, and bake for 30 minutes or until the crust is crisp and evenly golden brown. Serve warm.

Yield: 9 servings

Each with: 254 calories; 17 g fat; 14 g protein; 12 g carbohydrate; 1 g dietary fiber; 11 g usable carbs.

◎ Mock Apple Brown Betty

Here's a dessert made from Anne Logston's Mock Fried Apples (page 179)! This one will require that you get your hands on some Expert Foods Cake-ability, for which I know no good substitute. It's readily available from lots of low-carb e-tailers.

> 2 batches Mock Fried Apples (page 179)
> 1 cup (125 g) ground macadamia nuts
> 1/2 cup (60 g) wheat protein isolate or other protein powder
> 1/2 cup (55 g) Expert Foods Cake-ability
> 1 teaspoon salt
> 1 teaspoon cinnamon
> 1/2 cup (12 g) Splenda
> 1 stick (112 g) butter, chilled

Place Mock Fried Apples in ovenproof casserole dish. Preheat oven to 400°F (200°C).

Combine nut meal, protein powder, Cake-ability, salt, cinnamon, and sweetener in a bowl. Cut in butter thoroughly until mixture resembles coarse meal. Sprinkle this streusel evenly over Mock Apples.

Bake at 400°F (200°C) for 40 minutes. Serve hot.

Yield: 6 servings

Each with: 594 calories; 47 g fat; 30 g protein; 19 g carbohydrate; 11 g dietary fiber; 8 g usable carbs.

◎ Strawberries with Balsamic Vinegar

Light and flavorful! These are good without the cream cheese sauce, too.

>   2 pounds (1 kg) strawberries
>   1/4 cup (6 g) Splenda
>   1/4 cup (60 ml) balsamic vinegar
>   4 ounces (115 g) cream cheese, softened
>   4 tablespoons (60 g) plain yogurt
>   2 more teaspoons Splenda

Remove the green hulls from your strawberries, and halve them—if you have some really huge berries, quarter them. Place in a glass, plastic, or stainless steel mixing bowl. Sprinkle the 1/4 cup (6 g) Splenda over the berries, and toss to coat. Now sprinkle on the balsamic vinegar, and stir again. Stash the bowl in the fridge for at least a few hours, and a whole day would be fine.

Using an electric mixer, beat the cream cheese, yogurt or sour cream, and 2 teaspoons Splenda together until very smooth—you can do this in advance, too, if you'd like.

Simply spoon the berries into pretty dessert dishes, and drizzle some of the balsamic vinegar syrup in the bottom of the bowl over each serving. Top each serving with a dollop of the cream cheese sauce, and serve.

Yield: 8 servings

Each with: 89 calories; 6 g fat; 2 g protein; 9 g carbohydrate; 3 g dietary fiber; 6 g usable carbs.

◎ Strawberries with Orange Cream Dip

This will look fancy if you serve it on a pretty chip-and-dip tray. Good finger food for a party. You can drop the calorie count on this without increasing the carb count by using light (but not fat-free!) sour cream.

1 package (4-serving size) sugar-free instant vanilla pudding

1 cup (230 g) sour cream

1 1/2 cups (360 ml) heavy cream

2 teaspoons grated orange zest

2 pounds (1 kg) strawberries

Using your electric mixer, beat the pudding mix, sour cream, heavy cream, and orange zest together until smooth and fluffy. Put in the bowl of a chip-and-dip tray, surround with whole strawberries, and serve.

Yield: 10 servings

Each with: 362 calories; 34 g fat; 11 g protein; 15 g carbohydrate; 4 g dietary fiber; 11 g usable carbs.

◎ Tom Budlong's Crema di Mascherpone

This is an utterly elegant Italian-style dessert.

1 pound (455 g) cream cheese, softened

4 egg yolks

1/2 cup (12 g) Splenda, or to taste

2 or 3 tablespoons (30–45 ml) brandy, rum, or kirsch

Put cream cheese through a sieve and stir until smooth. In another bowl, beat egg yolks together with the Splenda, then add liqueur. Add this mixture gradually to the cream cheese until it is a thick cream. Chill for two to three hours. Great served alone or garnished with fresh berries.

Yield: 8 servings

Each will have: 241 calories; 22 g fat (87.3% calories from fat); 6 g protein; 2 g carbohydrate; 0 g dietary fiber; 2 g usable carbs. Analysis does not include any berries you might serve with it.

⊚ Lemon Mousse Cup

This is pretty darned simple, but delicious, with a sunny lemon flavor.

> 1 package (4-serving size) sugar-free lemon gelatin
> 3/4 cup (180 ml) boiling water
> 3 ounces (85 g) Neufchatel cheese or light cream cheese, softened
> 1/2 cup (120 ml) cold water
> 1 teaspoon grated lemon rind
> 3/4 cup (180 ml) heavy cream
> 2 teaspoons sugar-free vanilla instant pudding mix
> 2 tablespoons (15 g) almond meal
> 1/2 teaspoon polyol

Put the gelatin and the boiling water in your blender, and run the thing for a minute or so to dissolve the gelatin. Put the Neufchatel cheese in, cut into chunks, and run the blender again until the mixture is smooth, about 1 more minute. Now add the cold water and your teaspoon of grated lemon rind, and run it one more time, to blend.

Pour the gelatin mixture from the blender jar into a mixing bowl, and stick it in the fridge. You're going to chill it till it's just starting to thicken a bit. While that's happening . . .

Use your electric mixer to whip the heavy cream with the vanilla pudding mix until you have a good, thick whipped topping. (Don't overbeat, or you'll get vanilla butter!)

When the gelatin is starting to thicken, fold 1/2 cup (40 g) of the whipped topping gently into it, until everything is well blended. Pour into four pretty dessert dishes. Put the dessert dishes and the leftover whipped topping in the fridge. Let your mousse chill for at least a couple of hours.

Sometime before dinner, stir the almond meal with the polyol sweetener in a skillet over medium heat until it just gets a hint of golden color. Remove from heat.

When dessert time rolls around, top each serving of mousse with a little of the leftover whipped topping and 1 1/2 teaspoons of the toasted almond meal, and serve.

Yield: 4 servings

Each with: 249 calories; 22 g fat; 7 g protein; 4 g carbohydrate; trace dietary fiber; 4 g usable carbs.

◉ Eliot Sohmer'sChocolate Mousse

1 square unsweetened baking chocolate

1–2 cups (240 or 480 ml) whipping cream

1 teaspoon vanilla

4 packets sweetener (more or less according to taste)

Melt chocolate in microwave, stirring frequently. Meanwhile, whip the cream, vanilla, and sweetener with an electric mixer until soft peaks form. Add a little cream to chocolate to thin. Fold chocolate mixture into whipping cream.

Note: Use less whipping cream if you want a darker, more intense mousse with smaller servings, and more if you want a lighter mousse that's more like chocolate whipped cream.

Yield: Makes approximately 4 servings

Each with: 449 calories; 47 g fat; 2 g protein; 8 g carbohydrate; trace dietary fiber; 8 g usable carbs.

◉ Anne Logston's Raspberry Mousse

Here's an easy raspberry-cheese-cakey-mousse. This is low-carb enough for induction, and our tester gave it a 10! Feel free to vary the flavors of gelatin and of syrup.

1 cup (240 ml) Da Vinci Sugar-free raspberry syrup or other sugar-free coffee-flavoring syrup

1 package (4-serving size) sugar-free raspberry-flavored gelatin

2 cups (480 ml) heavy whipping cream

8 ounces (225 g) cream cheese, softened

In a saucepan, bring the syrup to a boil. Dissolve gelatin completely in boiling syrup; set aside while it's dissolving. Stir until every particle is dissolved.

In a good-sized bowl, whip cream until stable peaks form. Briefly mix in cream cheese. With mixer running, stir in gelatin mix. Pour into container and chill thoroughly.

Yield: 8 servings

Each with: 308 calories; 32 g fat; 4 g protein; 2 g carbohydrate; 0 g dietary fiber; 2 g usable carbs.

Sylvia Palmer's Pumpkin Mousse

2 ¼ teaspoons unflavored gelatin (1 envelope)

2 teaspoons cold water

1 ¾ cups (420 g) pumpkin puree (fresh or canned)

½ cup (12 g) Splenda

1 tablespoon (2 packets) stevia/FOS blend (find this in health food stores)

¼ teaspoon salt

½ teaspoon cinnamon

¼ teaspoon ground cloves

¼ teaspoon nutmeg

1 tablespoon (15 ml) spiced rum

1 tablespoon (15 ml) sugar-free vanilla coffee-flavoring syrup

1 ⅔ cups (400 ml) heavy cream

In a small bowl, sprinkle the gelatin over the cold water, stir, and let soften until opaque, about 3 minutes. In a saucepan over medium heat, combine about ½ cup of the pumpkin puree, Splenda, stevia/FOS, and salt, and heat, stirring, until the Splenda dissolves. Stir in the softened gelatin and let cool to room temperature.

In a bowl, stir the pumpkin mixture into the remaining pumpkin puree. Whisk in the cinnamon, cloves, nutmeg, and rum.

In another bowl, combine the vanilla syrup and the cream, and use your electric mixer to whip the mixture to soft peaks. Using a whip or large spatula, gently fold the whipped cream into the pumpkin to make a mousse.

Yield: 4 to 5 servings

Assuming 5, each will have: 319 calories; 30 g fat; 3 g protein; 11 g carbohydrate; 3 g dietary fiber; 8 g usable carbs.

◉ Eileene's Pumpkin Treat

Our tester, Julie, a real pumpkin lover, called it "decadent" and says, "It takes mere minutes to prepare and is sinfully delicious!"

    1 4-serving-size package instant vanilla pudding and pie filling mix,
        sugar- and fat-free
    1 12-ounce (355 ml) can 2% evaporated milk
    1 16-ounce (455 g) can pumpkin puree
    1 teaspoon pumpkin pie spice

Beat together pudding and milk. Refrigerate 5 minutes. Mix in pumpkin and spice. Refrigerate 10 minutes.

Yield: Makes 6 servings

Each with: 116 calories; 5 g fat; 5 g protein; 15 g carbohydrate; 2 g dietary fiber; 13 g usable carbs.

An Incredible Array of Cheesecakes

I was feeling a bit neglectful because I'd come up with only one cheesecake recipe for this book (the first one in this section). Then I started looking over the recipes that had come in from readers, and realized I was not going to have a shortage of cheesecake recipes!

Why so many cheesecake recipes? There are two really good reasons. First of all, because people like cheesecake. Indeed, it's one of those desserts that's a real passion with many people.

And second, because cheesecake is one of the easiest desserts to decarb. Why? Because very little of the texture comes from sugar—it's all from the protein and fat. So replacing the sugar with Splenda or other sweeteners yields a cheesecake that is virtually indistinguishable from the sugary kind.

So pick out a cheesecake recipe, and get to it!

◎ Chocolate Chocolate Chip Cheesecake

This cake happened because I found a bottle of white chocolate sugar-free coffee flavoring syrup on sale at TJ Maxx. My brain immediately cried, "Cheesecake!" Feel free to use cream cheese and full-fat sour cream, if you prefer—you'll raise the calorie count, but not the carb count.

> Crisp Chocolate Crust (page 524, but see instructions below)
> 24 ounces (680 g) Neufchatel cheese
> ¾ cup (180 ml) white chocolate sugar-free coffee-flavoring syrup
>   (Da Vinci makes this)
> 3 eggs
> ½ cup (115 g) light sour cream
> 5 ounces (140 g) sugar-free dark chocolate

Preheat oven to 325°F (170°C).

Make the Crisp Chocolate Crust first, only this time make it in a 9" (22.5 cm) springform pan. You won't be able to build it all the way up the sides, but be sure you cover the seam around the bottom of the pan, and press the crust mixture firmly in place. Prebake crust for 5 minutes. Remove from oven, and let it cool a bit while you make the filling.

In a big mixing bowl, use your electric mixer to beat the Neufchatel cheese and white chocolate syrup together until very smooth and creamy—scrape down the sides of the bowl often during this process.

Now beat in the eggs, one at a time, then the light sour cream. Turn off the mixer for the next step.

With a knife, or using the S-blade in your food processor, chop the sugar-free dark chocolate into little chunks, about the size of mini-chips. Add to the cheese mixture, and beat in. Pour the filling into the prepared crust.

Put a pan of water on the floor of the oven. Now place the cake on the rack above it, and bake for 50 to 60 minutes. Cool, then chill, before slicing.

Yield: 12 servings

Each with: 331 calories; 29 g fat; 13 g protein; 7 g carbohydrate; 3 g dietary fiber; 4 g usable carbs.

⊚ Eliot Sohmer's Most Wonderful Cheesecake

Our tester, Julie, called this cheesecake "Simply freaking fantastic"—and says she's made it seven times since she initially tested it!

2 pounds (1 kg) cream cheese

2 cups (50 g) Splenda

5 eggs

3 tablespoons (45 ml) heavy cream

Preheat oven to 375°F (190°C).

Mix everything together thoroughly with electric mixer. Fill a buttered 9" (22.5 cm) springform pan.

Bake cheesecake for 10 minutes. Reduce heat to 250°F (130°C) and bake an additional hour.

At the end of the hour, remove the cake and run a knife around the edge of the pan.

Return the cheesecake to the warm oven and let it sit until the oven cools (approximately another hour).

Chill in fridge overnight and enjoy!

Add ons:
- Top with Sergeant Brenda's Famous Sour Cream Topping: Simply sweeten sour cream to taste with Splenda, and spread over the top of the cake.
- Buy sugar-free coffee-flavoring syrups in your favorite flavors at any fancy coffee shop. Pour a little on your plate and dip the cheesecake in the syrup. Delicious.

Yield: 10 slices

Each with: 365 calories; 36 g fat; 10 g protein; 3 g carbohydrate; 0 g dietary fiber; 3 g usable carbs.

The Most Wonderful Pumpkin Cheesecake

As I've mentioned elsewhere, a good recipe deserves a varition! Here's Brenda's Pumpkin Cheesecake. Also known as "How to Impress the Family at Thanksgiving Dinner."

> 2 pounds (1 kg) cream cheese
> 2 cups (50 g) Splenda
> 5 eggs
> 3 tablespoons (45 ml) heavy cream
> 1 cup (240 g) pumpkin (not pumpkin pie filling, just canned pumpkin)
> 1 teaspoon cinnamon
> 1 teaspoon ground ginger
> ½ teaspoon nutmeg

Preheat oven to 375°F (190°C).

Mix everything together thoroughly with electric mixer. Fill a buttered 9" (22.5 cm) springform pan.

Bake cheesecake for 10 minutes. Reduce heat to 250°F (130°C) and bake an additional hour.

At the end of the hour remove the cake and run a knife around the edge of the pan.

Return the cheesecake to the warm oven and let it sit until the oven cools (approximately another hour).

Chill in fridge overnight and enjoy!

Yield: 10 slices

Each with: 375 calories; 36 g fat; 10 g protein; 5 g carbohydrate; 1 g dietary fiber; 4 g usable carbs.

Susan Case DeMari's Awesome Cheesecake

Here's another cheesecake. Our tester, Doris Courtney, said she would gladly pay for this in a restaurant. She also suggests sprinkling some chopped walnuts on top before baking.

Walnut Crust:
½ cup (75 g) walnuts

Cheesecake Filling:
3 8-ounce (225 g) packages cream cheese at room temperature
1 cup (25 g) Splenda
4 large eggs
1 ½ teaspoons vanilla extract
½ cup (60 ml) whipping cream

Preheat oven to 350°F (180°C). Grind the walnuts in your food processor, using the S-blade, and press into place in a greased 9" (22.5 cm) springform pan. Bake for 5 minutes, and cool completely before filling.

Beat the cream cheese and Splenda on medium speed for 4 minutes. Add the eggs and vanilla and beat well on high speed for 5 more minutes, making sure to scrape sides of bowl. On medium speed, add the cream and beat 3 more minutes.

Pour the batter into the pan and place the springform pan into a larger pan. Pour hot water into the larger pan until it reaches halfway up the sides of the springform pan. Bake for 45 minutes at 350°F (180°C). Then turn the oven off, leaving the oven door slightly opened for 1 hour. Remove from oven, cover, and refrigerate for several hours or overnight.

Optional sour cream topping:
1 cup (230 g) sour cream
1 tablespoon (1.5 g) Splenda
½ teaspoon vanilla extract

When the 45 minute cooking time is up, remove the cheesecake from the oven and let it cool for 5 minutes. In the meanwhile, blend together the sour cream, Splenda, and vanilla extract. Spread over the cake. Return cake to the oven, and bake for another 5 minutes before turning off the oven, cracking the oven door, and letting the cake cool for an hour. Then cover and refrigerate, of course!

Note: Susan says she serves the sour cream topping concoction cold and on the side, instead, and also serves Steel's brand Splenda-sweetened blueberry pie filling as an alternative topping.

Yield: Serves 10

Each with: 286 calories; 28 g fat (86.4% calories from fat); 7 g protein; 2 g carbohydrate; 0 g dietary fiber; 2 g usable carbs.

◎ Jill Taylor's No-Cook Cheesecake

Enjoy this plain, or dress it up with some berries or even sugar-free chocolate sauce.

1/2 stick (60 g) butter
1 cup (125 g) finely chopped pecans
4–6 packets artificial sweetener
  or 3–4 tablespoons (4.5–6 g) granular Splenda
16 ounces (455 g) cream cheese
1 cup (230 g) sour cream
1 teaspoon vanilla extract
2 tablespoons (20 g) sugar-free instant vanilla pudding
1/4 cup (60 ml) water

Melt butter over medium heat and gently brown the chopped pecans. Stir in sweetener to taste and press into the bottom of a lightly greased 9" (22.5 cm) springform pan. Chill in the freezer for 10 minutes.

Warm the cream cheese in the microwave for 1 minute to soften. Add artificial sweetener to taste and beat with an electric mixer until light and creamy. Mix in the sour cream and the vanilla extract.

In a separate container, mix the vanilla pudding with the water to make a loose paste. You have to work quickly as it will stiffen up fast. Immediately add it to the cheese mixture and beat it in for a few seconds until smooth. Pour the mixture over the pecan base and chill for at least an hour.

Yield: Makes 10 servings

Each with: 324 calories; 33 g fat; 5 g protein; 5 g carbohydrate; 1 g dietary fiber; 4 g usable carbs.

⦿ Linda Guiffre's
Marbled Cheesecake Muffins

For muffins:

5 eggs

1 cup (25 g) Splenda or equivalent sweetener of choice (Linda has been using 1/2 cup [12 g] granulated Splenda plus 12 Splenda packets)

1 8-ounce (225 g) package cream cheese, softened

16 ounces (455 g) ricotta

1/2 teaspoon vanilla

1 teaspoon almond extract

1 1/2 tablespoons cocoa powder

For topping:

1/2 cup (115 g) sour cream

1 tablespoon (1.5 g) Splenda

1/4 teaspoon vanilla

In a medium-sized bowl, with an electric mixer, briefly beat the eggs until blended. Add the rest of the muffin ingredients (except cocoa) to the bowl, and mix until completely blended.

Pour into muffin pan lined with cupcake liners until about a fifth of the batter remains in the bowl. Mix cocoa powder into the batter left in the bowl (there is no need to worry about or be exact with amount of batter left over in the bowl—this recipe is very forgiving). Slowly pour a dollop of the cocoa batter into the center of each cupcake compartment so that you have a two-toned design. Bake in a 350°F (180°C) oven for 30 to 35 minutes until the tops are puffy and slightly cracked, and a toothpick inserted in the center comes out relatively clean. Remove the cupcakes from the oven to cool for a couple of minutes, and while they're doing so, mix the topping ingredients together. Drop a rounded teaspoon of the topping onto the center of each cupcake (no need to flatten or shape) and return to the oven for another 5 minutes.

Cool and keep refrigerated. These freeze wonderfully well, so you can always have some on hand.

For an impressive dessert presentation I make this cheescake in a 7-inch springform pan, pouring the cocoa batter in a concentric design. I increase the topping to 3/4 cup (180 g) sour cream, 1 1/2 tablespoons (2.25 g) Splenda, and ⅓ teaspoon vanilla, and spread it over the cheescake. It's beautiful when sliced and gives the impression of being very labor intensive—only you will know differently.

Yield: Makes 12

Each with: 182 calories; 15 g fat; 8 g protein; 3 g carbohydrate; trace dietary fiber; 3 g usable carbs.

◉ AnaLisa K Moyers's Easy Pumpkin Cheesecake

Our tester, Barbo Gold, suggests taking the cheesecake out of the oven at the 30-minute mark, making a flower design of pecan halves on top, then putting it back to finish baking. Pretty! (Barbo also pronounced it "delicious!")

½ cup (75 g) almonds
½ cup (75 g) pecans
16 ounces (455 g) canned pumpkin (read label: Not pumpkin pie mix)
16 ounces (455 g) cream cheese, softened
⅓ cup (80 ml) half-and-half
¾ cup (18 g) Splenda
1 teaspoon vanilla
1 teaspoon pumpkin pie spice blend
2 teaspoon cinnamon
4 eggs, at room temperature

Preheat oven to 350°F (180°C).

Make nut meal with the almonds and the pecans. (AnaLisa puts them into 2 plastic bags and allows the kids to beat them with the bottom of any flat cooking pot [they love this].) Shake nut meal into a buttered 8" (20 cm) to 9" (22.5 cm) pie pan, then press down with the back of a large tablespoon.

Using an electric mixer or your blender, mix all the rest of the ingredients until smooth—this is easier if the cheese and eggs are at room temperature. Pour into prepared pie plate.

Yield: 10 slices

Each with: 214 calories; 19 g fat; 6 g protein; 6 g carbohydrate; 2 g dietary fiber; 4 g usable carbs.

Kimberly Lansdon's Chocolate Almond Cheesecake

Crust:

    1 cup (125 g) almond meal

    2 tablespoons (30 g) butter, melted

    1 tablespoon (1.5 g) Splenda

Filling:

    4 ounces (115 g) unsweetened baking chocolate

    16 ounces (455 g) cream cheese, softened

    1 cup (25 g) Splenda

    4 eggs

    1 teaspoon vanilla extract

    1/4 teaspoon almond extract

    1 1/2 cups (345 g) sour cream

Combine crust ingredients and press into the bottom of a greased 9" (22.5 cm) springform pan.

Melt chocolate in the top of a double boiler over hot water, or in the microwave on medium, then let cool.

Use your electric mixer to beat the cheese and Splenda until blended. Beat eggs and extracts and mix until smooth. Blend in chocolate and sour cream.

Pour into prepared pan. Bake in the middle of a preheated 300°F (150°C) oven for 35 minutes or until set. Turn off the oven, leave the door ajar, and let cool in the oven for 1 hour. Chill in refrigerator at least 3 hours or overnight.

When completely cooled, remove pan sides. Top with whipped cream sweetened with Splenda, and sprinkle with coarsely chopped almonds.

Yield: Makes 16 servings

Each with: 247 calories; 22 g fat; 8 g protein; 6 g carbohydrate; 1 g dietary fiber; 5 g usable carbs.

Mary Lou Theisen's Cheesecake Cupcakes

Cupcake:
   3 8-ounce (225 g) packages cream cheese, softened
   1 cup (25 g) Splenda
   3 jumbo eggs
   2 teaspoons vanilla extract

Topping:
   10 ounces (280 g) sour cream
   2 tablespoons (3 g) Splenda
   1/2 teaspoon vanilla extract

Put paper cupcake liners into cupcake pan—you'll need a dozen and a half.

Place cream cheese in a mixing bowl and start mixing on the medium setting of your electric mixer. Add one egg at a time, and beat in. Then beat in the Splenda and vanilla extract. Pour into paper cupcake liners to about 1/8" (3.125 mm) from the top. Bake in a 300°F (150°C) oven for 30 to 35 minutes. Remove from oven and let cool for 5 minutes.

For the topping, mix the Splenda and vanilla extract with the sour cream. Put a dollop—between a generous teaspoonful and a tablespoonful—on top of each cupcake and return to the oven for 5 minutes. Take cupcakes out, let cool. These can be frozen. (Can omit the topping above and just add a teaspoon of your favorite low-carb fruit spread. Mary Lou says her favorite is the Keto brand strawberry or raspberry—delicious!)

Yield: Assuming 12 cupcakes

Each will have: 268 calories; 26 g fat; 6 g protein; 3 g carbohydrate; 0 g dietary fiber; 3 g usable carbs.

Cherry Cheese Cupcakes

I know we've got some cherry cheesecake lovers out there! Ray Stevens came up with this recipe just for you. Well, okay, he really came up with it for a dinner party. But he sent it to me just for you.

> 8 ounces (225 g) cream cheese, softened
> 1/2 cup (12 g) Splenda
> 1/2 cup (115 g) sour cream
> 1/2 teaspoon vanilla
> 2 eggs
> 1 batch No-Sugar-Added Cherry Pie Filling (page 512)

Preheat oven to 350°F (180°C).

Using an electric mixer, beat everything but the cherry pie filling together until very smooth and well blended. Gently fold in the pie filling.

Spoon into a muffin tin you've lined with paper muffin cups. Fill them about to the top. (This does not expand much.)

Bake about 30 minutes, or till brown on top.

Yield: Makes about 12 cupcakes

Each with: 112 calories; 9 g fat; 3 g protein; 4 g carbohydrate; trace dietary fiber; 4 g usable carbs.

Connie Bishop's Sort-of Cheesecake

Here's a recipe for a cheesecake-flavored dessert that takes no baking.

> 1 cup (240 ml) heavy whipping cream, chilled
> 8 ounces (225 g) cream cheese, softened 1 teaspoon vanilla
> 1 4-serving package sugar-free gelatin, any flavor
>   (but lemon is Connie's favorite)

Whip the cream till it stands in soft peaks, then beat in the cream cheese, vanilla, and gelatin. You can spoon this into dessert dishes, or spread it in a nut crust.

Yield: 8 servings

Each of 8 servings will have: 213 calories; 21 g fat; 4 g protein; 2 g carbohydrate; 0 g dietary fiber.

Val's Cheesecake

Our tester, Diana Lee, says she'd make this for company—it'll serve a crowd!

Crust:

- 2 cups (250 g) ground nuts; almonds, pecans, or macadamias
- 2 egg whites
- 1/2 cup (12 g) Splenda

Mix together and press into a 10" x 10" (25 x 25 cm) parchment-lined pan. Wetting your hands helps a bit. Bake at 350°F (180°C) for 10 minutes. Remove from oven to cool, and turn oven down to 300°F (150°C).

Mix the batter while the crust is baking.

Batter:

- 7 8-ounce (225 g) packages cream cheese
- 4 eggs, plus the 2 egg yolks left from the crust
- 1/2 cup (120 ml) sugar-free vanilla coffee-flavoring syrup
- 1 cup (25 g) Splenda granular
- 1 tablespoon (15 ml) real vanilla
- 1/2 cup (115 c) sour cream

Using softened cream cheese, blend in a standing mixer at low speed, adding the eggs one at a time. On low speed, add the syrup, Splenda, vanilla, and sour cream. Don't beat the mixture on high or it will result in a cheesecake filled with air.

Pour batter into the crust you've prepared. Place the pan in a larger pan, and pour in water to a depth halfway up the cheesecake pan. Place the cake in its water bath in the oven, and bake for 2 hours and 15 minutes. Let set on the counter to cool, and then set in the fridge overnight. Cut with a wet knife.

Yield: 16 servings

Each with: 500 calories; 48 g fat; 13 g protein; 7 g carbohydrate; 2 g dietary fiber; 5 g usable carbs.

⊚ General Pam's Cheesecake

Pam is a general in the army of Protein Uber Alles, the tongue-in-cheek name for a group of online low-carb pals. She says she and her husband, Rod, finished this easy cheesecake off in two sittings!

> 2 8-ounce (225 g) packages cream cheese, softened
> 2 eggs (beat prior to adding to cheese)
> 3 1/2 teaspoons Equal
> 1 teaspoon vanilla (you can use any other flavored extract
> to vary the flavor of the cheesecake; lemon is a good choice)

Mix everything up. Grease an 8" x 8" (20 x 20 cm) pan (I used a glass pan) very well. Pour the cheese mixture into the pan and bake for 40 minutes at 350°F (180°C). Let cool.

Top with your favorite whipped cream and enjoy.

Yield: Assuming 10 servings

Each with: 181 calories; 17 g fat; 5 g protein; 4 g carbohydrate; 0 g dietary fiber; 4 g usable carbs.

Jennifer Krupp's Crustless Low-Carb Cheesecake

Here's a simple cheesecake that can be varied to your taste with toppings.

> 4 8-ounce (225 g) packages cream cheese, softened
> 2 cups (50 g) Splenda
> 1 teaspoon vanilla
> 6 large eggs, beaten
> 10 ounces (280 g) sour cream

Beat cream cheese with your electric mixer until very smooth. Add the Splenda and vanilla and beat well, then beat in the eggs and sour cream. Pour batter into a buttered 10"(25 cm) springform pan. Place pan in another pan of water about ½" (1.25 cm) deep and bake at 350°F (180°C) for 45 to 60 minutes or until top begins to turn a light toast color. The cake will not be set. Remove from oven and cool, then refrigerate for at least 2 hours before serving.

Good served with toppings: fresh fruit, low-carb sauce, or syrup of your choice.

Yield: With 10 servings

Each will have: 418 calories; 40 g fat; 11 g protein; 4 g carbohydrate; 0 g dietary fiber.

Sharon Frooshani's Cherry Cheesecake Dessert

2 pounds (1 kg) cream cheese, softened

3 tablespoons (4.5 g) Splenda

1 teaspoon vanilla

2 cups (160 g) whipped cream

1 can Lucky Leaf cherry low carb pie filling (Sharon buys it from Low Carb Connoisseur) or 1 batch No-Sugar-Added Cherry Pie Filling (page 512)

Mix together first 4 ingredients with a mixer. Pour into a glass dish. Top with cherry pie filling.

Yield: 12 servings

Each has: 348 calories; 34 g fat; 6 g protein; 6 g carbohydrate; trace dietary fiber; 1 g usable carbs.

Amy Pierce's Frozen Blueberries

Our tester said his didn't freeze too solid, but was yummy nonetheless.

1 cup (240 ml) heavy cream, chilled

1 cup (25 g) Splenda

2 teaspoons vanilla extract

1 1-pound (455 g) bag frozen unsweetened blueberries

Combine heavy cream, sugar substitute, and vanilla. Pour over frozen blueberries in a bowl big enough to stir the mix. Stir and watch the cream mixture "magically" adhere to the frozen blueberries! It's like ice cream!

Note: Amy says this also works well with frozen strawberries, just make sure the strawberries are cut into small pieces.

Yield: About 3 cups

With 6 servings, each will have: 223 calories; 22 g fat; 1 g protein; 5 g carbohydrate; 1 g dietary fiber; 4 g usable carbs.

Easy Low Carb Fudge

This recipe had a very special tester— my 7 year old friend Austin McIntosh.He gives this recipe a 10, and his mom, Julie, who helped, says it's quite easy to do, and really is doable for kids, especially since no heat is involved. She also says it's good without the nuts, too!

> 1 pound (455 g) cream cheese—softened
> 2 ounces bitter chocolate—melted
> 1/2 cup (12 g) Splenda
> 1 teaspoon vanilla extract
> 1/2 (63 g) cup chopped walnuts—or pecans

Beat the cream cheese until smooth, then beat in the chocolate, Splenda, and vanilla. Stir in the chopped nuts.

Line an 8"x8" pan with foil, and smooth the cream cheese mixture into it. Chill well, then cut in squares. Store in the fridge.

Yield: 64 1" squares

Each with: 36 calories; 4 g fat; 1 g protein; 1 g carbohydrate; trace dietary fiber; 1 gram carbohydrate.

Martha H. Harris's
Easy Almond Flour Lemon Pound Cake

Our tester, Ray, says this is great!

> Butter and oat flour for pan prep
> 2 cups (250 g) almond meal
> 1/2 teaspoon stevia-FOS blend
> 1 teaspoon baking powder
> Scant 1/2 teaspoon salt
> 1 cup (240 g) butter (2 sticks)
> 2/3 cup (16 g) Splenda
> 2 tablespoons lemon zest (about 2 medium lemons' worth)
> 1 teaspoon lemon juice
> 5 large eggs
> 1 teaspoon vanilla extract

Adjust oven rack to middle position and heat oven to 350°F (180°C). Grease 9" x 5" (22.5 x 13 cm) loaf pan with 1 tablespoon (15 g) softened butter; dust with 1 tablespoon oat flour, tapping out excess.

In medium bowl, whisk together almond meal, stevia-FOS blend, baking powder, and salt. (Our tester says you can just sift these things together just as easily in the sifting step below and save a dirty bowl.) Set aside. In a glass measuring cup or microwave-safe bowl, microwave butter, covered with plastic wrap, on high until melted, 1 to 2 minutes. Whisk melted butter thoroughly to reincorporate solids.

In food processor, process Splenda and zest until combined, about five 1-second pulses. Add lemon juice, eggs, and vanilla. Process about 5 seconds until combined.

With machine running, add melted butter through the feed tube in a steady stream. This should take about 20 seconds.

Transfer mixture to large bowl. Sift flour mixture over egg mixture in three steps, whisking gently after each addition until just combined.

Pour batter into prepared pan and bake 15 minutes. Reduce oven temperature to 325°F (170°C) and continue baking until done, about 35 minutes, rotating pan halfway through baking time. Cool in pan for 10 minutes, then turn onto wire rack.

Martha notes: "The key to the natural sweet taste is using both Splenda and SteviaPlus (stevia-FOS blend). Instead of the combination indicated, you can omit the SteviaPlus and increase the Splenda to 1 cup (25 g), but the taste will not be as true to sugar taste."

Note: You can also put this in a muffin tin to make snack cakes. Cooking time will be shorter. Also good to know this travels well in a cooler.

Yield: 12 servings

Each of 12 servings has: 292 calories; 27 g fat; 6 g protein; 6 g carbohydrate; 2 g dietary fiber; 4 g usable carbs.

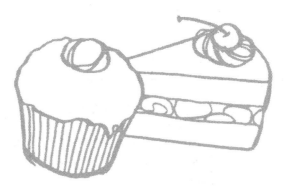

◎ Italian Walnut Cake

This traditional Italian cake is a clear demonstration that a few simple ingredients, properly combined, can yield extraordinary results. If it takes you a few days to eat up all of your Italian Walnut Cake, the Splenda on top will melt, leaving a glazed look instead of powdery whiteness, but it will still taste wonderful. This would be fabulous with a simple cup of espresso.

> 12 ounces (340 g) walnuts
> ½ cup (100 g) polyol sweetener, divided
> 4 eggs
> 1 pinch cream of tartar
> ¾ cup (18 g) Splenda
> 2 teaspoons lemon zest
> 1 pinch salt
> 2 tablespoons (30 g) extra Splenda for topping

Preheat oven to 350°F (180°C). Spray a 9" (22.5 cm) springform pan with nonstick cooking spray, and line the bottom with a circle of baking parchment, or a reusable Teflon pan liner.

Put the walnuts in your food processor with the S-blade in place. Pulse till nuts are chopped medium-fine. Add 2 tablespoons (25 g) of the polyol sweetener, and pulse until nuts are finely ground but not oily. (Don't overprocess. You don't want nut butter!)

Separate your eggs. Since even the tiniest speck of egg yolk will cause the whites to stubbornly refuse to whip, do yourself a big favor and separate each one into a small dish or cup before adding the white to the bowl you plan to whip them in! Then, if you break one yolk, you've only messed up that white. (Give that one to the dog, or save it for scrambled eggs for breakfast.) Put the whites in a deep, narrow mixing bowl, and put the yolks in a larger mixing bowl.

Add the pinch of cream of tartar to the whites, and using your electric mixer (not a blender or food processor!), whip egg whites until they stand in stiff peaks. Set aside.

In a larger bowl, beat the yolks with the rest of the polyol sweetener, and all of the Splenda, until the mixture is pale yellow and very creamy—at least 3 to 4 minutes. Beat in the lemon zest and the salt.

Stir the ground walnuts into the yolk mixture—you can use the electric mixer, but the mixture will be so thick, I think a spoon is easier. When that's well combined, gently fold in the egg whites, using a rubber scraper, a third at a time, incorporating each third well before adding the next. When all the egg whites are folded in, gently pour batter into the prepared pan.

Bake for 45 minutes. Sprinkle top with the 2 additional tablespoons Splenda while cake is hot, then let cool before serving. Cut in thin wedges to serve.

Yield: 12 servings

Each with: 194 calories; 18 g fat; 9 g protein; 4 g carbohydrate; 1 g dietary fiber; 3 g usable carbs. Carb count does not include polyol sweetener.

◉ Better Than S-X!

The Jell-O company invented this quite spectacular special-occasion dessert, which I had to alter in numerous ways to make it fit for low carbers. They're responsible for the name, too. Cryptic, isn't it? Better than the Sox? Better than playing the sax? Better than any other six desserts? Who knows? Since the nice folks at Jell-O came up with the original recipe (though the chocolate sauce was my idea!), it would be nice to use their sugar-free pudding to make this.

1 ½ cups (225 g) almonds
3 tablespoons (40 g) polyol
3 tablespoons (4.5 g) Splenda
1 stick (112 g) butter, melted
½ cup (75 g) pecan halves
8 ounces (225 g) cream cheese, softened
3 cups (720 ml) Carb Countdown Dairy Beverage, divided
2 4-serving-size packages sugar-free instant vanilla pudding mix
1 batch Angel-Type Coconut (page 518)
1 batch Maltitol-Splenda Chocolate Sauce (page 519) or Sugar-Free
    Chocolate Sauce (page 539)
1 ½ cups (360 ml) heavy cream, chilled
1 ½ tablespoons (15 g) sugar-free instant vanilla pudding mix

Preheat your oven to 350°F (180°C). Put your almonds in the food processor, with the S-blade in place, and run it until they're fairly finely ground. Add the polyol and Splenda, and pulse to combine.

 Now pour in the melted butter and the pecan halves, and pulse until the butter is melted in, and the pecans are chopped medium-fine.

Spray a 9" x 13" (22.5 x 32.5 cm) pan with nonstick cooking spray. Dump the almond mixture into it, and press it firmly and evenly into place. Bake for 12 to 15 minutes, or until golden. You'll want a little time for this to cool before you put the filling on top.

Beat the softened cream cheese until it's smooth. Beat in ½ cup (120 ml) of the Carb Countdown Dairy Beverage. Now add the 2 packages of pudding mix and the rest of the Carb Countdown. Beat for about 2 minutes, scraping down the sides of the bowl often. Now beat in 1 cup of your Angel-Type Coconut. Spread this mixture over your crust.

Spread your Maltitol-Splenda Chocolate Sauce over the pudding layer.

Whip the cream with the 1 ½ tablespoons of extra pudding mix, making whipped topping. Spread this over the chocolate layer.

Take the remaining coconut, and stir it in a dry skillet over medium heat until it acquires just a touch of gold. Sprinkle the toasted coconut evenly over the whipped topping. Chill for at least 2 hours before serving.

Yield: 12 servings

Each with: 515 calories; 49 g fat; 10 g protein; 14 g carbohydrate; 4 g dietary fiber; 10 g usable carbs.

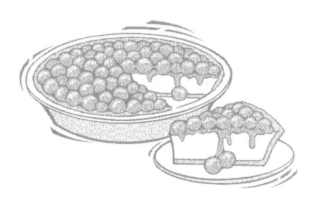

◉ Layered Chocolate-and-Vanilla Decadence

I adapted this recipe, and my sister, Kim, tested it for me one night when she was having company. She said that they threatened to eat the whole thing—and it makes a lot! A good choice if you want to take a dessert to a gathering.

Crust:
  1 ¼ cup (190 g) pecans
  1 cup (120 g) vanilla whey protein powder
  ½ cup (12 g) Splenda
  ½ cup (120 g) melted butter

Chop pecans in food processor, add other ingredients, pulse to blend thoroughly.

Pour into a 9" x 13" (22.5 x 32.5 cm) baking pan; press down to make firm so that it covers the bottom.

Bake at 350°F (180°C) for 15 minutes.

While the crust is cooling, make your **layers:**
  2 ½ cups (600 ml) heavy cream, chilled
  2 ½ tablespoons (25 g) sugar-free instant vanilla pudding mix
  8 ounces (225 g) cream cheese, softened
  ½ cup (12 g) Splenda
  2 tablespoons (30 ml) Carb Countdown Dairy Beverage
  1 package (6-serving size) sugar-free instant chocolate pudding mix
  2 ½ cups (600 ml) Carb Countdown Dairy Beverage

With your electric mixer, whip the heavy cream with the instant sugar-free vanilla pudding powder. Set aside.

In another bowl, beat the cream cheese, Splenda, and 2 tablespoons (30 ml) of Carb Countdown Dairy Beverage together until smooth. Fold in a little less than half of the whipped cream. Spread cream cheese mixture over the crust.

In the same bowl from which you've removed the cream cheese mixture, mix the package of chocolate sugar-free instant pudding mix with 2 ½ cups (600 ml) of Carb Countdown Dairy Beverage. Beat until smooth and creamy and beginning to thicken. Spread over the top of the cream cheese layer.

Put the 9" x 13" (22.5 x 32.5 cm) pan in the refrigerator to set. Store the leftover whipped cream in the refrigerator. In about 2 ½–3 hours, spread the remaining whipped cream over the top of the pudding as the top layer. Chill for at least another hour. Serve.

Yield: About 12 to 16 servings

Assuming 16 servings, each will have: 370 calories; 32 g fat; 15 g protein; 7 g carbohydrate; 1 g dietary fiber; 6 g usable carbs.

◉ Jenny's Silly Strawberry Surprise

This recipe made our tester feel like she was cheating!

- 1 4-serving-size package sugar-free Jell-O brand white chocolate pudding
- 2 cups (460 g) plain yogurt
- 6 packets of artificial sweetener (Splenda, Sweet'n Low, etc.), divided or 4 tablespoons (6 g) Splenda granular, divided
- 1/3 cup (80 ml) heavy cream
- 2 cups (340 g) quartered strawberries
- 1 cup (240 ml) water
- 1 batch Whipped Topping (page 540)

Combine pudding mix, yogurt, and 2 packets artificial sweetener or 4 teaspoons Splenda granular. Add the heavy cream. Mix together by hand. This mixture should have the consistency of thick pudding. (Add a little more cream if necessary.)

Place the strawberries in a separate microwave-safe dish with the water and 4 packets of artificial sweetener or 8 teaspoons (4 g) Splenda granular. Cover. Microwave on high for 2 1/2 minutes. Drain off the water. Chill the berries before serving.

Serve in individual bowls—strawberries on bottom, then pudding mixture, then add Whipped Topping.

Yield: Serves 6 to 8

Assuming 8, each serving has: 145 calories; 11 g fat; 3 g protein; 9 g carbohydrate; 1 g dietary fiber; 8 g usable carbs.

◉ No-Sugar-Added Cherry Pie Filling

Our tester, Ray Stevens, made this when he couldn't find the Lucky Leaf cherry low-carb pie filling. Very, very simple.

> 1 14.5-ounce (411 g) can sour cherries packed in water
> ½ cup (12 g) Splenda
> 2 teaspoons guar or xanthan
> Red food coloring (optional)

Open the can of cherries and dump the whole thing, water and all, into a bowl. Stir in the Splenda and thickener, plus 4 to 6 drops of red food coloring if you want a pretty color. Let stand 5 minutes before using.

Yield: 6 to 8 servings

Assuming 6, each will have: 28 calories; 0 g fat; 1 g protein; 6 g carbohydrate; 1 g dietary fiber; 5 g usable carbs.

◉ Laura Cottom's Strawberry Fluff

Laura and her sister invented this quick and easy dessert, and our tester, Stacy Sims, gave it a 10. Feel free to vary the flavor of gelatin.

> 8 ounces (225 g) cream cheese, softened
> 1 package (4-serving size) sugar-free strawberry gelatin
> 2–3 batches Whipped Topping (page 540)
> Chopped nuts

With a mixer, beat the cheese until creamy. (Easier to do if room temperature.) Beat in the gelatin powder. Fold in whipped topping and then the nuts. You can serve right away or chill, covered, for several days.

Variations: Add fresh chopped strawberries (or any berry!) in season. Unsweetened frozen berries are fine, too.

Yield: 8 servings (assuming 2 batches of the topping)

Each will have: 338 calories; 34 g fat; 5 g protein; 4 g carbohydrate; trace dietary fiber; 4 g usable carbs.

Bonnie Morrison's Finger Gelatin

A kid-friendly favorite! Try mixing flavors of gelatin to customize, but be careful you don't mix flavors with clashing colors—you could end up with muddy brown Finger Gelatin!

3 .3-ounce (8.5 g) packages sugar-free gelatin—pick your flavor(s)!
2 packets unflavored gelatin
4 cups (960 ml) boiling water

Dissolve both kinds of gelatin well and pour into a 9" x 13" (22.5 x 32.5 cm) pan you've sprayed with nonstick cooking spray. Refrigerate until gelled, and cut into squares.

Yield: Assuming 1" (2.5 cm) squares (117 squares)

Each will have: 1 calorie; 0 g fat; trace protein; 0 g carbohydrate; 0 g dietary fiber; 0 g usable carb. And it wiggles!

Marilyn Schroer's Finger Gelatin

Marilyn's recipe uses your favorite sugar-free soda to give really interesting flavor variations.

4 envelopes unsweetened, unflavored gelatin
2 cups (480 ml) sugar-free soda
2 1/2 cups (600 ml) water
2 .6-ounce (17 g) packages sugar-free gelatin, any flavor

Dissolve unflavored gelatin in cold sugar-free soda. Set aside.

Bring water to a boil in a saucepan and add sugar-free gelatin. Stir until dissolved. Add the gelatin-soda mixture to the pan with the hot gelatin mixture. Stir to combine. Pour into a 9" x 13" (22.5 x 32.5 cm) pan you've sprayed with nonstick cooking spray. Refrigerate until solid (about 2 hours). Cut into squares.

Marilyn's note: "I like to use Fresca. Diet Cherry 7UP is also good. Any of the Diet Rite sodas are excellent, as they will cut down on the amount of aspartame in the recipe!" [Our tester used Fresca and liked the results.]

Yield: Assuming 1" (2.5 cm) squares (117 squares)

Each will have: 1 calorie; 0 g fat; trace protein; 0 g carbohydrate; 0 g dietary fiber; 0 g usable carb. And it wiggles!

◎ German Chocolate Pie

My tester Julie claims that the true name of this recipe is, "OH SWEET MOTHER OF ALL THAT IS HOLY, THIS IS LIKE A SYMPHONY IN MY MOUTH!" and rates it a 15 on the 1–10 scale. She also says it looks "gorgeous!" Hope you like it just as much!

Crust:

1 cup (70g) Angel-type coconut (recipe page 518)
1 cup (125 g) finely chopped pecans
6 tablespoons (84 g) butter, melted
1/3 cup (40 g) vanilla whey protein powder
3 tablespoons (4.5 g) Splenda

Preheat oven to 325°F (170°C).

Combine everything well. Turn out into a 10" pie plate you've sprayed with non-stick cooking spray, and press firmly into place, building all the way up the sides. Bake for 12-15 minutes, or until it browns a little. Let cool before filling.

Filling:

4 ounces cream cheese, softened
1 package, 4-serving size, sugar-free chocolate instant pudding
1 package, 4 serving size, sugar-free vanilla instant pudding 2 3/4 cups
Carb Countdown Dairy Beverage 1/2 cup Angel-type coconut
(see recipe page xx)

Beat the cream cheese till smooth. Now beat in the two pudding mixes, and the Carb Countdown, then fold in the coconut. Spread this in the pie shell.

Topping:

1/2 cup (70 g) Angel-type Coconut
1/2 cup (63 g) chopped pecans
2 tablespoons (28 g) butter
1 teaspoon vanilla
3 tablespoons (4.5 g) Splenda

Garnish:

1/2 cup (120 ml) heavy cream, chilled

In a big skillet, over medium-low heat, saute the the coconut and pecans in the butter until the coconut is golden. Stir in the vanilla and the Splenda, and let the mixture cool. Now scatter it evenly over the pie.

Chill the pie for several hours.

Whip the cream, and use it to decorate the pie before serving.

Yield: 8-12 servings.

Each will have: (assuming 12) 341 calories; 31 g fat ; 10g protein; 10 g carbohydrate; 2 g dietary fiber; 8 grams usable carbs.

◎ Slow Cooker Maple Pumpkin Pudding

This is a great dessert for any of you pumpkin pie freaks out there!

15 ounces (455 g) canned pumpkin
1 cup (240 ml) Carb Countdown Dairy Beverage
3 eggs
¼ cup (60 ml) sugar free pancake syrup
½ cup (12 g) Splenda
1 tablespoon (7 g) pumpkin pie spice
½ teaspoon maple flavoring
½ cup (63 g) chopped pecans — toasted
Cinnamon

This is simple: Combine everything but the pecans in a mixing bowl, and whisk together well. Pour it into a 1 ½ quart Pyrex casserole or other heat-proof dish that fits into your slow cooker — spray the dish with non-stick cooking spray first. Now put the casserole in your slow cooker, and carefully pour water around it, to within 1" of the rim.

Cover, set the slow cooker to high, and let it cook for 4 hours. When the time's up, turn off the pot, uncover it, and let the whole thing cool till you can remove the casserole without scalding your fingers. You can chill this, or serve it warm. Either way, scatter those toasted pecans over each serving, and dust each with just a little cinnamon. You can also add whipped cream if you like, but it's not essential.

Yield: 6 servings,

Each with: 216 calories; 18 g fat; 7 g protein; 10 g carbohydrate; 3 g dietary fiber; 7 g usable carbs.

Coconut Cream Pie

My decarbed version of the old-time favorite!

1 1/2 cups (225 g) almonds
1/4 cup (30 g) vanilla whey protein powder
3 tablespoons (4.5 g) Splenda
4 tablespoons (55 g) butter, melted
1 1/3 cups (120 g) Angel-type Coconut (see recipe page 518)
2 2/3 cups (157 ml) Carb Countdown Dairy Beverage
1 1/2 packages vanilla sugar free instant pudding mix
1 cup (240 ml) heavy cream, chilled
1 tablespoon (10 g) vanilla sugar free instant pudding mix

Preheat your oven to 325°F (170°C).

In your food processor, using the S-blade, grind the almonds fine. Add the vanilla whey and Splenda, and pulse to combine. Now add the butter, and pulse till it's all well-mixed. Turn this out into a 9" pie plate you've sprayed with non-stick cooking spray. Press firmly into place, building up the sides. Bake for 12-15 minutes, or until starting to turn golden. Cool before filling.

Put 2/3 cup of the Angel-type Coconut in the pie shell, spreading evenly. Set aside.

Pour the Carb Countdown into a mixing bowl, and add the first pudding mix. Whisk until smooth, about 2 minutes. Pour over the coconut in the pie shell. Chill for at least 1 hour.

While the pie is chilling, stir the remaining coconut in a dry skillet over medium heat, unti it's touched with gold. Set aside to cool.

Using your electric mixer, whip the heavy cream with the 1 tablespoon of pudding mix until you have whipped topping (then turn off the mixer fast! You don't want vanilla butter!) Spread over the pie, and top with the toasted coconut before serving.

Yield: 10-12 servings.

Each will have: (assuming 12) 296 calories; 25 g fat; 11 g protein; 9 g carbohydrate; 3 g dietary fiber; 6 grams usable carbs.

◉ Easy Key Lime Pie

Julie calls this "Yummy, light, and summery." She also says it couldn't be easier to make!

> 1 ½ cups (225 g) almonds
> ¼ cup (30 g) vanilla whey protein powder
> ⅓ cup (8 g) Splenda
> 1 teaspoon ground ginger
> 4 tablespoons (55 g) butter, melted
> 2 packages sugar-free lime gelatin
> 2 cups (470 ml) boiling water
> 2 limes, grated zest and juice
> 1 pint no sugar added vanilla ice cream (I use Breyer's Carb Smart) 1 cup
>   heavy cream, chilled 1 tablespoon vanilla sugar free instant pudding mix

Preheat your oven to 325°F (170°C).

In your food processor, with the S-blade in place, grind the almonds fine. Add the vanilla whey protein, the Splenda, and the ground ginger, and pulse to mix. Now add the butter, and pulse until everything's blended. Turn the mixture out into a 9" pie plate you've sprayed with non-stick cooking spray. Press firmly into place, building up the sides, and bake for 12 minutes, or until golden. Cool before filling.

In a big mixing bowl, dissolve the gelatin in the boiling water. Add the grated lime zest and the juice. Now stir in the ice cream, until the ice cream is melted, and the mixture is smooth. Chill until the mixture is thickened, but not set.

Spoon the lime mixture into the prepared crust. Chill until firm. In the meanwhile, whip the cream with the pudding mix until you have whipped topping—but don't overbeat, or you'll get butter! Serve the pie with the whipped topping.

Yield: 8 servings,

Each with: 365 calories; 31 g fat; 14 g protein; 9g carbohydrate; 3 g dietary fiber; 6 grams usable carbs.

Angel-Type Coconut

You'll need this to make the extraordinary dessert we call Better Than S-X (page 508)! You could use it over fresh fruit, for that matter, or anywhere you think a little coconut might be nice.

> 3 tablespoons (40 g) polyol sweetener
> 1/3 cup (80 ml) boiling water
> 2 cups (140 g) shredded coconut meat

In a medium-sized mixing bowl, dissolve polyol sweetener in water. Stir in coconut, making sure coconut is evenly damp. Cover bowl, and let sit for 10 to 15 minutes.

Yield: 2 cups (180 g), or 16 servings of 2 tablespoons each

Each with: 35 calories; 3 g fat; trace protein; 2 g carbohydrate; 1 g dietary fiber; 1 g usable carb. Carb count does not include polyol sweetener.

Dipping Chocolate

> 12 ounces (340 g) sugar-free dark chocolate
> 2 tablespoons (40 g) sugar-free imitation honey or 2 tablespoons (25 g)
>   granular polyol
> 2 tablespoons (30 ml) heavy cream
> 1/4 cup (60 ml) plus 1 tablespoon (15 ml) water

In a double boiler, over hot, not boiling, water, melt the chocolate. Stir in the sugar-free imitation honey, the cream, and the water. Keep hot over water while dipping cookies, fruit, or what have you.

Yield: It's hard to know how many things you're going to dip! But assuming you make 36 Chocolate Dip cookies, or dip three dozen strawberries, the dip will add to each of them:

3 calories; trace fat; trace protein; trace carbohydrate; trace dietary fiber; no usable carb. Carb count does not include polyols in the sugar-free chocolate.

◉ Maltitol-Splenda Chocolate Sauce

I actually think that chocolate sauce made with only maltitol is a little better than this, but this version is less likely to cause, er, social offensiveness. Anyway, maltitol makes Splenda look cheap! Do use maltitol, not any of the other polyols, in this recipe. When I tried isomalt and erythritol in chocolate sauce, they turned grainy on me as they cooled. Maltitol makes a sauce with an excellent texture.

> ½ cup (120 ml) water
> 2 ounces (55 g) bitter chocolate
> ¼ cup (50 g) maltitol
> ¼ cup (6 g) Splenda
> 3 tablespoons (45 g) butter
> ¼ teaspoon vanilla
> Guar or xanthan

Put the water and the chocolate in a 4-cup glass measuring cup (I tried a 2-cup jobbie, and my sauce cooked over), and microwave on high for 45 to 60 seconds. Stir, and microwave for another 30 seconds, or until chocolate is melted.

Stir in the maltitol, and microwave on high for 1 minute. Stir, and microwave on high for 1 more minute. Stir in the Splenda, butter, and vanilla—keep stirring till the butter is melted. If you find your chocolate sauce a trifle thin, or find that a little of the butter refuses to be incorporated into the sauce, use just a tiny bit of guar or xanthan to thicken further. Serve right away, or store in a closed container in the fridge.

Yield: 1 cup (240 ml), or 8 servings of 2 tablespoons (30 ml)

Each: 76 calories; 8 g fat; 1 g protein; 2 g carbohydrate; 1 g dietary fiber; 1 g usable carb. Carb count does not include maltitol.

◉ Cyndy Riser's Spiced Tea

This is a low-carb version of an old favorite.

> 1 package sugar-free Tang (makes 6-quarts [5.7 L])
> 2/3 cup (80 g) instant tea mix2 packages sugar-free lemonade
>   (each makes 2 quarts [1.9 L])
> 1 tablespoon (7 g) ground cloves
> 1 tablespoon (7 g) ground cinnamon
> 2 cups (50 g) Splenda

Mix all ingredients. Store in airtight container. Add 1 heaping teaspoon
to 1 cup (240 ml) hot water.

Note: Spices can be adjusted to taste. Cindy likes a little more cinnamon and
cloves than indicated. However, my family likes it just the way it is.

Yield: 40 servings

Each with: 2 calories; trace fat; trace protein; 1 g carbohydrate; trace dietary
fiber; 1 g usable carb.

◉ Laure's Homemade LC "Bailey's Mae"

This is named in honor of Laure's chocolate lab! Barbo Gold, our tester, had, er,
a good time testing this recipe, and says it's tops.

> 2 cups (480 ml) any booze
>   (rum, vodka, bourbon, Southern Comfort, or brandy)
> 14 ounces (415 ml) heavy cream
> 1 cup (240 ml) half-and-half
> 2 tablespoons (15 ml) no-sugar chocolate syrup (Laur uses Walden
>   Farms brand)
> 2 teaspoons instant coffee crystals
> 1 teaspoon vanilla
> 1/2 cup (12 g) Splenda
> 1/2 teaspoon almond extract

Combine all in blender. Put in a tall jar. Store in fridge. Stir before serving. YUM!

Yield: 10 servings, 1/2 cup each

Each with: 274 calories; 17 g fat; 2 g protein; 2 g carbs; no fiber; 2 g usable carbs.

Dana Massey's
Low-Carb Irish Cream Liqueur

Our tester, Barbo Gold, loved this. (Come to think of it, how come Barbo gets all the really fun recipes?)

1 ¼ cups (300 ml) heavy whipping cream
3 egg yolks
¼ cup (6 g) Splenda
¼ cup (60 g) erythritol (can be replaced with another ¼ cup (6 g) Splenda)
1 tablespoon DiabetiSweet

Whisk all ingredients together in the order given in a saucepan over low heat. Stir constantly until thickened and be careful not to overcook. Cool completely and set aside.

3 eggs (or equivalent egg substitute, if you prefer not to use raw egg)
2 tablespoons (30 ml) sugar-free chocolate syrup (like Hershey's syrup; Walden Farms makes one and so does Sorbee)
2 tablespoons (30 ml) vanilla extract
1 tablespoon (15 g) instant coffee powder (not granular)
⅓ cup (80 ml) water
1 ⅓ cups (320 ml) Irish Whiskey

In a blender, blend eggs, chocolate syrup, vanilla, coffee powder, and water until well mixed. Stir in whipping cream mixture and whiskey (don't blend). Pour into container with a tight-fitting lid. Refrigerate up to 3 weeks. Enjoy!

Dana's note: Feel free to use a combined 5 tablespoons of any polyol sweetener in place of the erythritol and DiabetiSweet.

Yield: About 20 1 ½-ounce (40 ml) "shots"

Each with: 112 calories; 7 g fat; 2 g protein; 1 g carbohydrate; 0 g dietary fiber; 1 g usable carb. Carb count does not include the polyol in the syrup.

◎ Sugar-Free Eggnog

This festive libation by Sylvia Palmer is for those of you who are not afraid of raw eggs. Take care to use fresh, uncracked eggs that have been properly refrigerated!

> 1 cup (240 ml) heavy cream, chilled
> 6 eggs, separated
> 1/2 cup (12 g) Splenda
> 2 cups (480 ml) whole milk or Carb Countdown Dairy Beverage
> 3/4–1 cup (180–240 ml) good brandy (Sylvia likes Korbel)
> Nutmeg to garnish

First whip your cream, using an electric mixer. Beat till stiff, but don't overbeat—you don't want butter! You'll end up with 2 cups of whipped cream.

Be careful separating your eggs—if you get even a tiny speck of yolk in the whites, they'll refuse to whip. So separate each egg into a little custard cup before adding the white to the bowl you plan to whip them in. Put the yolks in another bowl.

Make sure you've washed the beaters of your electric mixer! Whip the egg whites until soft peaks form. Now fold the whipped egg whites into the whipped cream. Beat the egg yolks until light in color and add the Splenda. Carefully blend in the milk. Add the brandy. Fold the egg yolk mixture into the whipped egg whites/cream until blended. Serve with a sprinkle of nutmeg as desired.

Yield: Makes 20 small servings, according to our tester

Each with: 103 calories; 7 g fat; 3 g protein; 2 g carbohydrate; 0 g dietary fiber; 2 g usable carbs.

Dana Massey's Low-Carb Strawberry Daiquiris

Okay, this recipe isn't really a dessert. But it is a sweet indulgence, so have fun!

> 3–4 cups (330–440 g) fresh or frozen unsweetened strawberries, thawed if using frozen
>
> ½–¾ cup (120–180 ml) light rum
>
> ¼ cup (60 ml) lime juice (don't use Rose's bottled lime juice—it has sugar added)
>
> ¼–⅓ cup (6-8 g) Splenda (you may use a different sugar substitute, adjust measurements accordingly)
>
> Crushed ice

Place strawberries, rum, lime juice, and sugar substitute in a blender. Blend until smooth. Add ice; continue to blend until well combined.

To make Low-Carb Strawberry Margaritas, replace rum with tequila.

Dana Massey's note: "We use erythritol in this recipe."

Dana Carpender's note: I'd probably use Splenda, myself.

Yield: 4 to 6 servings

Assuming 4, each will have: 138 calories; trace fat; 1 g protein; 11 g carbohydrate; 3 g dietary fiber; 8 g usable carbs.

◎ Crisp Chocolate Crust

1 ½ cups (225 g) almonds
¼ cup (6 g) Splenda
2 squares bitter chocolate, melted
3 tablespoons (45 g) butter, melted
2 tablespoons (15 g) vanilla whey protein powder

Preheat oven to 325°F (170°C).

Using the S-blade of your food processor, grind the almonds until they're the texture of corn meal. Add the Splenda and pulse to combine. Pour in the melted chocolate, then the melted butter, and run processor till evenly distributed—you may need to stop the processor and run the tip of a knife blade around the outer edge to get everything to combine properly. Then add the vanilla whey protein, and pulse again to combine.

Turn out into a 10" (25 cm) pie plate you've coated with nonstick cooking spray. Press firmly and evenly into place. Bake for 8 minutes. Cool before filling.

Yield: 10 servings

Each with: 197 calories; 18 g fat; 7 g protein; 6 g carbohydrate; 3 g dietary fiber; 3 g usable carbs.

◎ Ice Cream!

These two ice cream recipes come from Diana Lee's book *Low Carb Ice Cream: Drinks, Desserts,* and are used with her permission. Diana was also one of our last-minute recipe testers for this book. We couldn't have done it without her! If you don't have her three books (the other two are *Baking Low Carb* and *Bread and Breakfast: Baking Low Carb II*), go to Amazon.com and order them right now. Diana provides the following freezing and storage suggestions for low-carb ice cream:

When the machine quits processing, serve immediately or use one of the following suggestions for storing. Because homemade, sugar free ice cream freezes harder than store purchased, you may want to store it differently. My favorite is to spoon it into muffin cups, add sticks, and freeze. Set muffin tin in sink, in cold water, for a minute to loosen ice cream and then place in plastic bags. Freeze.

You can also freeze in single serving containers. Remove from freezer ten minutes before you are ready to eat. Or use one large container, but then you will have to allow for longer thawing before you can scoop it out. Thaw for at least 20 to 30 minutes in the refrigerator. If you forget to remove before serving, you can use the defrost cycle on your microwave for a couple minutes.

◎ Eggnog Ice Cream

1 package unflavored, unsweetened gelatin
1 cup (240 ml) hot water
1 teaspoon vanilla extract
3/4–1 teaspoon brandy extract (optional)
1 1/2 cups (360 ml) heavy cream
1/3 cup (8 g) Splenda
1/4 teaspoon nutmeg
1/4 teaspoon cinnamon
1/2 teaspoon liquid sweetener (Sweet'n Low)
1/4 cup (30 g) egg white protein

Sprinkle gelatin over hot water and let it set for a minute. Stir until gelatin is dissolved. With a mixer, blender, or food processor, combine extracts, cream, Splenda, nutmeg, cinnamon, Sweet'n Low, egg protein, and gelatin water. Mix well and chill for at least 1/2 hour. Stir and pour into your ice cream maker, following manufacturer's directions for making ice cream. Makes 1 quart (.95 L).

Yield: 4 servings

Each with: 344 calories; 33 g fat; 9 g protein; 3 g carbohydrate; trace dietary fiber; 3 g usable carbs.

Peanut Butter Dough Ice Cream

1 package unflavored, unsweetened gelatin

1 cup (240 ml) hot water

2 teaspoons peanut butter extract

1 teaspoon vanilla extract

1 1/2 cups (360 ml) heavy cream

1/2 cup (12 g) Splenda

1/2 teaspoon liquid sweetener (Sweet'n Low)

1/4 cup (30 g) egg white protein

1/4 cup (60 g) natural peanut butter

Sprinkle gelatin over hot water and let it set for a minute. Stir until gelatin is dissolved. With a mixer, blender, or food processor, combine extracts, cream, Splenda, Sweet'n Low, egg protein, gelatin water, and peanut butter. Mix well and chill for at least 1/2 hour. Stir and pour into your ice cream maker, following manufacturer's directions for making ice cream. Makes 1 quart (.95 L).

Yield: 4 servings

Each with: 435 calories; 40 g fat; 13 g protein; 6 g carbohydrate; 1 g dietary fiber; 5 g usable carb.

chapter fifteen

The BONUS CHAPTER!

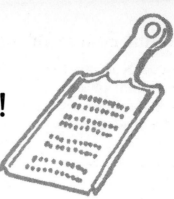

Why is this the bonus chapter? Because you get these recipes *in addition* to the 500 you paid for!

These are recipes I'm repeating from previous books, because I think you need them. Some of them, like the ketchup recipe, are for things that are called for in other recipes in the book. Others I just think of as something you ought to have. So here they are!

We'll start with the single most-repeated recipe I've come up with—so far, it's in every cookbook I've written. Low-carb ketchup is starting to appear; I know Heinz is test-marketing one. But it's hardly universally available yet—as I know, because I can't get it here in Bloomington. However, if you can get commercial low-carb ketchup, feel free to use it in place of this in any recipe that calls for it.

Dana's No-Sugar Ketchup

Store-bought ketchup has more sugar in it per ounce than ice cream does! This great-tasting ketchup has all the flavor of your favorite brand, without the high carb count. The guar or xanthan isn't essential, but it makes your ketchup a little thicker and helps keep the water from separating out if you don't use it up quickly.

1 6-ounce (170 g) can tomato paste

2/3 cup (160 ml) cider vinegar

1/3 cup (80 ml) water

1/3 cup (8 g) Splenda

2 tablespoons (20 g) finely minced onion

2 cloves garlic, crushed

1 teaspoon salt or Vege-Sal

1/8 teaspoon ground allspice

1/8 teaspoon ground cloves

1/8 teaspoon pepper

1/4 teaspoon guar or xanthan

Assemble everything in a blender, and run the blender—you'll have to scrape down the sides; this mixture is thick—until the bits of onion disappear. Store in a tightly lidded container in the refrigerator.

Yield: Makes 1 1/2 cups (360 g) of ketchup, or 24 1-tablespoon (15 g) servings

Each with: 2.25 g carb per tablespoon, with a trace of fiber and protein.

⦾ Reduced-Carb Spicy Barbecue Sauce

Ketchup is bad enough, but barbecue sauce has even more sugar!
Make your own.

1 small onion, minced fine

1 clove garlic, crushed

¼ cup (60 g) butter or oil

4 tablespoons (6 g) Splenda

1 teaspoon salt or Vege-Sal

1 teaspoon dry mustard

1 teaspoon paprika

1 teaspoon chili powder

½ teaspoon black pepper

2 teaspoons blackstrap molasses

1 ½ cups (360 ml) water

¼ cup (60 ml) cider vinegar

1 tablespoon (15 ml) Worcestershire sauce

1 tablespoon (15 g) prepared horseradish

1 6-ounce (170 g) can tomato paste

1 tablespoon (15 ml) liquid smoke
   (Most big grocery stores carry this. A company called Colgin makes it.)

In a saucepan, cook the onion and garlic in the butter or oil for a few minutes.
Stir in all the dry ingredients, then stir in everything else but the tomato paste
and the liquid smoke. Let it simmer for about 15 to 20 minutes. Then whisk in
the tomato paste and smoke flavoring, and let it simmer another 5 to 10 minutes.
Store in a jar in the refrigerator.

Yield: This makes about 2 ⅔ cups (640 g) of sauce, or about 21 1-ounce
(2 tablespoon; 30 g) servings

Each serving has: 3 g carbohydrate, 1 g of which is fiber, for a usable
carb count of 2 g.

Kansas City Barbecue Sauce

This is it—what most of us think of when we think of barbecue sauce: tomato-y, spicy, and sweet. Unbelievably close to a top-flight commercial barbecue sauce—and my Kansas City–raised husband agrees. If you like a smoky note in your barbecue sauce, add 1 teaspoon of liquid smoke flavoring to this.

2 tablespoons (30 g) butter

1 clove garlic

¼ cup (40 g) chopped onion

1 tablespoon (15 ml) lemon juice

1 cup (240 g) Dana's No-Sugar Ketchup (page 528)

⅓ cup (8 g) Splenda

1 tablespoon (15 ml) blackstrap molasses

2 tablespoons (30 ml) Worcestershire sauce

1 tablespoon (7 g) chili powder

1 tablespoon (15 ml) white vinegar

1 teaspoon pepper

¼ teaspoon salt

Just combine everything in a saucepan over low heat. Heat until the butter melts, stir the whole thing up, and let it simmer for five minutes or so. That's it!

Yield: Roughly 1 ¾ cups (420 g), or 14 servings of 2 tablespoons (30 g) each

Each serving will have: 7 g carbohydrate, with 1 g fiber, for a usable carb count of 6 g; 1 g protein.

Hoisin Sauce

This Chinese sauce is usually made from fermented soy bean paste, but fermented soy bean paste has bunches of sugar in it. Peanut butter is inauthentic, but it tastes quite good here.

4 tablespoons (60 ml) soy sauce
2 tablespoons (30 g) creamy natural peanut butter
2 tablespoons (3 g) Splenda
2 teaspoons white vinegar
1 clove garlic, crushed
2 teaspoons toasted sesame oil
$1/8$ teaspoon Chinese five-spice powder

Just assemble everything in your blender, and run it until smooth and everything is well combined. Store in a snap-top container.

Yield: Makes roughly $1/3$ cup (80 ml)

Each tablespoon will contain: 2 g carbohydrate, a trace fiber, and 2 g protein.

Teriyaki Sauce

Good on chicken, beef, fish—just about anything!

$1/2$ cup (120 ml) soy sauce
$1/4$ cup (60 ml) dry sherry
1 clove garlic, crushed
2 tablespoons (3 g) Splenda
1 tablespoon (10 g) grated fresh gingerroot

Simply combine all ingredients.

Yield: Makes just over $3/4$ cup (180 ml)

About 3 g carbohydrate per tablespoonful.

Hollandaise for Sissies

An easy sauce for asparagus, artichokes, broccoli, whatever you like.

    4 egg yolks
    1 cup (230 g) sour cream
    1 tablespoon (15 ml) lemon juice
    1/2 teaspoon salt or Vege-Sal
    Dash Tabasco or other hot sauce

You'll need either a double boiler or a heat diffuser for this—it needs very gentle heat. If you're using a double boiler, you want the water in the bottom hot, but not boiling. If you're using a heat diffuser, use the lowest possible heat under the diffuser.

Put all your ingredients in a heavy-bottomed saucepan or in the top of a double boiler. Whisk everything together well. Let it heat through, and serve it over vegetables or whatever you like.

Yield: 6 to 8 servings

Each with: 2 g carbohydrate, a trace fiber, and 3 g protein in each.

Raspberry Vinegar

Commercial raspberry vinegar has as much as 4 g of carbohydrate per tablespoon!

    1/2 cup (120 ml) white vinegar
    1/4 teaspoon raspberry cake flavoring
        —this is a highly concentrated oil in a teeny little bottle
    3 tablespoons (4.5 g) Splenda

Just combine these ingredients, and pour it into any handy small bottle with a lid.

Yield: Makes about 1/2 cup (120 ml)

The whole batch has 11.5 g carbohydrate, for 1.5 g carbohydrate per tablespoon. No fiber, no protein.

◉ Cauliflower Puree, aka Fauxtatoes

This is a wonderful substitute for mashed potatoes if you want something to put a fabulous sour cream gravy on! Feel free, by the way, to use frozen cauliflower instead; it works quite well here.

> 1 head cauliflower or 1 ½ pounds (680 g) frozen cauliflower
> 4 tablespoons (60 g) butter
> Salt and pepper

Steam or microwave the cauliflower until it's soft. Drain it thoroughly, and put it through the blender or food processor until it's well pureed. Add butter, salt, and pepper to taste.

Yield: At least 6 servings—and they're generous servings

Each will have: 72 calories; 8 g fat; trace protein; 1 g carbohydrate; trace dietary fiber; 1 g usable carb.

◉ Adele Hite's Fauxtatoes Deluxe

> 1 large head cauliflower
> About ⅓ cup (80 ml) cream
> 4 ounces (115 g) cream cheese
> 1 tablespoon (15 g) butter
> Salt and pepper to taste

Simmer cauliflower in water with about ⅓ cup (80 ml) cream added to it (this keeps the cauliflower sweet and prevents it from turning an unappetizing gray color) until very soft. Drain thoroughly. Throw in food processor with rest of ingredients while still warm (you may have to do this in more than one batch). Process until smooth.

Options: Add a few cloves of sliced garlic to the cooking water, or add some roasted garlic to the food processor when blending the cauliflower with the other ingredients. Add 1 gram of carbohydrate to the carb count for the total batch for each clove of garlic added.

Yield: At least 6 servings

If you serve 6, each serving will have: 6 g carbohydrate, of which 2 are fiber, for a usable carbohydrate count of 4 g; 4 g protein.

⦿ Cauliflower Rice

With thanks to Fran McCullough! I got this idea from her book *Living Low Carb,* and it's served me very well indeed.

>   1/2 head cauliflower

Simply put the cauliflower through your food processor, using the shredding blade. This gives a texture that is remarkably similar to rice. You can steam this or microwave it or even sauté it in butter. Whatever you do, though, don't overcook it!

Yield: This is about 3 cups (500 g), or at least 3 to 4 servings

Assuming 3 servings, each will have: 5 g carbohydrate, 2 g of which will be fiber, for a usable carb count of 3 g; 2 g protein.

⦿ Cauliflower Rice Deluxe

This is higher carb than plain cauliflower rice, but the wild rice adds a grain flavor that makes it quite convincing, and wild rice has about 25 percent less carbohydrate than most other kinds of rice do. I use this only for special occasions, but it's wonderful.

>   3 cups (500 g) cauliflower rice—about 1/2 head's worth
>   1/4 cup (50 g) wild rice
>   3/4 cup (180 ml) water

Cook your cauliflower rice as you please—I microwave mine for making this— taking care not to overcook it to mushiness; you want it just tender. Put the wild rice and water in a saucepan, cover it, and set it on a burner on lowest heat until all the water is gone—at least half an hour, maybe a bit more. Toss together the cooked cauliflower rice and wild rice, and season as you please.

Yield: 8 servings

Even with the wild rice, this has only 6 g carb, with 1 g fiber, for 5 g usable carb per 1/2 cup (85 g) serving.

◉ Taco Seasoning

Many store-bought seasoning blends include sugar or cornstarch—my food counter book says that several popular brands have 5 grams of carb in 2 teaspoons! This is very easy to put together, and it tastes great. It's even cheaper than the premixed stuff.

> 2 tablespoons (14 g) chili powder
> 1 1/2 tablespoons (10 g) cumin
> 1 1/2 tablespoons (10 g) paprika
> 1 tablespoon onion (9 g) powder
> 1 tablespoon (9 g) garlic powder
> 1/8 teaspoon cayenne pepper (mild)
>   or 1/4 teaspoon cayenne (a bit hotter)

Simply combine all ingredients, blending well, and store in an airtight container. Use 2 tablespoons of this mixture to a pound of ground beef, ground turkey, or chicken.

Yield: This makes about 8 tablespoons (70 g), or 4 batches worth

Using 2 tablespoons of this seasoning will add just under 2 g carbohydrate to a 4-ounce (115 g) serving of taco meat.

Cajun Seasoning

This New Orleans–style seasoning is good sprinkled over chicken, steak, pork, fish—just about anything.

2 ½ tablespoons (17 g) paprika

2 tablespoons (32 g) salt

2 tablespoons (18 g) garlic powder

1 tablespoon (7 g) black pepper

1 tablespoon (9 g) onion powder

1 tablespoon (7 g) cayenne pepper

1 tablespoon (3 g) dried oregano

1 tablespoon (2.5 g) dried thyme

Combine all ingredients thoroughly, and keep in an airtight container.

Yield: Makes ⅔ (100 g) cup

This has 37 g carbohydrate in the entire batch, of which 9 g are fiber, for a usable carb count of 28 g in the batch. Considering how spicy this is, you're unlikely to use more than a teaspoon or two at a time. One teaspoon has 1 g carbohydrate, with a trace fiber.

◉ Jerk Seasoning

Sprinkle this over chicken, pork chops, or fish before cooking for an instant hit of flavor! Hot, sweet, and spicy.

- 1 tablespoon (3 g) onion flakes
- 2 teaspoons ground thyme
- 1 teaspoon ground allspice
- 1/4 teaspoon ground cinnamon
- 1 teaspoon black pepper
- 1 teaspoon cayenne pepper
- 1 tablespoon (9 g) onion powder
- 2 teaspoons salt
- 1/4 teaspoon ground nutmeg
- 2 tablespoons (3 g) Splenda

Combine all ingredients, and store in an airtight container.

Yield: Makes about 1/3 cup (50 g)

If you use 1 teaspoon, it will have 1 g carbohydrate, with a trace fiber.

◎ Classic Barbecue Rub

As the name suggests, this is the rub that cries "classic barbecue"! A great combo with the Kansas City Barbecue Sauce, but use it with any sauce—and on any meat!

¼ cup (6 g) Splenda
1 tablespoon (18 g) seasoned salt
1 tablespoon (9 g) garlic powder
1 tablespoon (18 g) celery salt
1 tablespoon (9 g) onion powder
2 tablespoons (14 g) paprika
1 tablespoon (7 g) chili powder
2 teaspoons pepper
1 teaspoon (7 g) lemon pepper
1 teaspoon sage
1 teaspoon mustard
½ teaspoon dried thyme
½ teaspoon cayenne

Combine everything, stir well, and store in a shaker. Sprinkle heavily over just about anything, but especially over pork ribs and chicken.

Yield: Makes just over ⅔ cup (100 g), or roughly 12 tablespoons

3 g carbohydrate, with 1 g fiber, for a usable carb count of 2 g; 1 g protein.

◉ Sugar-Free Chocolate Sauce

This is as good as any sugar-based chocolate sauce you've ever had, if I do say so myself. Which I do. Don't try to make this with Splenda, it won't work—the polyol sweetener somehow makes the water and the chocolate combine. It's chemistry, or magic, or some darned thing.

> 1/3 cup (80 ml) water
> 2 ounces (55 g) bitter baking chocolate
> 1/2 cup (100 g) maltitol
> 3 tablespoons (45 g) butter
> 1/4 teaspoon vanilla

Put the water and bitter chocolate in a glass measuring cup, and microwave on high for 1–1 1/2 minutes or until chocolate is melted. Stir in the maltitol and microwave on high for another 3 minutes, stirring halfway through. Stir in the butter and vanilla, and it's ready to serve (or make into a pie!).

Note: This worked beautifully with maltitol. However, when I tried to make it with erythritol, it started out fine but crystallized and turned grainy as it cooled— though it would still have been okay used hot over ice cream, it wouldn't have worked for the frozen pies in this chapter.

Yield: Makes roughly 1 cup (240 ml), or 8 servings of 2 tablespoons (30 g) each

2 g carbohydrate and 1 g fiber, not including the maltitol, for a usable carb count of 1 g; 1 g protein; 75 calories.

◎ Whipped Topping

This has a wonderful flavor and texture.

> 1 cup (240 ml) heavy cream, well chilled
> 1 tablespoon (10 g) vanilla sugar-free instant pudding powder

Simply whip them together until the cream is stiff. The pudding adds a very nice texture and helps the whipped cream "stand up." Also adds a slightly vanilla/sweet flavor to the cream, of course.

Note: This is incredible with berries, as a simple but elegant dessert. I like to serve strawberries and whipped cream in my nice chip-and-dip—looks so pretty! And makes the whole thing engagingly informal. This whipped topping is also great on any dessert, and terrific on Irish coffee!

Yield: This makes about 2 cups (240 g), or 16 2-tablespoon servings

Each with only a trace carbohydrate, no fiber, and a trace protein.

◎ Mockahlua

My sister, a longtime Kahlua fan, says this is addictive. And my husband demanded to know, "How did you do that?!" You can make this with decaf if caffeine bothers you.

> 2 1/2 cups (600 ml) water
> 3 cups (75 g) Splenda
> 3 tablespoons (25 g) instant coffee crystals
> 1 teaspoon vanilla
> 1 750 ml bottle 100-proof vodka (use the cheap stuff)

In a large pitcher or measuring cup combine water, Splenda, coffee crystals, and vanilla. Stir until coffee and Splenda are completely dissolved. Pour through funnel into a 1.5–2 liter bottle—a clean 1.5 liter wine bottle works fine, so long as you've saved the cork. Pour in the whole contents of the bottle of vodka. Cork, and shake well.

Yield: This makes 32 1 1/2-ounce (40 ml) servings—a standard shot

Each shot will have: 2 g carbohydrate, no fiber, and the merest trace protein.

appendix A

A Refresher
on Measurements

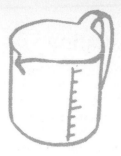

Just in case these details have slipped your mind since junior high school home economics class!

Please note that these do not apply to the metric system; all ingredient measurements in this book contain the metric equivalent inside parentheses.

3 teaspoons = 1 tablespoon

2 tablespoons = 1 fluid ounce

2 ounces = ¼ cup

4 ounces = ½ cup

8 ounces = 1 cup

2 cups = 1 pint

4 cups = 1 quart

2 pints = 1 quart

4 quarts = 1 gallon

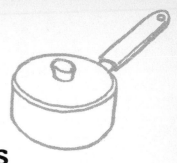

Where to Find a Few Less-Common Ingredients

Sugar-Free Imitation Honey

HoneyTree brand imitation honey is available from the HoneyTree Company:
    HoneyTree, Inc.
    8570 Monroe Rd., Onsted, MI 49265
    Phone: (517) 467-2482

At this writing, the minimum order is twelve bottles, but that will set you back only $22, not too bad, and it'll keep. Consider getting a group of low-carbing friends together to share an order!

At this writing, CarbSmart is also planning to carry HoneyTree Sugar Free Imitation Honey: http://www.carbsmart.com.

Steel's brand of imitation honey is available from:
    Synergy Diet: http://www.synergydiet.com
    Low Carb Outfitters: http://www.lowcarboutfitters.com

I've had readers report that they've found sugar-free imitation honey at Wal-Mart!

Polyols

DiabetiSweet (isomalt blended with the artificial sweetener acesulfame-K) is available through:
    http://www.puritans.com (This is also where I buy most of my vitamins.)
    http://www.diabeticproducts.com
    http://www.focuspharmacy.com
    http://www.diabetesstore.com

And, according to some of my contacts, DiabetiSweet is also available at some Wal-Mart stores! It's generally worth looking at any pharmacy in the diabetic-supplies section. This makes DiabetiSweet the easiest polyol sweetener to obtain.

Erythritol is available through:

    http://www.carbsmart.com

    http://www.lowcarbgrocery.com

    http://www.lowcarbnexus.com

(**Note:** Erythritol didn't work out for the chocolate sauce recipe in this book, so if that's what you want to make, go for maltitol instead.)

Maltitol is available through:

    http://www.carbsmart.com

    http://www.lowcarbnexus.com

Xylitol is available through:

    http://www.synergydiet.com

(**Note:** I have no personal experience cooking with xylitol.)

Wheat Protein Isolate

I know of two sources of wheat protein isolate:

    http://www.locarber.com

    http://www.carbsmart.com

I have done business with both, and had no trouble.

Index

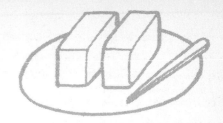

A

Adele Hite's Fauxtatoes Deluxe, 533
Adobe Seasoning, 448
Albondigas, 353
Alcoholic beverages. *See* Drinks
Almond meal/ground almonds, 22–23
Almonds
    Almond-Parmesan Crust, 132
    Better Than S-X!, 508–9
    Ginger-Almond Chicken Salad, 382
    Kimberly Lansdon's Chocolate
        Almond Cheesecake, 496
    Lorraine Achey's Dilled Almonds, 67
    Orange Swordfish Steaks with
        Almonds, 271
    Ruth Green's Cinnaamon Crackers, 122
    Ruth Green's Coconut Crackers, 123
    Sesame-Almond Napa Slaw, 200
    Smoked Almonds, 68
    Susan Higgs's Chicken Salad
        Surprise, 393
Amanda's Sugar Cookies, 463
Amy Dungan's Broccoli, Ham, and Cheese
    Soup, 437
Amy K. Crawford's Easy Chicken Cordon
    Bleu, 245
Amy Pierce's Frozen Blueberries, 502
AnaLisa K. Moyers's Easy Pumpkin
    Cheesecake, 495
Angel-Type Coconut, 518
Anne Logston's Cheesy Broccoli
    Casserole, 149
Anne Logston's Mock-Fried Apples, 179
Anne Logston's Raspberry Mousse, 486
Appetizers. *See* Snacks
Apples, Anne Logston's Mock-Fried, 179
Apricots
    Apricot-Chipotle Glaze, 439
    Spice-Rubbed Leg of Lamb with
        Apricot-Chipotle Glaze, 378
Artichokes
    Artichoke and Friends Frittata, 94
    Artichoke Chicken Salad, 380

Artichokes with Chipotle
    Mayonnaise, 175
Artichokes with Curried Mock
    Hollandaise, 174
Grace Brown's Spinach and
    Artichoke Casserole, 173
Shrimp and Artichoke "Risotto", 279
Asian dishes
    See also Curried dishes
    Asian Chicken Salad, 383
    Cathy Kayne's Chinese Beef Soup, 407
    Chicken Teriyaki Stir-Fry, 252
    Chinese Chicken Salad, 387
    Chinese Five-Spice Roasted Chicken,
        227
    Chinese Soup with Bok Choy and
        Mushrooms, 406–7
    Fiery Indian Lamb and Cauliflower, 370
    Five-Spice Lamb Steaks, 373
    Ginger Sesame Pork, 344
    Orange-Five-Spice Roasted Chicken,
        225
    Oriental Chicken, "Rice," and Walnut
        Salad Wrapped in Lettuce, 386
    Robin Loiselle's Teriyaki Chicken
        Wings, 243
    Thai Beef Lettuce Wraps, 322
    Thai Chicken Soup, 406
    Thai Turkey Burgers, 258
    Vietnamese Salad, 186
Asparagus
    Asparagus with Chipotle
        Mayonnaise, 190
    Asparagus with Curried Walnut
        Butter, 158–59
    Asparagus with Sun-Dried
        Tomatoes, 160
    Audra Olsen's Asparagus/Salami
        Roll-Ups, 76
    Barbo Gold's To-Die-For Asparagus
        Skillet, 161
    Grilled Asparagus with Balsamic
        Vinegar, 159
    Karen Sonderman's Roasted
        Asparagus, 162

    Springtime Scramble, 85
    Stir-Fried Scallops and Asparagus, 276
Audra Olsen's Asparagus/Salami Roll-Ups,
    76
Avocados, 36
    Avocado, Egg, and Blue Cheese
        Salad, 395
    Avocado-Walnut Salad, 189
    Cauliflower Avocado Salad, 192–93
    Guacamole Eggs, 48
    Mexican Avocado and Ham Omelet, 80
    Orange, Avocado, and Bacon Salad,
        189
    Pat Best's Guacamole, 64
    Ruth Lambert's Avocado Mousse, 180
    Shrimp and Avocado Salad, 401
    Sopa Tlalpeno, 405

B

Bacon
    Bacon Chili Burgers, 300
    Blue Bacon Burgers, 301
    Broccoli Sunshine Salad Low-Carb, 199
    Club Omelet, 79
    Eliot Sohmer's Bacon Cheese
        Frittata, 93
    Jody Leimbek's Low-Carb Wraps, 260
    Jody's Breakfast Wrap, 101
    Kristy Howell's Chicken Carbonara,
        251
    Orange, Avocado, and Bacon Salad,
        189
    Orange Bacon Dressing, 207
    Quiche Lorraine, 87
    Stephanie Hill's Creamy Cauliflower
        and Bacon Casserole, 147
Baked goods
    Buttermilk Drop Biscuits, 124
    Cranberry Nut Muffins, 107
    Dinner Rolls, 126
    Elizabeth Dean's Next Best Thing to
        Cornbread, 129
    Exceedingly Crisp Waffles, 111
    Gingerbread Waffles, 110

Graham Crackers, 118–19
Jeanette Wiese's Best Pancakes I've Ever Had, 114
Jill Taylor's Soy Pancakes, 113
John Smolinski's Low-Carb Dutch Baby, 117
Julie Sandell's Low-Carb Blueberry Pancakes, 112–13
Libby Sinback's Peach Sour Cream Muffins, 109
Maple Oat Bread, 127
Mary Lou Theisen's Best Low-Carb Waffle, 112
Oat Bran Pancakes, 115
Parmesan Garlic Crackers, 120
Poppy Seed Bread, 128
Pumpkin Muffins, 108
Ruth Green's Cinnamon Crackers, 122
Ruth Green's Coconut Crackers, 123
Sharyn Taylor's Granny's Spoon Bread, 130
Sunflower Wheat Crackers, 121
"Whole Wheat" Buttermilk Pancakes, 116
Zucchini Bread, 106
Baked Sole in Creamy Curry Sauce, 267
Balsamic-Mint Lamb Steak, 376
Barb Thompson's Meatballs Arrabiata, 314
Barbecued Pumpkin Seeds, 68
Barbo Gold's To-Die-For Asparagus Skillet, 161
Bean Sprout Scramble, Marilee Wellersdick's, 86
Beans
    See also Green beans
    black soy beans, 19–20
    Pat Best's Chili Con Carne, 329
    Pat Best's Hearty Black Soy Bean Soup, 422
    Pat Best's Hearty Black Soy Bean Soup, the Short-Cooking Version, 423
    Pat Best's Refried Black Soy Beans, 63
    Pat Best's Seven Layer Bean Dip, 66
    Sopa De Frijoles Negros, 421
Beef
    burgers
        Bacon Chili Burgers, 300
        Blue Bacon Burgers, 301
        Linda Magsasay's Chili Burgers, 302

Debbie White's Colorado Chipped Beef Appetizer, 61
    ground
        Albondigas, 353
        Cherie Johnson's Cheeseburger Soup, 414
        George Hollenbeck's Hamburger Stroganoff, 328
        Hamburger Curry, 309
        Holly Holder's Cheesy Chipotle Soup, 417
        Kathryn Luzardo's Stuffed Poblano Peppers, 306
        Kathy Monahon's Baked Penne, 330
        Kristy Howell's Zucchini Moussaka, 307–8
        Marcelle Flint's Zucchini Lasagna, 332
        Melisa McCurley's Good Stuff Casserole, 308
        Nanci Messersmith's Low-Carb Lasagna Recipe Using Zucchini for Noodles, 331
        Nancy O'Connor's Greek Shepherd's Pie, 325
        Nancy O'Connor's Low-Carb Moussaka, 326
        Pat Best's Chili Con Carne, 329
        Rita Eichman's Shepherd's Pie, 334
        Ropa Vieja, 319
        Ropa Vieja Chili, 320
        Ropa Vieja Hash, 321
        Salisbury Steak, 303
        Sesame Orange Beef, 318
        Sheryl McKenney's Stuffed Tomatoes, 305
        Southwestern Stuffed Peppers, 304
        Susan Higgs's Piquant Ground Beef, 327
        Tee's Taco Soup, 408
        Thai Beef Lettuce Wraps, 322
        Tracy Lohr's Quick Taco Salad, 397
    Inauthentic Machaca Eggs, 83
    Janette Kling's Bourbon Glazed Cajun Tenderloin, 341–42
    Kim's Boeuf Bourguignonne, 323–24
    meat loafs
        Chili-Glazed Meat Loaf, 310
        Famous Meat Loaf, 312–13

Homestyle Meat Loaf, 312
        Jen Holling's Cream Cheese Meat Loaf Surprise, 313
        Philippa's Meat Loaf, 311
    meatballs
        Barb Thompson's Meatballs Arrabiata, 314
        Cranberry Meatballs, 316
        Spicy Orange Meatballs, 315
        Swedish Meatballs, 317
    Portobello Fillets, 292
    roasts
        Dorothy Keefe's Marinated Chuck Roast, 338
        Nancy Machinton's Pot Roast, 336
        Pamela Merritt's Marinated Pot Roast, 337
        Patty Southard's Festiva Beef Italiano, 335
        Rho's Slow-Cooker Chuck Roast, 339
    Ropa Vieja Omelet, 82
    Sharon Palmer-Brownstein's Fantastic Brisket of Beef, 340
    soups
        Cathy Kayne's Chinese Beef Soup, 407
        Cathy Kayne's Spicy Garlic Ginger Beef Soup, 426
        Cherie Johnson's Cheeseburger Soup, 414
        Holly Holder's Cheesy Chipotle Soup, 417
        Tee's Taco Soup, 408
    steaks
        Cajun Steak Caesar Salad, 396
        Gwen Meehan's Delicious Peppers and Onions with Cheesy steak, 297
        Lori Herbel's Country Fried Steak, 296
        Marco Polo Steak, 293
        Orange Tequila Steak, 294
        Pepper Steak with Whiskey Sauce, 295
        Smoky Marinated Steak, 298
        Steak with Brandy-Stilton Cream Sauce, 299
        Susan Higgs's Imperial Beef, 333
Beer, 27
Betsy Calvin's Breakfast Casserole, 97
Better Than S-X!, 508–9
Beverages. See Drinks

Big Italian Restaurant Dressing, 208
Black and Bleu Chicken, 229
Black Forest Parfaits, 470
Black soy beans
    about, 19–20
    Pat Best's Chili Con Carne, 329
    Pat Best's Hearty Black Soy Bean
        Soup, 422
    Pat Best's Hearty Black Soy Bean
        Soup, the Short-Cooking
        Version, 423
    Pat Best's Refried Black Soy Beans, 63
    Sopa De Frijoles Negros, 421
Blackstrap molasses, 32
Bland oils, 20
Blue cheese
    Avocado, Egg, and Blue Cheese
        Salad, 395
    Black and Bleu Chicken, 229
    Blue Bacon Burgers, 301
    Broccoli Blue Cheese Soup, 409
    Gratin of Cauliflower and
        Turnips, 144
    Sally Waldron's Spicy Blue Cheese
        Dressing and Dip, 60
Blueberries
    Amy Pierce's Frozen Blueberries, 502
    Grandma's Blueberry Cobbler, 480
    Julie Sandell's Low-Carb Blueberry
        Pancakes, 112–13
Bok Choy and Mushrooms, Chinese Soup
    with, 406–7
Bonnie Morrison's Finger Gelatin, 513
Bouillon, 30
Brans, 22
Breads
    See also Baked goods
    Dinner Rolls, 126
    Elizabeth Dean's Next Best Thing to
        Cornbread, 129
    Leslie's Low-Carb Broccoli
        Cornbread, 151
    Maple Oat Bread, 127
    Poppy Seed Bread, 128
    Sharyn Taylor's Granny's Spoon
        Bread, 130
    Zucchini Bread, 106
Brie and Walnut Quesadillas, 58
Broccoli
    Amy Dungan's Broccoli, Ham, and
        Cheese Soup, 437
    Anne Logston's Cheesy Broccoli
        Casserole, 149

Broccoli Blue Cheese Soup, 409
Broccoli Dijon, 150
Broccoli Sunshine Salad Low-Carb, 199
Eleanor Monfett's Cheddar Broccoli
    Salad, 198, 402
Joan Wilson's Turkey on Spaghetti
    Squash, 255
Leslie's Broccoli and Cauliflower
    Casserole, 148
Leslie's Low-Carb Broccoli
    Cornbread, 151
Lisa Bousson's Fantastic Creamy
    Broccoli Soup, 424
Marco Polo Stir-Fried Vegetables, 158
Melissa Miller's Ham and Broccoli
    Cheese Soup, 414–15
Michele Holbrook's Broccoli Bake, 152
Poppy Seed Chicken, 236
Sharon Marlow's Broccoli Cashew
    Salad, 198–99
Susan Higgs's Broccoli and
    Cauliflower Salad, 197
Swiss Cheese and Broccoli Soup, 412
Broiled Orange Chili Lobster, 273
Broths/Broth concentrates, 27, 30
Brownies
    Brownie Mocha Fudge Pie, 472–73
    Dana's Brownies, 467
    Espresso Chocolate Chip Brownies,
        466
    Pam's Brownies, 469
    Sara Driver's Brownies, 468
Brussels sprouts
    Jennie's Bodacious Brussels Sprouts,
        177
    Orange Mustard Glazed Sprouts, 178
    Susan Higgs's Brussels Sprouts in
        Browned Butter, 176
Bubble and Squeak, 138
Burgers
    Bacon Chili Burgers, 300
    Blue Bacon Burgers, 301
    Linda Magsasay's Chili Burgers, 302
    Thai Turkey Burgers, 258
    Turkey Feta Burgers, 256
Butter, 20–21
Buttermilk
    about, 38–39
    Buttermilk Drop Biscuits, 124

C
Cabbage
    See also Coleslaw

Bubble and Squeak, 138
Chinese Chicken Salad, 387
Curried Swordfish and Cabbage, 272
Dragon's Teeth, 165
Lauren Zizza's Mustard Chicken
    Dish, 239
Linda Carroll-King's Red Cabbage
    Recipe, 167
Mexican Cabbage Soup, 434
Roasted Cabbage with Balsamic
    Vinegar, 166
Susan Higgs's Skillet Cabbage, 168
Cajun Nut Mix, 55
Cajun Seasoning, 536
Cajun Steak Caesar Salad, 396
Cake-ability, 22
Cakes
    See also Cheesecakes
    Italian Walnut Cake, 506–7
    Martha H. Harris's Easy Almond
        Flour Lemon Pound Cake,
        504–5
Cannery Row UnPotato Salad, 192
Carb Countdown Dairy Beverage, 27
Carb counts
    about, 10–12
    calculation of, 14
    usable, 12–13, 15
Caribbean Grilled Chicken Salad, 381
Carnitas, 344–45
Carol Tessman's Raspberry Pie, 478
Carol Tessman's Skillet Supper, 246
Carrots, 36
    Kristy Howell's Carrot and Cottage
        Cheese Salad, 206
    Sesame Orange Beef, 318
Cashews
    Cajun Nut Mix, 55
    Sharon Marlow's Broccoli Cashew
        Salad, 198–99
Catalina Dressing, 210
Cathy Kayne's Chinese Beef Soup, 407
Cathy Kayne's Spicy Garlic Ginger Beef
    Soup, 426
Cathy Sparks's Creamed Onions, 183
Cat's Chili, 258–58
Cauliflower
    Adele Hite's Fauxtatoes Deluxe, 533
    Bubble and Squeak, 138
    Cannery Row UnPotato Salad, 192
    Cauliflower Avocado Salad, 192–93
    Cauliflower Puree, aka Fauxtatoes, 533

Cauliflower Rice, 534
Cauliflower Rice Deluxe, 534
Cheesy Cauliflower, 143
Cheesy Cauliflower Soup, 410
Chicken Sancocho, 222–23
Chipotle-Cheese Fauxtatoes, 137
Ensalada de "Arroz", 193
Fiery Indian Lamb and Cauliflower, 370
Gratin of Cauliflower and Turnips, 144
Hellzapoppin Cheese "Rice", 139
Irene Haldeman's Czech Unpotato Salad, 194
Jansonn's Temptation, 145
Japanese Fried "Rice", 140
Leslie's Broccoli and Cauliflower Casserole, 148
Lonestar "Rice", 141
Melissa Wright's Two-Cheese Cauliflower, 146
Nancy O'Connor's Creamy Garlic-Chive Fauxtatoes, 137
Oriental Chicken, "Rice," and Walnut Salad Wrapped in Lettuce, 386
Pat Resler's Cauliflower and Cheese Salad, 195
Stephanie Hill's Creamy Cauliflower and Bacon Casserole, 147
Susan Higgs's Broccoli and Cauliflower Salad, 197
Susan Higgs's Cauliflower Mexican Salad, 196
Teresa Egger's Calcutta Chicken and "Rice" Salad, 394
Ultimate Fauxtatoes, The, 136
UnPotato and Sausage Soup, 420
Venetian "Rice", 142
Wendy Kaess's Cauliflower Salad, 197
Celery, Susan Higgs's Salmon Stuffed, 72
Celeste's Chicken with Creamy Mushroom Sauce, 247
Celia Volk's Portobello Mushroom Pizza, 366
Ceviche, 262–63
Cheese
    Amy Dungan's Broccoli, Ham, and Cheese Soup, 437
    Anne Logston's Cheesy Broccoli Casserole, 149
    Betsy Calvin's Breakfast Casserole, 97

Black and Bleu Chicken, 229
Brie and Walnut Quesadillas, 58
Broccoli Blue Cheese Soup, 409
Cheese "Danish", 99
Cheese-Pecan Nibbles, 54
Cheesy Cauliflower, 143
Cheesy Cauliflower Soup, 410
Cheesy Onion Soup, 411
Chicken Chili Cheese Salad, 384
Chipotle-Cheese Fauxtatoes, 137
Diane Lyon's Savory Cheese and Ham Torte, 95
Dorothy Markuske's Chicken Stuffed with Spinach and Goat Cheese, 248–49
Dorothy Markuske's Pork Chops in Cream Sauce Topped with Seasoned Goat Cheese, 356–57
Eleanor Monfett's Cheddar Broccoli Salad, 198, 402
Eliot Sohmer's Bacon Cheese Frittata, 93
Garlic Cheese Stuffed Mushrooms, 52
Gratin of Cauliflower and Turnips, 144
Gwen Meehan's Delicious Peppers and Onions with Cheesy Steak, 297
Ham and Cheese Salad, 398
Holly Holder's Cheesy Chipotle Soup, 417
Jill Taylor's Chili Relleno Casserole, 104
Jill Taylor's Fried Cheese Taco Shells, 70
Kristy Howell's Carrot and Cottage Cheese Salad, 206
Lynn Avery's Pimiento Cheese, 67
Lynn Avery's Provolone "Chips", 69
Lynn Davis's Cottage Cheese Spinach Chicken, 234
Margaret King's Cheese Crisps, 69
Melissa Wright's Two-Cheese Cauliflower, 146
Pat Best's Jalapeno Cheese Spread, 65
Pat Resler's Cauliflower and Cheese Salad, 195
Sally Miller's Awesome Pimento Cheese, 62
Sally Waldron's Spicy Blue Cheese Dressing and Dip, 60
Sheryl McKenney's Easy Cheese Soup, 413
Sonlight Mom's Cheesy Chicken, 250
Strawberry Cheese Pie, 471
Swiss Cheese and Broccoli Soup, 412
Swiss Puff, 103

Tracie Jansen's Cheesy Spinach Pie, 91
Turkey Feta Burgers, 256
Warm Brie with Sticky Nuts, 50
Cheesecakes
    AnaLisa K. Moyers's Easy Pumpkin Cheesecake, 495
    Cherry Cheese Cupcakes, 498
    Chocolate Chocolate Chip Cheesecake, 489
    Connie Bishop's Sort-of Cheesecake, 498
    Eliot Sohmer's Most Wonderful Cheesecake, 490
    General Pam's Cheesecake, 500
    Jennifer Krupp's Crustless Low-Carb Cheesecake, 501
    Jill Taylor's No-Cook Cheesecake, 493
    Kimberly Lansdon's Chocolate Almond Cheesecake, 496
    Linda Guiffre's Marbled Cheesecake Muffins, 494–95
    Mary Lou Theisen's Cheesecake Cupcakes, 497
    Most Wonderful Pumpkin Cheesecake, 491
    Sharon Frooshani's Cherry Cheesecake Dessert, 502
    Susan Case DeMarti's Awesome Cheesecake, 492–93
    Val's Cheesecake, 499
Cherie Johnson's Cheeseburger Soup, 414
Cherries
    Cherry Cheese Cupcakes, 498
    Grandma's Cherry Cobbler, 481
    No-Sugar-Added Cherry Pie Filling, 512
    Sharon Frooshani's Cherry Cheesecake Dessert, 502
Chewy Oatmeal Cookies, 454–55
Chicken
    Amy K. Crawford's Easy Chicken Cordon Bleu, 245
    Black and Bleu Chicken, 229
    Carol Tessman's Skillet Supper, 246
    Celeste's Chicken with Creamy Mushroom Sauce, 247
    Chicken Kampama, 218
    Chicken "Risotto" alla Milanese, 233
    Chicken Sancocho, 222–23
    Chicken Teriyaki Stir-Fry, 252
    Chunky Chicken Pie, 228–29
    Curried Chicken Dip, 60
    Curried Chicken "Pilau", 230

Debbie Murawski's BBQ Chicken Breast, 250–51

Donna Nisleit's Garlic Parmesan Chicken Breasts, 238

Dorothy Markuske's Chicken Stuffed with Spinach and Goat Cheese, 248–49

Easy Italian Skillet Chicken, 231

Greek Chicken with Yogurt, 219

Gwen Meehan's Yummy Chicken Casserole, 240

Italian Chicken with White Wine, Peppers, and Anchovy, 221

Jody Leimbek's Low-Carb Wraps, 260

Kristy Howell's Chicken Carbonara, 251

Lauren Zizza's Mustard Chicken, 239

Laurence Erhili's Tagine of Chicken and Olives, 224–25

Lemon Mustard Herb Chicken, 232

Lynn Davis's Cottage Cheese Spinach Chicken, 234

Melissa Cathey's Jalepeno Lime Chicken, 244

Patti Shreiner's Chicken Continental, 249

Pollo en Jugo de Naranja (Mexican Chicken in Orange Juice), 220

Poppy Seed Chicken, 236

roasted
    Chinese Five-Spice Roasted Chicken, 227
    Citrus Chicken, 226–27
    Orange-Five-Spice Roasted Chicken, 225

salads
    Artichoke Chicken Salad, 380
    Asian Chicken Salad, 383
    Avocado, Egg, and Blue Cheese Salad, 395
    Caribbean Grilled Chicken Salad, 381
    Chicken Chili Cheese Salad, 384
    Chinese Chicken Salad, 387
    Cobb Salad, 389
    Ginger-Almond Chicken Salad, 382
    Jerk Chicken Salad, 385
    Mexican Chicken Salad, 391
    Oriental Chicken, "Rice," and Walnut Salad Wrapped in Lettuce, 386
    Pat Best's Deviled Chicken Salad, 392
    Susan Higgs's Chicken Salad Surprise, 393

Teresa Egger's Calcutta Chicken and "Rice" Salad, 394

Tex-Mex Chicken Salad, 388

Thai Cobb Salad, 390

Sally Waldron's Buffalo Chicken and Slaw, 242

Sonlight Mom's Cheesy Chicken, 250

Sophia Loren Chicken, 241

soups
    Chicken and Andouille Gumbo, 418–19
    Chunky Cream of Chicken and Portobello Soup, 430
    Karen Sonderman's Cream of Chicken Mushroom Soup, 431
    Linda Blackburn's Cream of Chicken Soup, 432
    Sopa Tlalpeno, 405
    Thai Chicken Soup, 406

Tee's Cajun Chicken and Spinach, 235

Tee's Crockpot Jambalaya, 416–17

Terrie Shortsleeve's Lemon-Garlic Chicken, 237

wings
    Chili Lime Wings, 42
    Chinese Sticky Wings, 43
    Lemon-Mustard Chicken Wings, 44–45
    Lemon Soy Chicken Wings, 44
    Robin Loiselle's Teriyaki Chicken Wings, 243
    Winnie Spicer's Chicken in Raspberry Cream Sauce, 238–39

Chili/Chilies
    Bacon Chili Burgers, 300
    Cat's Chili, 258–59
    Chicken Chili Cheese Salad, 384
    Chile garlic paste, 30
    Chili-Glazed Meat Loaf, 310
    Chili Lime Mayo, 447
    Chili Lime Pumpkin, 163
    Chili Lime Wings, 42
    Linda Magsasay's Chili Burgers, 302
    Pat Best's Chili Con Carne, 329
    Pork Chili, 346
    Ropa Vieja Chili, 320

Chinese Chicken Salad, 387

Chinese Five-Spice Roasted Chicken, 227

Chinese Soup with Bok Choy and Mushrooms, 406–7

Chinese Sticky Wings, 43

Chipotle-Cheese Fauxtatoes, 137

Chipotle Mayonnaise, 446

Chocolate
    Better Than S-X!, 508–9
    Black Forest Parfaits, 470
    brownies
        Dana's Brownies, 467
        Espresso Chocolate Chip Brownies, 466
        Pam's Brownies, 469
        Sara Driver's Brownies, 468
    cheesecakes
        Chocolate Chocolate Chip Cheesecake, 489
        Kimberly Lansdon's Chocolate Almond Cheesecake, 496
    Chocolate Coconut Rum Balls, 476
    Chocolate Dips, 459
    Chocolate Walnut Balls, 457
    Crisp Chocolate Crust, 524
    Dipping Chocolate, 518
    Easy Low Carb Fudge, 503
    Eliot Sohmer's Chocolate Mousse, 486
    Jan Tucker's Chocolate Shortbread Cookies, 465
    Layered Chocolate-and-Vanilla Decadence, 510–11
    pies
        Brownie Mocha Fudge Pie, 472–73
        Chocolate Raspberry Pie, 472
        German Chocolate Pie, 514–15
        Maria Marshall's Low-Carb Chocolate Pecan Pie, 475
    sauces
        Maltitol-Splenda Chocolate Sauce, 519
        Sugar-Free Chocolate Sauce, 539

Chowders. See soups

Chunky Chicken Pie, 228–29

Chunky Cream of Chicken and Portobello Soup, 430

Cindy Shield's BBQ Green Bean Casserole, 157

Citrus Chicken, 226–27

Citrus Dressing, 209

Clams
    Tee's Crockpot Jambalaya, 416–17

Classic Barbecue Rub, 538

Club Omelet, 79

Cobb Salad, 389

Cobb Salad Dressing, 213

Cocktail Ham Tartlets, 59

Coconut
    Angel-Type Coconut, 518
    Better Than S-X!, 508–9
    Chocolate Coconut Rum Balls, 476
    Coconut Cream Pie, 516
    Nancy Harrigan's Coconut Ginger
        Sauce, 445
    Ruth Green's Coconut Crackers, 123
Coconut oil, 21
Coleslaw
    Jill Taylor's Coleslaw, 201
    Marcelle Flint's Buttermilk Coleslaw,
        202
    Napa Mint Slaw, 191
    Sally Waldron's Buffalo Chicken and
        Slaw, 242
    Sesame-Almond Napa Slaw, 200
    Tee's Cajun Dirty UnRice, 148–49
Condiments
    Chili Lime Mayo, 447
    Chipotle Mayonnaise, 446
    Dana's No-Sugar Ketchup, 528
    Major Grey's Chutney, 442
    Simple No-Sugar Pickle Relish, 441
Connie Bishop's Sort-of Cheesecake, 498
Cookies
    Amanda's Sugar Cookies, 463
    Chewy Oatmeal Cookies, 454–55
    Chocolate Coconut Rum Balls, 476
    Chocolate Dips, 459
    Chocolate Walnut Balls, 457
    Gingersnaps, 456
    Hermits, 461–62
    Jan Tucker's Chocolate Shortbread
        Cookies, 465
    Nut Butter Balls, 460
    Peanut Butter Cookies, 458
    Ray's Peanut Butter Cookies, 464
    Tee's Butter Pecan Bars, 462
Coquilles St. Jacques, 274
Cornbread
    Elizabeth Dean's Next Best Thing to
        Cornbread, 129
    Leslie's Low-Carb Broccoli
        Cornbread, 151
Crab
    Debra Rodriguez's Crab Chowder,
        433
    Leslie's Crab-Stuffed Poblano
        Peppers, 284–85
    Susan Higgs's Deviled Crab, 286

Winnie Spicer's Favorite Imperial
    Crab Casserole, 285
Crackers
    Graham Crackers, 118–19
    Parmesan Garlic Crackers, 120
    Ruth Green's Cinnamon Crackers,
        122
    Ruth Green's Coconut Crackers, 123
    Sunflower Wheat Crackers, 121
Cranberries
    Cranberry Meatballs, 316
    Cranberry Nut Muffins, 107
    Pat Best's Gingered Cranberry
        Sauce, 443
Creole Seasoning, 449
Crusts
    Almond-Parmesan Crust, 132
    Crisp Chocolate Crust, 524
    Pie Crust, 132–33
Crystal Caskey's Deviled Eggs, 49
Cumin Vinaigrette, 213
Curried dishes
    Baked Sole in Creamy Curry Sauce,
        267
    Curried Chicken Dip, 60
    Curried Chicken "Pilau," 230
    Curried Mock Hollandaise, 447
    Curried Pumpkin Soup, 427
    Curried Shrimp in Coconut Milk,
        277
    Curried Swordfish and Cabbage,
        272
    Hamburger Curry, 309
Cybdy Riser's Spiced Tea, 520

D
Dana Massey's Low-Carb Irish Cream
    Liqueur, 521
Dana Massey's Low Carb Strawberry
    Daiquiris, 523
Dana's Brownies, 467
Dana's Easy Omelet Method, 77–78
Dana's No-Sugar Ketchup, 528
Dean's Granola, 131
Deb Gajewski's Zucchini Quiche, 89
Debbie Murawski's BBQ Chicken Breast,
    250–51
Debbie White's Colorado Chipped Beef
    Appetizer, 61
Debra Rodriguez's Crab Chowder, 433
Debra Rodriguez's Green Bean Casserole,
    156–57

Desserts
    See also cheesecakes; ice cream; pies
    Amy Pierce's Frozen Blueberries,
        502
    Angel-Type Coconut, 518
    Anne Logston's Raspberry Mousse,
        486
    Better Than S-X!, 508–9
    Black Forest Parfaits, 470
    Bonnie Morrison's Finger Gelatin,
        513
    Easy Low Carb Fudge, 503
    Eileene's Pumpkin Treat, 488
    Eliot Sohmer's Chocolate Mousse,
        486
    Grandma's Blueberry Cobbler, 480
    Grandma's Cherry Cobbler, 481
    Grandma's Peach Cobbler, 479
    Italian Walnut Cake, 506–7
    Jenny's Silly Strawberry Surprise,
        511
    Laura Cottom's Strawberry Fluff, 512
    Layered Chocolate-and-Vanilla
        Decadence, 510–11
    Lemon Mousse Cup, 485
    Marilyn Schroer's Finger Gelatin,
        513
    Martha H. Harris's Easy Almond
        Flour Lemon Pound Cake, 504–5
    Mock Apple Brown Betty, 482
    No-Sugar-Added Cherry Pie Filling,
        512
    Slow Cooker Maple Pumpkin
        Pudding, 515
    Strawberries with Balsamic Vinegar,
        483
    Strawberries with Orange Cream
        Dip, 484
    Sylvia Palmer's Pumpkin Mousse,
        487
    Tom Budlong's Crema di
        Mascherpone, 484
    Whipped Topping, 540
Diane Kingsbury's Spicy Chops, 358
Diane Lyon's Savory Cheese and Ham
    Torte, 95
Dinner Rolls, 126
Dipping Chocolate, 518
Dips and spreads
    Lynn Avery's Pimiento Cheese, 67
    Marcie Vaughn's Sausage Dip, 64
    Pat Best's Guacamole, 64
    Pat Best's Jalapeno Cheese Spread, 65

Pat Best's Seven Layer Bean Dip, 66
Sally Miller's Awesome Pimento Cheese, 62
Sally Waldron's Spicy Blue Cheese Dressing and Dip, 60
Donna Barton's Pumpkin Mousse Casserole, 164
Donna Nisleit's Garlic Parmesan Chicken Breasts, 238
Dorothy Keefe's Marinated Chuck Roast, 338
Dorothy Markuske's Chicken Stuffed with Spinach and Goat Cheese, 248–49
Dorothy Markuske's Pork Chops in Cream Sauce, 356–57
Dragon's Teeth, 165
Dressings
    Big Italian Restaurant Dressing, 208
    Catalina Dressing, 210
    Citrus Dressing, 209
    Cobb Salad Dressing, 213
    Cumin Vinaigrette, 213
    Ginger Salad Dressing, 211
    Honey-Lime-Mustard Dressing, 212
    Lemon-Mustard Dressing, 215
    Orange Bacon Dressing, 207
    Sally Waldron's Spicy Blue Cheese Dressing and Dip, 60
    Soy and Sesame Dressing, 207
    Spicy Peanut Dressing, 216
    Sun-Dried Tomato-Basil Vinaigrette, 214
    Sweet Poppy Seed Vinaigrette, 214
Drinks
    Cybdy Riser's Spiced Tea, 520
    Dana Massey's Low-Carb Irish Cream Liqueur, 521
    Dana Massey's Low-Carb Strawberry Daiquiris, 523
    Laure's Homemade LC "Bailey's Mae", 520
    Mockahlua, 540
    Sugar-Free Eggnog, 522

E

Easy Italian Skillet Chicken, 231
Easy Key Lime Pie, 517
Easy Low Carb Fudge, 503
Easy Orange Salsa, 440
Easy Shrimp in Garlic Herb Cream Sauce, 278
Eggnog Ice Cream, 525

Eggplant
    Nancy O'Connor's Low-Carb Moussaka, 326
Eggs
    about, 20
    Artichoke and Friends Frittata, 94
    Avocado, Egg, and Blue Cheese Salad, 395
    Betsy Calvin's Breakfast Casserole, 97
    Eliot Sohmer's Bacon Cheese Frittata, 93
    Grandma Mel's Egg and Olive Salad, 395
    Inauthentic Machaca Eggs, 83
    Irene Haldeman's Czech Unpotato Salad, 194
    Jill Boelsma's Scottish Eggs, 100
    Jody's Breakfast Wrap, 101
    omelets
        Club Omelet, 79
        Dana's Easy Omelet Method, 77–78
        Mexican Avocado and Ham Omelet, 80
        Roman Mushroom Omelet, 80–81
        Ropa Vieja Omelet, 82
        Sloppy Tom Omelet, 81
    quiches
        Deb Gajewski's Zucchini Quiche, 89
        Jan Carmichael's Sausage Mushroom Quiche, 90
        Quiche Lorraine, 87
        Spinach Mushroom Quiche, 88
        Tracie Jansen's Cheesy Spinach Pie, 91
    scrambled
        Italian Sausage and Mushroom Scramble, 84
        Marilee Wellersdick's Bean Sprout Scramble, 86
        Spring Ham and Mushroom Scramble, 84–85
        Springtime Scramble, 85
    Sharon Walsh's Mushroom-Spinach-Egg-Muffin Thing or Something Like That, 102
    Stephanie H.'s French Toasty Eggs, 98
    stuffed
        Crystal Caskey's Deviled Eggs, 49
        Guacamole Eggs, 48
        Pâté' Eggs, 47
        Southwestern Stuffed Eggs, 45
        Stilton Eggs, 46
        Tuna Stuffed Eggs, 46–47
    Swiss Puff, 103
    Turkey Chorizo with Eggs, 257
    UnPotato Tortilla, 92
Eileene's Pumpkin Treat, 488
Eleanor Monfett's Cheddar Broccoli Salad, 198, 402
Eliot Sohmer's Bacon Cheese Frittata, 93
Eliot Sohmer's Chocolate Mousse, 486
Eliot Sohmer's Most Wonderful Cheesecake, 490
Eliot Sohmer's Spinach Soufflé, 96
Elizabeth Dean's Next Best Thing to Cornbread, 129
Ensalada de "Arroz", 193
Erythritol, 33–34
Espresso Chocolate Chip Brownies, 466
Exceedingly Crisp Waffles, 111

F

Famous Meat Loaf, 312–13
Fats and oils, 20–21
Fiber, 12–13
Fiery Indian Lamb and Cauliflower, 370
Fish
    See also Seafood
    Ceviche, 262–63
    Grilled Fish with Caper Sauce, 287
    salmon
        Flo Conklin's Salmon with Heavenly Topping, 264
        Leslie's Pickled Salmon, 266
        Nancy Zarr's Pan-Seared Salmon, 265
        Orange-Sesame Salmon, 263
        Salmon Stuffed with Lime, Cilantro, Anaheim Peppers, and Scallions, 266–67
        Susan Higgs's Salmon Stuffed Celery, 72
    sea bass
        Pan-Barbecued Sea Bass, 270
        Zijuatenejo Sea Bass, 270–71
    sole
        Baked Sole in Creamy Curry Sauce, 267
        Sautéed Sole in White Wine, 268
    Susan Higgs's Broiled Fish with Creamy Topping, 290
    Susan Higgs's Shrimp-Stuffed Fish, 288–89
    swordfish

Curried Swordfish and Cabbage, 272
Orange Swordfish Steaks with Almonds, 271
tilapia
　Kim's Tilapia Provençal, 268–69
　Susan Higgs's Tilapia in Browned Butter, 269
tuna
　Marlene D. Wurdeman's Easy Tuna Casserole, 283
　Susan Higgs's Tuna Roll-Ups, 284
　Tuna Puffs, 51
　Tuna Stuffed Eggs, 46–47
Fish sauce (nuoc mam), 30
Five-Spice Lamb Steaks, 373
Flax seed, 28–29
Flo Conklin's Salmon with Heavenly Topping, 264
Flour substitutes, 21–26
Food labels, 17
FOS (fructooligosaccharide), 35
French dishes
　Coquilles St. Jacques, 274
　Kim's Boeuf Bourguignonne, 323–24
　Kim's Tilapia Provenc,al, 268–69

G

Garlic, 30–31
Garlic Cheese Stuffed Mushrooms, 52
General Mike's Finger-Lickin' Ribs, 350
General Pam's Cheesecake, 500
George Fairchild's Low-Carb Peanut Butter Pie, 474
George Hollenbeck's Hamburger Stroganoff, 328
German Chocolate Pie, 514–15
Ginger-Almond Chicken Salad, 382
Ginger Salad Dressing, 211
Ginger Sesame Pork, 344
Gingerbread Waffles, 110
Gingerroot, 31
Gingersnaps, 456
Glazes
　See also Sauces
　Apricot-Chipotle Glaze, 439
　Maple-Orange Ham Glaze, 440
Grace Brown's Spinach and Artichoke Casserole, 173
Graham Crackers, 118–19
Grandma Angelica's Catsurra, 351
Grandma Mel's Egg and Olive Salad, 395

Grandma's Blueberry Cobbler, 480
Grandma's Cherry Cobbler, 481
Grandma's Peach Cobbler, 479
Granola, Dean's, 131
Gratin of Cauliflower and Turnips, 144
Greek dishes
　Greek Chicken with Yogurt, 219
　Greek Meatza, 371
　Nancy O'Connor's Greek Shepherd's Pie, 325
　Nancy O'Connor's Low-Carb Moussaka, 326
Green beans
　Cindy Shield's BBQ Green Bean Casserole, 157
　Debra Rodriguez's Green Bean Casserole, 156–57
　Holiday Green Bean Casserole, 152–53
　Janet Hoy's Twice-Fried Green Beans, 155
　Nancy O'Connor's Greek Shepherd's Pie, 325
　Sesame Orange Beef, 318
　Stephanie H.'s Green Beans Old Roman Style, 156
　Stir-Fried Green Beans and Water Chestnuts, 154
　Tom Budlong's Italian Olive Salad, 205
Grilled Asparagus with Balsamic Vinegar, 159
Grilled Fish with Caper Sauce, 287
Ground beef. See Beef
Guacamole Eggs, 48
Guar, 23
Gwen Meehan's Delicious Peppers and Onions with Cheesy Steak, 297
Gwen Meehan's Yummy Chicken Casserole, 240

H

Ham
　Amy Dungan's Broccoli, Ham, and Cheese Soup, 437
　Amy K. Crawford's Easy Chicken Cordon Bleu, 245
　Cocktail Ham Tartlets, 59
　Diane Lyon's Savory Cheese and Ham Torte, 95
　Ham and Cheese Salad, 398
　Ham Kedgeree, 363
　Melissa Miller's Ham and Broccoli Cheese Soup, 414–15
　Mexican Avocado and Ham Omelet, 80

Orange-Maple Ham Slice, 364
　Spring Ham and Mushroom Scramble, 84–85
　Submarine Salad, 400
　Tee's Crockpot Jambalaya, 416–17
Hamburger Curry, 309
Health food stores, 16
Hellzapoppin Cheese "Rice", 139
Herbert D. Focken's Sweetened Jalapeno Bites, 73
Hermits, 461–62
Hoisin Sauce, 531
Holiday Green Bean Casserole, 152–53
Hollandaise for Sissies, 532
Holly Holder's Cheesy Chipotle Soup, 417
Homestyle Meat Loaf, 312
Honey, imitation, 35–36, 543
Honey-Lime-Mustard Dressing, 212
Hot Paprika Shrimp, 278

I

Ice cream
　Eggnog Ice Cream, 525
　Peanut Butter Dough Ice Cream, 526
Inauthentic Machaca Eggs, 83
Indy Airport Tuna Salad, 399
Ingredients, sources of, 543–44
Irene Haldeman's Czech Unpotato Salad, 194
Irish Stew, 372
Island Pork Steaks, 345
Italian dishes
　Barb Thompson's Meatballs Arrabiata, 314
　Chicken "Risotto" alla Milanese, 233
　Easy Italian Skillet Chicken, 231
　Italian Chicken with White Wine, Peppers, and Anchovy, 221
　Italian Sausage and Mushroom Scramble, 84
　Kathy Monahon's Baked Penne, 330
　Kristy Howell's Chicken Carbonara, 251
　Marcelle Flint's Zucchini Lasagna, 332
　Nanci Messersmith's Low-Carb Lasagna Recipe Using Zucchini for Noodles, 331
　Patty Southard's Festiva Beef Italiano, 335
　Pork and Provolone with White Wine and Mushrooms, 352–53
　Sautéed Sole in White Wine, 268
　Tom Budlong's Italian Sausage and Peppers, 367

Tuscan Soup, 404
Italian Seasoned Crumbs, 452
Italian Walnut Cake, 506–7

J

Jan Carmichael's Sausage Mushroom Quiche, 90
Jan Tucker's Chocolate Shortbread Cookies, 465
Jane's Pumpkin Pie, 476–77
Janet Hoy's Twice-Fried Green Beans, 155
Janette Kling's Bourbon Glazed Cajun Tenderloin, 341–42
Jansonn's Temptation, 145
Japanese Fried "Rice", 140
Jeanette Wiese's Best Pancakes I've Ever Had, 114
Jeannie Aromi's Pernil, 359
Jen Holling's Cream Cheese Meat Loaf Surprise, 313
Jen Wardell's Low-Carb Cocktail Weenie Sauce, 443
Jen Wardell's Low-Carb Spinach Bisque Soup, 436
Jennie's Bodacious Brussels Sprouts, 177
Jennifer Krupp's Crustless Low-Carb Cheesecake, 501
Jenny's Silly Strawberry Surprise, 511
Jerk Chicken Salad, 385
Jerk Seasoning, 537
Jill Boelsma's "Breaded" Pork Tenderloin, 362
Jill Boelsma's Pork Loin Roast, 360
Jill Boelsma's Scottish Eggs, 100
Jill Taylor's Chili Relleno Casserole, 104
Jill Taylor's Coleslaw, 201
Jill Taylor's Fried Cheese Taco Shells, 70
Jill Taylor's No-Cook Cheesecake, 493
Jill Taylor's Soy Pancakes, 113
Joan Wilson's Turkey on Spaghetti Squash, 255
Jody Leimbek's Low-Carb Wraps, 260
Jody's Breakfast Wrap, 101
John Smolinski's Low-Carb Dutch Baby, 117
Julie Sandell's Low-Carb Blueberry Pancakes, 112–13

K

Kale
    Mary Anne Ward's Sausage Soup with Kale, 429
    Tuscan Soup, 404

Kansas City Barbecue Sauce, 530
Karen Sonderman's Cream of Chicken Mushroom Soup, 431
Karen Sonderman's Roasted Asparagus, 162
Karen Sonderman's Strawberry Romaine Salad, 188
Kathryn Luzardo's Stuffed Poblano Peppers, 306
Kathy Monahon's Baked Penne, 330
Ketatoes, 26
Kimberly Lansdon's Chocolate Almond Cheesecake, 496
Kim's Boeuf Bourguignonne, 323–24
Kim's Tilapia Provenc,al, 268–69
Kishke, Leslie's Mock, 182
Kristy Howell's Carrot and Cottage Cheese Salad, 206
Kristy Howell's Chicken Carbonara, 251
Kristy Howell's Zucchini Moussaka, 307–8

L

Labels, reading, 17
Lamb
    Balsamic-Mint Lamb Steak, 376
    Fiery Indian Lamb and Cauliflower, 370
    Five-Spice Lamb Steaks, 373
    Greek Meatza, 371
    Irish Stew, 372
    Kristy Howell's Zucchini Moussaka, 307–8
    Lamb Steak with Walnut Sauce, 374
    Orange-Rosemary Lamb Steak, 375
    Spanish Skillet Lamb, 377
    Spice-Rubbed Leg of Lamb with Apricot-Chipotle Glaze, 378
    steaks, about, 373
    Susan Higgs's Lamb Florentine, 369
    Susan Higgs's Lemon-Rosemary Lamb Chops, 368
Laura Cottom's Strawberry Fluff, 512
Lauren Zizza's Mustard Chicken Dish, 239
Laurence Erhili's Tagine of Chicken and Olives, 224–25
Laure's Homemade LC "Bailey's Mae", 520
Layered Chocolate-and-Vanilla Decadence, 510–11
Lemon-Ginger Pork Chops, 355
Lemon Mousse Cup, 485
Lemon-Mustard Chicken Wings, 44–45
Lemon-Mustard Dressing, 215
Lemon Mustard Herb Chicken, 232

Lemon Soy Chicken Wings, 44
Leslie's Broccoli and Cauliflower Casserole, 148
Leslie's Crab-Stuffed Poblano Peppers, 284–85
Leslie's Low-Carb Broccoli Cornbread, 151
Leslie's Mock Kishke, 182
Leslie's Pickled Salmon, 266
Libby Sinback's Peach Sour Cream Muffins, 109
Linda Blackburn's Cream of Chicken Soup, 432
Linda Carroll-King's Red Cabbage Recipe, 167
Linda Guiffre's Marbled Cheesecake Muffins, 494–95
Linda Guiffre's Pizza Muffin Appetizers, 74
Linda Magsasay's Chili Burgers, 302
Linda Wagner's Any Way You Want It BBQ Sauce, 444
Lisa Bousson's Fantastic Creamy Broccoli Soup, 424
Lobster, Broiled Orange Chili, 273
Lonestar "Rice", 141
Lori Herbel's Country Fried Steak, 296
Lorraine Achey's Dilled Almonds, 67
Lorraine Achey's Parmesan-Dill Seasoning Mix, 450–51
Low-carb baking, 105
Low-carb specialty foods
    about, 14–16
    availability of, 16–17
Low-carbohydrate diets, 10–12
Low-sugar preserves, 31
Lynn Avery's Pimiento Cheese, 67
Lynn Avery's Provolone "Chips", 69
Lynn Davis's Cottage Cheese Spinach Chicken, 234

M

M. E. Grundman's Salad Soup, 425
Major Grey's Chutney, 442
Maltitol-Splenda Chocolate Sauce, 519
Maple Oat Bread, 127
Maple-Orange Ham Glaze, 440
Marcelle Flint's Buttermilk Coleslaw, 202
Marcelle Flint's Zucchini Lasagna, 332
Marcie Vaughn's Sausage Dip, 64
Marco Polo Marinade, 445
Marco Polo Steak, 293
Marco Polo Stir-Fried Vegetables, 158
Margaret King's Cheese Crisps, 69

Margaret King's Tortilla Chips, 70
Maria Marshall's Low-Carb Chocolate Pecan Pie, 475
Marilee Wellersdick's Bean Sprout Scramble, 86
Marilyn Olshansky's Creamed Spinach, 172
Marilyn Olshansky's Pumpkin-Coconut Bisque, 428
Marilyn Olshansky's Spicy Pecans, 57
Marilyn Schroer's Finger Gelatin, 513
Marinades. See Sauces
Marlene D. Wurdeman's Easy Tuna Casserole, 283
Martha H. Harris's Easy Almond Flour Lemon Pound Cake, 504–5
Mary Anne Ward's Sausage Soup with Kale, 429
Mary Beth Wilson's Pork Tenderloin Medallions in Garlic Cream Reduction, 361
Mary Lou Theisen's Best Low-Carb Waffle, 112
Mary Lou Theisen's Cheesecake Cupcakes, 497
Mary Lou Theisen's Three Cheese Spinach Bake, 170
Mary's Pepperonu Pizza Soup, 435
Measurements, 541
Meat loafs
    Chili-Glazed Meat Loaf, 310
    Famous Meat Loaf, 312–13
    Homestyle Meat Loaf, 312
    Jen Holling's Cream Cheese Meat Loaf Surprise, 313
    Philippa's Meat Loaf, 311
Meatballs
    Albondigas, 353
    Barb Thompson's Meatballs Arrabiata, 314
    Cranberry Meatballs, 316
    Spicy Orange Meatballs, 315
    Swedish Meatballs, 317
Melisa McCurley's Good Stuff Casserole, 308
Melissa Cathey's Jalepeno Lime Chicken, 244
Melissa Miller's Ham and Broccoli Cheese Soup, 414–15
Melissa Wright's Two-Cheese Cauliflower, 146
Mexican dishes
    Albondigas, 353
    Carnitas, 344–45

Inauthentic Machaca Eggs, 83
Jill Taylor's Chili Relleno Casserole, 104
Mexican Avocado and Ham Omelet, 80
Mexican Cabbage Soup, 434
Mexican Chicken Salad, 391
Pat Best's Refried Black Soy Beans, 63
Pat Best's Seven Layer Bean Dip, 66
Pepitas Calientes, 56
Piernas de Guatalote en Mole de Cacahuates (Mexican Turkey Legs in Peanut Sauce), 253
Pollo en Jugo de Naranja (Mexican Chicken in Orange Juice), 220
Ropa Vieja, 319
Ropa Vieja Chili, 320
Ropa Vieja Hash, 321
Ropa Vieja Omelet, 82
Sopa De Frijoles Negros, 421
Sopa Tlalpeno, 405
Susan Higgs's Cauliflower Mexican Salad, 196
Tee's Taco Soup, 408
Tracy Lohr's Quick Taco Salad, 397
Turkey Chorizo with Eggs, 257
Zijuatenejo Sea Bass, 270–71
Michele Holbrook's Broccoli Bake, 152
Michele S.'s Chunky Salad, 204
Mindy Sauve's Low-Carb Nachos Supreme, 71
Mock Apple Brown Betty, 482
Mockahlua, 540
Molasses, 32
Most Wonderful Pumpkin Cheesecake, 491
Muffins
    Cranberry Nut Muffins, 107
    Libby Sinback's Peach Sour Cream Muffins, 109
    Pumpkin Muffins, 108
Mushrooms
    Celeste's Chicken with Creamy Mushroom Sauce, 247
    Celia Volk's Portobello Mushroom Pizza, 366
    Chinese Soup with Bok Choy and Mushrooms, 406–7
    Chunky Cream of Chicken and Portobello Soup, 430
    Garlic Cheese Stuffed Mushrooms, 52
    Italian Sausage and Mushroom Scramble, 84

Jan Carmichael's Sausage Mushroom Quiche, 90
Joan Wilson's Turkey on Spaghetti Squash, 255
Karen Sonderman's Cream of Chicken Mushroom Soup, 431
Lonestar "Rice", 141
Marco Polo Stir-Fried Vegetables, 158
Pork and Provolone with White Wine and Mushrooms, 352–53
Portobello Fillets, 292
Roman Mushroom Omelet, 80–81
Sharon Walsh's Mushroom-Spinach-Egg-Muffin Thing or Something Like That, 102
Spinach Mushroom Kugel, 169
Spinach Mushroom Quiche, 88
Spinach Stuffed Mushrooms, 53
Spring Ham and Mushroom Scramble, 84–85
Stephanie H.'s Mushroom-Spinach Casserole, 171–72
Venetian "Rice", 142
Mustard-Horseradish Dipping Sauce, 446

N
Nachos Supreme, Mindy Sauve's Low-Carb, 71
Naked Shrimp Stir-Fry, 289
Nanci Messersmith's Low-Carb Lasagna Recipe Using Zucchini for Noodles, 331
Nancy Harrigan's Coconut Ginger Sauce, 445
Nancy Harrigan's Spinach Balls, 75
Nancy Machinton's Pot Roast, 336
Nancy O'Connor's Creamy Garlic-Chive Fauxtatoes, 137
Nancy O'Connor's Greek Shepherd's Pie, 325
Nancy O'Connor's Low-Carb Moussaka, 326
Nancy Zarr's Pan-Seared Salmon, 265
Napa Mint Slaw, 191
New Orleans Gold, 450
No-Sugar-Added Cherry Pie Filling, 512
nuoc mam (fish sauce), 30
Nut Butter Balls, 460
Nut butters, 29
Nuts
    See also Almonds; Pecans; Walnuts
    about, 29–30
    Cajun Nut Mix, 55

Dean's Granola, 131
Val's Cheesecake, 499
Warm Brie with Sticky Nuts, 50

O

Oat Bran Pancakes, 115
Oat flour, 23
Oats, rolled
    about, 24
    Chewy Oatmeal Cookies, 454–55
    Dean's Granola, 131
    Maple Oat Bread, 127
Oils, 20–21
Okra
    Chicken and Andouille Gumbo,
        418–19
    Tee's Crockpot Jambalaya, 416–17
Olive oil, 21
Olives
    Grandma Mel's Egg and Olive Salad,
        395
    Tom Budlong's Italian Olive Salad, 205
    Tuna Salad with Mustard-Mayo and
        Olives, 399
Omelets
    Club Omelet, 79
    Dana's Easy Omelet Method, 77–78
    Mexican Avocado and Ham Omelet, 80
    Roman Mushroom Omelet, 80–81
    Ropa Vieja Omelet, 82
    Sloppy Tom Omelet, 81
Onions
    about, 37
    Cathy Sparks's Creamed Onions, 183
    Cheesy Onion Soup, 411
    Gwen Meehan's Delicious Peppers and
        Onions with Cheesy Steak, 297
Oranges
    Broiled Orange Chili Lobster, 273
    Easy Orange Salsa, 440
    Maple-Orange Glaze, 440
    Orange, Avocado, and Bacon Salad, 189
    Orange Bacon Dressing, 207
    Orange-Five-Spice Roasted Chicken,
        225
    Orange-Maple Ham Slice, 364
    Orange Mustard Glazed Sprouts, 178
    Orange-Rosemary Lamb Steak, 375
    Orange-Sesame Salmon, 263
    Orange Swordfish Steaks with
        Almonds, 271
    Orange Tequila Steak, 294

Sesame Orange Beef, 318
Spicy Orange Meatballs, 315
Oriental Chicken, "Rice," and Walnut Salad
    Wrapped in Lettuce, 386
Oven Barbecued Ribs, 349

P

Pamela Merritt's Marinated Pot Roast, 337
Pam's Brownies, 469
Pan-Barbecued Sea Bass, 270
Pancake syrup, sugar-free, 36
Pancakes
    Jeanette Wiese's Best Pancakes I've
        Ever Had, 114
    Jill Taylor's Soy Pancakes, 113
    John Smolinski's Low-Carb Dutch
        Baby, 117
    Julie Sandell's Low-Carb Blueberry
        Pancakes, 112–13
    Oat Bran Pancakes, 115
    "Whole Wheat" Buttermilk Pancakes,
        116
Parmesan Garlic Crackers, 120
Pat Best's Chili Con Carne, 329
Pat Best's Deviled Chicken Salad, 392
Pat Best's Gingered Cranberry Sauce, 443
Pat Best's Guacamole, 64
Pat Best's Hearty Black Soy Bean Soup,
    422
Pat Best's Hearty Black Soy Bean Soup,
    the Short-Cooking Version, 423
Pat Best's Jalapeno Cheese Spread, 65
Pat Best's Refried Black Soy Beans, 63
Pat Best's Seven Layer Bean Dip, 66
Pat Resler's Cauliflower and Cheese Salad,
    195
Pâté Eggs, 47
Patti Shreiner's Chicken Continental, 249
Patty Southard's Festiva Beef Italiano, 335
Peaches
    Grandma's Peach Cobbler, 479
    Libby Sinback's Peach Sour Cream
        Muffins, 109
    Major Grey's Chutney, 442
Peanuts/peanut butter
    Cajun Nut Mix, 55
    George Fairchild's Low-Carb Peanut
        Butter Pie, 474
    Peanut Butter Cookies, 458
    Peanut Butter Dough Ice Cream, 526
    Ray's Peanut Butter Cookies, 464
    Spicy Peanut Dressing, 216

Thai Cobb Salad, 390
Peas
    Japanese Fried "Rice", 140
    Springtime Scramble, 85
Pecans
    Better Than S-X!, 508–9
    Cajun Nut Mix, 55
    Cheese-Pecan Nibbles, 54
    Jill Taylor's No-Cook Cheesecake, 493
    Maria Marshall's Low-Carb Chocolate
        Pecan Pie, 475
    Marilyn Olshansky's Spicy Pecans, 57
    Nut Butter Balls, 460
    Tee's Butter Pecan Bars, 462
Pepitas Calientes, 56
Pepper Steak with Whiskey Sauce, 295
Peppers
    Gwen Meehan's Delicious Peppers and
        Onions with Cheesy Steak, 297
    Herbert D. Focken's Sweetened
        Jalapeno Bites, 73
    Italian Chicken with White Wine,
        Peppers, and Anchovy, 221
    Kathryn Luzardo's Stuffed Poblano
        Peppers, 306
    Leslie's Crab-Stuffed Poblano Peppers,
        284–85
    Southwestern Stuffed Peppers, 304
    Tom Budlong's Italian Sausage and
        Peppers, 367
Philippa's Meat Loaf, 311
Pie Crust, 132–33
Pie crusts. See Crusts
Piernas de Guatalote en Mole de
    Cacahuates (Mexican Turkey Legs in
    Peanut Sauce), 253
Pies
    Brownie Mocha Fudge Pie, 472–73
    Carol Tessman's Raspberry Pie, 478
    Chocolate Raspberry Pie, 472
    Chunky Chicken Pie, 228–29
    Coconut Cream Pie, 516
    Easy Key Lime Pie, 517
    George Fairchild's Low-Carb Peanut
        Butter Pie, 474
    German Chocolate Pie, 514–15
    Jane's Pumpkin Pie, 476–77
    Maria Marshall's Low-Carb Chocolate
        Pecan Pie, 475
    Nancy O'Connor's Greek Shepherd's
        Pie, 325
    Rita Eichman's Shepherd's Pie, 334
    Strawberry Cheese Pie, 471

Pizza
    Celia Volk's Portobello Mushroom Pizza, 366
    Greek Meatza, 371
    Linda Guiffre's Pizza Muffin Appetizers, 74
    Mary's Pepperoni Pizza Soup, 435
Pollo en Jugo de Naranja (Mexican Chicken in Orange Juice), 220
Polyol sweeteners, 15, 32–34, 543–44
Poppy Seed Bread, 128
Poppy Seed Chicken, 236
Pork
    See also ham; sausage
    Albondigas, 353
    Carnitas, 344–45
    chops
        Diane Kingsbury's Spicy Chops, 358
        Dorothy Markuske's Pork Chops in Cream Sauce Topped with Seasoned Goat Cheese, 356–57
        Lemon-Ginger Pork Chops, 355
        Sara Emmert's "The Last Pork Chop Recipe You'll Ever Need", 354
    Ginger Sesame Pork, 344
    Island Pork Steaks, 345
    loin
        Jill Boelsma's Pork Loin Roast, 360
        Pork and Provolone with White Wine and Mushrooms, 352–53
    Marcie Vaughn's Sausage Dip, 64
    Pork Chili, 346
    Pork Stew, 347
    ribs
        General Mike's Finger-Lickin' Ribs, 350
        Grandma Angelica's Catsurra, 351
        Oven Barbecued Ribs, 349
        Seriously Simple Roasted Ribs, 348
    roasts
        Jeannie Aromi's Pernil, 359
        Jill Boelsma's Pork Loin Roast, 360
    tenderloins
        Jill Boelsma's "Breaded" Pork Tenderloin, 362
        Mary Beth Wilson's Pork Tenderloin Medallions in Garlic Cream Reduction, 361

Pork rinds
    Italian Seasoned Crumbs, 452
    Trish Z.'s Pork Rind Stuffing, 138–39
Portobello Fillets, 292
Pudding, Slow Cooker Maple Pumpkin, 515
Pumpkin
    AnaLisa K. Moyers's Easy Pumpkin Cheesecake, 495
    Barbecued Pumpkin Seeds, 68
    Chicken Sancocho, 222–23
    Chili Lime Pumpkin, 163
    Curried Pumpkin Soup, 427
    Donna Barton's Pumpkin Mousse Casserole, 164
    Eileene's Pumpkin Treat, 488
    Jane's Pumpkin Pie, 476–77
    Marilyn Olshansky's Pumpkin-Coconut Bisque, 428
    Most Wonderful Pumpkin Cheesecake, 491
    Pepitas Calientes, 56
    Pumpkin Muffins, 108
    Slow Cooker Maple Pumpkin Pudding, 515
    Sylvia Palmer's Pumpkin Mousse, 487
Pumpkin seed meal, 24

Q
Quiches
    Deb Gajewski's Zucchini Quiche, 89
    Jan Carmichael's Sausage Mushroom Quiche, 90
    Quiche Lorraine, 87
    Spinach Mushroom Quiche, 88
    Tracie Jansen's Cheesy Spinach Pie, 91

R
Raspberries
    Anne Logston's Raspberry Mousse, 486
    Carol Tessman's Raspberry Pie, 478
    Chocolate Raspberry Pie, 472
    Raspberry Vinegar, 532
    Winnie Spicer's Chicken in Raspberry Cream Sauce, 238–39
Ray's Peanut Butter Cookies, 464
Reader recipes, 9–10
Recipes
    carb counts of, 10–12, 14
    reader, 9–10

Reduced-Carb Spicy Barbecue Sauce, 529
Rho's Slow-Cooker Chuck Roast, 339
Rice
    Hellzapoppin Cheese "Rice", 139
    Japanese Fried "Rice", 140
    Lonestar "Rice", 141
    Venetian "Rice", 142
Rice protein powder, 24
Rita Eichman's Shepherd's Pie, 334
Roasted Cabbage with Balsamic Vinegar, 166
Robin Loiselle's Teriyaki Chicken Wings, 243
Rolls, Dinner, 126
Roman Mushroom Omelet, 80–81
Ropa Vieja, 319
Ropa Vieja Chili, 320
Ropa Vieja Hash, 321
Ropa Vieja Omelet, 82
Ruth Green's Cinnamon Crackers, 122
Ruth Green's Coconut Crackers, 123
Ruth Lambert's Avocado Mousse, 180

S
Salads
    Avocado, Egg, and Blue Cheese Salad, 395
    Avocado-Walnut Salad, 189
    beef
        Cajun Steak Caesar Salad, 396
        Tracy Lohr's Quick Taco Salad, 397
    Broccoli Sunshine Salad Low-Carb, 199
    Cannery Row UnPotato Salad, 192
    Cauliflower Avocado Salad, 192–93
    chicken
        Artichoke Chicken Salad, 380
        Asian Chicken Salad, 383
        Caribbean Grilled Chicken Salad, 381
        Chicken Chili Cheese Salad, 384
        Chinese Chicken Salad, 387
        Cobb Salad, 389
        Ginger-Almond Chicken Salad, 382
        Jerk Chicken Salad, 385
        Mexican Chicken Salad, 391
        Oriental Chicken, "Rice," and Walnut Salad Wrapped in Lettuce, 386
        Pat Best's Deviled Chicken Salad, 392

Susan Higgs's Chicken Salad Surprise, 393

Teresa Egger's Calcutta Chicken and "Rice" Salad, 394

Tex-Mex Chicken Salad, 388

Thai Cobb Salad, 390

Cobb Salad, 389

Eleanor Monfett's Cheddar Broccoli Salad, 198, 402

Ensalada de "Arroz", 193

Grandma Mel's Egg and Olive Salad, 395

Ham and Cheese Salad, 398

Irene Haldeman's Czech Unpotato Salad, 194

Karen Sonderman's Strawberry Romaine Salad, 188

Kristy Howell's Carrot and Cottage Cheese Salad, 206

Marcelle Flint's Buttermilk Coleslaw, 202

Michele S.'s Chunky Salad, 204

Napa Mint Slaw, 191

Orange, Avocado, and Bacon Salad, 189

Pat Resler's Cauliflower and Cheese Salad, 195

Sesame-Almond Napa Slaw, 200

Sharon Marlow's Broccoli Cashew Salad, 198–99

Shrimp and Avocado Salad, 401

Snow Pea Salad Wraps, 203

Spinach-Strawberry Salad, 187

Submarine Salad, 400

Susan Higgs's Broccoli and Cauliflower Salad, 197

Susan Higgs's Cauliflower Mexican Salad, 196

Tom Budlong's Italian Olive Salad, 205

tuna

Indy Airport Tuna Salad, 399

Tuna Salad with Mustard-Mayo and Olives, 399

Vietnamese Salad, 186

Wendy Kaess's Cauliflower Salad, 197

Salisbury Steak, 303

Sally Miller's Awesome Pimento Cheese, 62

Sally Waldron's Buffalo Chicken and Slaw, 242

Sally Waldron's Spicy Blue Cheese Dressing and Dip, 60

Salmon

Flo Conklin's Salmon with Heavenly Topping, 264

Leslie's Pickled Salmon, 266

Nancy Zarr's Pan-Seared Salmon, 265

Orange-Sesame Salmon, 263

Salmon Stuffed with Lime, Cilantro, Anaheim Peppers, and Scallions, 266–67

Susan Higgs's Salmon Stuffed Celery, 72

Salmonella, 20

Sara Driver's Brownies, 468

Sara Emmert's "The Last Pork Chop Recipe You'll Ever Need", 354

Sauces

See also Glazes

Curried Mock Hollandaise, 447

Easy Orange Salsa, 440

Hoisin Sauce, 531

Hollandaise for Sissies, 532

Jen Wardell's Low-Carb Cocktail Weenie Sauce, 443

Kansas City Barbecue Sauce, 530

Linda Wagner's Any Way You Want It BBQ Sauce, 444

Maltitol-Splenda Chocolate Sauce, 519

Marco Polo Marinade, 445

Mustard-Horseradish Dipping Sauce, 446

Nancy Harrigan's Coconut Ginger Sauce, 445

Pat Best's Gingered Cranberry Sauce, 443

Reduced-Carb Spicy Barbecue Sauce, 529

Sugar-Free Chocolate Sauce, 539

Teriyaki Sauce, 531

Sausage

Audra Olsen's Asparagus/Salami Roll-Ups, 76

Betsy Calvin's Breakfast Casserole, 97

Carol Tessman's Skillet Supper, 246

Celia Volk's Portobello Mushroom Pizza, 366

Italian Sausage and Mushroom Scramble, 84

Jan Carmichael's Sausage Mushroom Quiche, 90

Jill Boelsma's Scottish Eggs, 100

Marcie Vaughn's Sausage Dip, 64

Mary Anne Ward's Sausage Soup with Kale, 429

Tee's Cajun Dirty UnRice, 148–49

Tee's Crockpot Jambalaya, 416–17

Tom Budlong's Italian Sausage and Peppers, 367

Tuscan Soup, 404

UnPotato and Sausage Soup, 420

Winter Night Sausage Bake, 365

Sautéed Sole in White Wine, 268

Scallops

Coquilles St. Jacques, 274

Scallops Vinaigrette, 275

Scallops with Morroccan Spices, 281

Stir-Fried Scallops and Asparagus, 276

Sea bass

Pan-Barbecued Sea Bass, 270

Zijuatenejo Sea Bass, 270–71

Seafood

See also Fish

clams

Tee's Crockpot Jambalaya, 416–17

crab

Debra Rodriguez's Crab Chowder, 433

Leslie's Crab-Stuffed Poblano Peppers, 284–85

Susan Higgs's Deviled Crab, 286

Winnie Spicer's Favorite Imperial Crab Casserole, 285

lobster

Broiled Orange Chili Lobster, 273

scallops

Coquilles St. Jacques, 274

Scallops Vinaigrette, 275

Scallops with Morroccan Spices, 281

Stir-Fried Scallops and Asparagus, 276

shrimp

Curried Shrimp in Coconut Milk

Easy Shrimp in Garlic Herb Cream Sauce, 278

Hot Paprika Shrimp, 278

Naked Shrimp Stir-Fry, 289

Shrimp and Artichoke "Risotto", 279

Shrimp and Avocado Salad, 401

Shrimp in Sherry, 280

Spicy Shrimp in Beer Batter, 280–81

Susan Higgs's Shrimp-Stuffed Fish, 288–89

Sweet and Spicy Shrimp, 282

Tee's Crockpot Jambalaya, 416–17

Seasonings
    about, 30–32
    Adobe Seasoning, 448
    Cajun Seasoning, 536
    Classic Barbecue Rub, 538
    Creole Seasoning, 449
    Jerk Seasoning, 537
    Lorraine Achey's Parmesan-Dill
      Seasoning Mix, 450–51
    New Orleans Gold, 450
    Taco Seasoning, 535
    Tee's Cajun Seasoning Mix, 451
Seeds, 29–30
Seriously Simple Roasted Ribs, 348
Serving sizes, 13
Sesame-Almond Napa Slaw, 200
Sesame Orange Beef, 318
Sharon Frooshani's Cherry Cheesecake
    Dessert, 502
Sharon Marlow's Broccoli Cashew Salad,
    198–99
Sharon Palmer-Brownstein's Fantastic
    Brisket of Beef, 340
Sharon Walsh's Mushroom-Spinach-Egg-
    Muffin Thing, 102
Sharyn Taylor's Granny's Spoon Bread,
    130
Sheryl McKenney's Easy Cheese Soup,
    413
Sheryl McKenney's Stuffed Tomatoes, 305
Shrimp
    Curried Shrimp in Coconut Milk, 277
    Easy Shrimp in Garlic Herb Cream
      Sauce, 278
    Hot Paprika Shrimp, 278
    Naked Shrimp Stir-Fry, 289
    Shrimp and Artichoke "Risotto", 279
    Shrimp and Avocado Salad, 401
    Shrimp in Sherry, 280
    Spicy Shrimp in Beer Batter, 280–81
    Susan Higgs's Shrimp-Stuffed Fish,
      288–89
    Sweet and Spicy Shrimp, 282
    Tee's Crockpot Jambalaya, 416–17
Simple No-Sugar Pickle Relish, 441
Sloppy Tom Omelet, 81
Sloppy Toms, 259
Slow Cooker Maple Pumpkin Pudding, 515
Smoked Almonds, 68
Smoky Marinated Steak, 298
Snacks
    Audra Olsen's Asparagus/Salami Roll-
      Ups, 76

Barbecued Pumpkin Seeds, 68
Brie and Walnut Quesadillas, 58
Cajun Nut Mix, 55
Cheese-Pecan Nibbles, 54
Chili Lime Wings, 42
Chinese Sticky Wings, 43
Cocktail Ham Tartlets, 59
Crystal Caskey's Deviled Eggs, 49
Curried Chicken Dip, 60
Debbie White's Colorado Chipped
    Beef Appetizer, 61
Garlic Cheese Stuffed Mushrooms, 52
Guacamole Eggs, 48
Herbert D. Focken's Sweetened
    Jalapeno Bites, 73
Jill Taylor's Fried Cheese Taco Shells, 70
Lemon-Mustard Chicken Wings, 44–45
Lemon Soy Chicken Wings, 44
Linda Guiffre's Pizza Muffin Appetizers,
    74
Lorraine Achey's Dilled Almonds, 67
Lynn Avery's Pimiento Cheese, 67
Lynn Avery's Provolone "Chips", 69
Marcie Vaughn's Sausage Dip, 64
Margaret King's Cheese Crisps, 69
Margaret King's Tortilla Chips, 70
Marilyn Olshansky's Spicy Pecans, 57
Mindy Sauve's Low-Carb Nachos
    Supreme, 71
Nancy Harrigan's Spinach Balls, 75
Pat Best's Guacamole, 64
Pat Best's Jalapeno Cheese Spread, 65
Pat Best's Refried Black Soy Beans, 63
Pat Best's Seven Layer Bean Dip, 66
Pâté Eggs, 47
Pepitas Calientes, 56
Sally Miller's Awesome Pimento
    Cheese, 62
Sally Waldron's Spicy Blue Cheese
    Dressing and Dip, 60
Smoked Almonds, 68
Southwestern Stuffed Eggs, 45
Spinach Stuffed Mushrooms, 53
Stilton Eggs, 46
Susan Higgs's Salmon Stuffed Celery,
    72
Tuna Puffs, 51
Tuna Stuffed Eggs, 46–47
Warm Brie with Sticky Nuts, 50
Snow Pea Salad Wraps, 203
Sole
    Baked Sole in Creamy Curry Sauce, 267

Sautéed Sole in White Wine, 268
Sonlight Mom's Cheesy Chicken, 250
Sopa De Frijoles Negros, 421
Sopa Tlalpeno, 405
Sophia Loren Chicken, 241
Soufflé, Eliot Sohmer's Spinach, 96
Soups
    bean
      Pat Best's Hearty Black Soy Bean
        Soup, 422
      Pat Best's Hearty Black Soy Bean
        Soup, the Short-Cooking
        Version, 423
    beef
      Cathy Kayne's Chinese Beef Soup,
        407
      Cathy Kayne's Spicy Garlic Ginger
        Beef Soup, 426
      Cherie Johnson's Cheeseburger
        Soup, 414
    broccoli
      Amy Dungan's Broccoli, Ham, and
        Cheese Soup, 437
      Broccoli Blue Cheese Soup, 409
      Lisa Bousson's Fantastic Creamy
        Broccoli Soup, 424
      Melissa Miller's Ham and Broccoli
        Cheese Soup, 414–15
      Swiss Cheese and Broccoli Soup,
        412
    cabbage
      Mexican Cabbage Soup, 434
    cauliflower
      Cheesy Cauliflower Soup, 410
    chicken
      Chicken and Andouille Gumbo,
        418–19
      Chunky Cream of Chicken and
        Portobello Soup, 430
      Karen Sonderman's Cream of
        Chicken Mushroom Soup, 431
      Linda Blackburn's Cream of
        Chicken Soup, 432
      Thai Chicken Soup, 406
    Chinese Soup with Bok Choy and
      Mushrooms, 406–7
    Debra Rodriguez's Crab Chowder, 433
    Holly Holder's Cheesy Chipotle Soup,
      417
    Jen Wardell's Low-Carb Spinach Bisque
      Soup, 436
    M. E. Grundman's Salad Soup, 425
    Mary Anne Ward's Sausage Soup with
      Kale, 429

Mary's Pepperoni Pizza Soup, 435
onions
  Cheesy Onion Soup, 411
pumpkin
  Curried Pumpkin Soup, 427
  Marilyn Olshansky's Pumpkin-Coconut Bisque, 428
Sheryl McKenney's Easy Cheese Soup, 413
Sopa De Frijoles Negros, 421
Sopa Tlalpeno, 405
Tee's Taco Soup, 408
Tuscan Soup, 404
UnPotato and Sausage Soup, 420
Southwestern Stuffed Eggs, 45
Southwestern Stuffed Peppers, 304
Soy and Sesame Dressing, 207
Soy beans. See Black soy beans
Soy flour, 24–25
Spaghetti squash, Joan Wilson's Turkey on, 255
Spanish Skillet Lamb, 377
Specialty foods, low-carb, 14–16
Spice-Rubbed Leg of Lamb with Apricot-Chipotle Glaze, 378
Spicy Orange Meatballs, 315
Spicy Peanut Dressing, 216
Spicy Shrimp in Beer Batter, 280–81
Spinach
  Dorothy Markuske's Chicken Stuffed with Spinach and Goat Cheese, 248–49
  Eliot Sohmer's Spinach Soufflé, 96
  Grace Brown's Spinach and Artichoke Casserole, 173
  Jen Wardell's Low-Carb Spinach Bisque Soup, 436
  Lynn Davis's Cottage Cheese Spinach Chicken, 234
  Marilyn Olshansky's Creamed Spinach, 172
  Mary Lou Theisen's Three Cheese Spinach Bake, 170
  Melisa McCurley's Good Stuff Casserole, 308
  Nancy Harrigan's Spinach Balls, 75
  Sharon Walsh's Mushroom-Spinach-Egg-Muffin Thing or Something Like That, 102
  Spinach Mushroom Kugel, 169
  Spinach Mushroom Quiche, 88
  Spinach-Strawberry Salad, 187
  Spinach Stuffed Mushrooms, 53

Stephanie H.'s Mushroom-Spinach Casserole, 171–72
Susan Higgs's Lamb Florentine, 369
Tee's Cajun Chicken and Spinach, 235
Tracie Jansen's Cheesy Spinach Pie, 91
Splenda, 34–35
Spring Ham and Mushroom Scramble, 84–85
Springtime Scramble, 85
Steak with Brandy-Stilton Cream Sauce, 299
Steaks. See beef
Stephanie Hill's Creamy Cauliflower and Bacon Casserole, 147
Stephanie H.'s French Toasty Eggs, 98
Stephanie H.'s Green Beans Old Roman Style, 156
Stephanie H.'s Mushroom-Spinach Casserole, 171–72
Stevia, 35
Stews
  See also Soups
  Chicken Sancocho, 222–23
  Irish Stew, 372
  Pork Stew, 347
  Tee's Crockpot Jambalaya, 416–17
Stilton Eggs, 46
Stir-Fried Green Beans and Water Chestnuts, 154
Stir-Fried Scallops and Asparagus, 276
Strawberries
  Dana Massey's Low-Carb Strawberry Daiquiris, 523
  Jenny's Silly Strawberry Surprise, 511
  Karen Sonderman's Strawberry Romaine Salad, 188
  Spinach-Strawberry Salad, 187
  Strawberries with Balsamic Vinegar, 483
  Strawberries with Orange Cream Dip, 484
  Strawberry Cheese Pie, 471
Stuffing, Trish Z.'s Pork Rind, 138–39
Submarine Salad, 400
Sugar alcohols. See Polyol sweeteners
Sugar-Free Chocolate Sauce, 539
Sugar-Free Eggnog, 522
Sugar-free imitation honey, 35–36, 543
Sugar-free pancake syrup, 36
Sun-Dried Tomato-Basil Vinaigrette, 214
Sunflower seeds
  Parmesan Garlic Crackers, 120
  Sunflower Wheat Crackers, 121

Susan Case DeMarti's Awesome Cheesecake, 492–93
Susan Higgs's Skillet Cabbage, 168
Susan Higgs's Broccoli and Cauliflower Salad, 197
Susan Higgs's Broiled Fish with Creamy Topping, 290
Susan Higgs's Brussels Sprouts in Browned Butter, 176
Susan Higgs's Cauliflower Mexican Salad, 196
Susan Higgs's Chicken Salad Surprise, 393
Susan Higgs's Deviled Crab, 286
Susan Higgs's Imperial Beef, 333
Susan Higgs's Lamb Florentine, 369
Susan Higgs's Lemon-Rosemary Lamb Chops, 368
Susan Higgs's Piquant Ground Beef, 327
Susan Higgs's Salmon Stuffed Celery, 72
Susan Higgs's Shrimp-Stuffed Fish, 288–89
Susan Higgs's Spicy Zucchini and Tomato Sauté, 181
Susan Higgs's Tilapia in Browned Butter, 269
Susan Higgs's Tuna Roll-Ups, 284
Swedish Meatballs, 317
Sweet and Spicy Shrimp, 282
Sweet Poppy Seed Vinaigrette, 214
Sweeteners, 32–36
Swiss Cheese and Broccoli Soup, 412
Swiss Puff, 103
Swordfish
  Curried Swordfish and Cabbage, 272
  Orange Swordfish Steaks with Almonds, 271
Sylvia Palmer's Pumpkin Mousse, 487

T

Taco Seasoning, 535
Tee's Butter Pecan Bars, 462
Tee's Cajun Chicken and Spinach, 235
Tee's Cajun Dirty UnRice, 148–49
Tee's Cajun Seasoning Mix, 451
Tee's Crockpot Jambalaya, 416–17
Tee's Taco Soup, 408
Teresa Egger's Calcutta Chicken and "Rice" Salad, 394
Teriyaki Sauce, 531
Terrie Shortsleeve's Lemon-Garlic Chicken, 237
Tex-Mex Chicken Salad, 388

Thai Beef Lettuce Wraps, 322
Thai Chicken Soup, 406
Thai Cobb Salad, 390
Thai Turkey Burgers, 258
Tilapia
    Kim's Tilapia Provençal, 268–69
    Susan Higgs's Tilapia in Browned
        Butter, 269
Tom Budlong's Crema di Mascherpone,
    484
Tom Budlong's Italian Olive Salad, 205
Tom Budlong's Italian Sausage and
    Peppers, 367
Tomatoes
    about, 37–38
    Asparagus with Sun-Dried Tomatoes,
        160
    Sheryl McKenney's Stuffed Tomatoes,
        305
    Susan Higgs's Spicy Zucchini and
        Tomato Sauté', 181
Tortilla Chips, Margaret King's, 70
Tracie Jansen's Cheesy Spinach Pie, 91
Tracy Lohr's Quick Taco Salad, 397
Trish Z.'s Pork Rind Stuffing, 138–39
Tuna
    Indy Airport Tuna Salad, 399
    Marlene D. Wurdeman's Easy Tuna
        Casserole, 283
    Susan Higgs's Tuna Roll-Ups, 284
    Tuna Puffs, 51
    Tuna Salad with Mustard-Mayo and
        Olives, 399
    Tuna Stuffed Eggs, 46–47
Turkey
    Cat's Chili, 258–59
    Club Omelet, 79
    Cobb Salad, 389
    Joan Wilson's Turkey on Spaghetti
        Squash, 255
    Jody Leimbek's Low-Carb Wraps, 260
    Piernas de Guatalote en Mole de
        Cacahuates (Mexican Turkey Legs
        in Peanut Sauce), 253
    Sloppy Tom Omelet, 81
    Sloppy Toms, 259
    Thai Turkey Burgers, 258
    Turkey Chorizo with Eggs, 257
    Turkey Feta Burgers, 256
    Turkey Tetrazzini, 254–55
Turnips
    Gratin of Cauliflower and Turnips, 144
    Jansonn's Temptation, 145

Tuscan Soup, 404

U
Ultimate Fauxtatoes, The, 136
UnPotato and Sausage Soup, 420
UnPotato Tortilla, 92
Usable carb count, 12–13, 15

V
Val's Cheesecake, 499
Vege-Sal, 31–32
Vegetables
    See also specific types
    Chicken Teriyaki Stir-Fry, 252
    frozen, 36–37
    Marco Polo Stir-Fried Vegetables, 158
Venetian "Rice", 142
Vietnamese Salad, 186
Vinegar
    about, 28
    Raspberry Vinegar, 532

W
Waffles
    Exceedingly Crisp Waffles, 111
    Gingerbread Waffles, 110
    Mary Lou Theisen's Best Low-Carb
        Waffle, 112
Walnuts
    Avocado-Walnut Salad, 189
    Brie and Walnut Quesadillas, 58
    Chocolate Walnut Balls, 457
    Italian Walnut Cake, 506–7
    Lamb Steak with Walnut Sauce, 374
Warm Brie with Sticky Nuts, 50
Water Chestnuts, Stir-Fried Green Beans
    with, 154
Weight loss, 11
Wendy Kaess's Cauliflower Salad, 197
Wheat germ, 25
Wheat gluten, 25
Wheat protein isolate, 26, 544
Whey protein powder, 26
Whipped Topping, 540
"Whole Wheat" Buttermilk Pancakes, 116
Wine, 28
Winnie Spicer's Chicken in Raspberry
    Cream Sauce, 238–39
Winnie Spicer's Favorite Imperial Crab
    Casserole, 285
Winter Night Sausage Bake, 365

X
Xanthan gum, 23

Y
Yeast, 38
Yogurt, 38–39

Z
Zijuatenejo Sea Bass, 270–71
Zucchini
    Albondigas, 353
    Artichoke and Friends Frittata, 94
    Deb Gajewski's Zucchini Quiche, 89
    Holly Holder's Cheesy Chipotle Soup,
        417
    Kristy Howell's Zucchini Moussaka,
        307–8
    Marcelle Flint's Zucchini Lasagna, 332
    Nanci Messersmith's Low-Carb
        Lasagna Recipe Using Zucchini for
        Noodles, 331
    Susan Higgs's Spicy Zucchini and
        Tomato Sauté', 181
    Zucchini Bread, 106